GENDER AND WELL-BEING

Gender and Well-Being

Series Editors: Cristina Borderías, Professor of Contemporary History, University of Barcelona, Spain and Bernard Harris, Professor of the History of Social Policy, University of Southampton, UK

The aim of this series is to enhance our understanding of the relationship between gender and well-being by addressing the following questions:

- How can we compare levels of well-being between women and men?
- Is it possible to develop new indicators which reflect a fuller understanding of the nature of well-being in the twenty-first century?
- How have women and men contributed to the improvement of individual well-being at different times and in different places?
- What role should institutions play in promoting and maintaining well-being?
- In what ways have different social movements contributed to the improvement of well-being over the last 300 years?

The volumes in this series are designed to provide rigorous social-scientific answers to these questions. The series emerges from a series of symposia, organized as part of COST Action 34 on 'Gender and Well-being: Work, Family and Public Policies'. Participants were drawn from disciplines including economics, demography, history, sociology, social policy and anthropology and they represent more than 20 European countries.

Also in this series

Transforming Gendered Well-Being in Europe
The Impact of Social Movements
Edited by Alison E. Woodward, Jean-Michel Bonvin and Mercè Renom
ISBN 978-1-4094-0283-1

Gender Inequalities, Households
and the Production of Well-Being in Modern Europe
Edited by Tindara Addabbo, Marie-Pierre Arrizabalaga, Cristina Borderías
and Alastair Owens
ISBN 978-0-7546-7968-4

Gender and Well-Being in Europe
Historical and Contemporary Perspectives
Edited by Bernard Harris, Lina Gálvez and Helena Machado
ISBN 978-0-7546-7264-7

Gender and Well-Being
The Role of Institutions

Edited by

ELISABETTA ADDIS
University of Sassari, Italy

PALOMA DE VILLOTA,
Complutense University of Madrid, Spain

FLORENCE DEGAVRE
Catholic University, Louvain, Belgium

and

JOHN ERIKSEN
Norwegian Social Research Institute, Norway

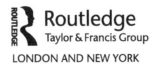
LONDON AND NEW YORK

First published 2011 by Ashgate Publishing

Published 2016 by Routledge
2 Park Square, Milton Park, Abingdon, Oxfordshire OX14 4RN
711 Third Avenue, New York, NY 10017, USA

First issued in paperback 2016

Routledge is an imprint of the Taylor & Francis Group, an informa business

British Library Cataloguing in Publication Data
Gender and well-being : the role of institutions. – (Gender and well-being)
 1. Well-being–Sex differences–Europe–Congresses. 2. Equality–Europe–Congresses.
 3. Human services–Government policy–Europe–Congresses. 4. Family policy–Europe–Congresses. 5. Sexual division of labor–Europe–Congresses. 6. Caregivers–Europe–Congresses. 7. Work and family–Europe–Congresses. 8. Europe–Social policy–Congresses.
 I. Series II. Addis, E. (Elisabetta)
 361.9'4–dc22

Library of Congress Control Number
2011930688

ISBN 13: 978-1-138-25448-0 (pbk)
ISBN 13: 978-1-4094-0705-8 (hbk)

Contents

List of Figures

List of Tables

Notes on Contributors

Tindara Addabbo is Associate Professor of Economic Policy and Labour Economics at the University of Modena and Reggio Emilia, Italy. Her recent publications include 'Gender auditing in a capability approach' (co-authored with D. Lanzi and A. Picchio), *Journal of Human Development and Capabilities*, vol. 11, no. 4 (2010) and *Gender Inequalities, Households and the Production of Well-being in Modern Europe* (co-edited with M.P. Arrizabalaga, C. Borderías and A. Owens) (Ashgate, 2010).

Elisabetta Addis is Professor of Economics at the University of Sassari and fellow of GenderCAPP (Centre for the Analysis of Public Policies), University of Modena, Italy. Her research interests include aspects of gender differences in the economy: wage differentials, effects of taxation and welfare state provisions, economic consequences of being a soldier, gender and science, and most recently the economic consequences of the financial crisis on women. Her recent publications include the report on *Gender and Scientific Excellence* in the 7th Framework Programme, "A Meta-analysis of Gender and Science Research".

Laura Alipranti-Maratou, PhD in Sociology, is a Researcher at the National Centre for Social Research in Athens, Greece. Her publications include *Female Migration in Greece* (KETHI, Centre for Studies on Gender Equality, Athens, 2007). She was co-editor (with Margaret Abraham, Esther Ngan-ling Chow and Evangelia Tastsoglou) of *Contours of Citizenship: Women, Diversity and Practices of Citizenship* (Ashgate, 2010). She has been the National Representative for Greece in the COST European research system, Domain Committee on Individuals, Society, Culture and Health, since 2005. She is an elected Member of the Executive Board of RC32, Women in Society, of the International Sociological Association.

Margareta Bäck-Wiklund is Professor of Social Work and Family Policy at the University of Gothenburg, Sweden. Her research interests are modern family life and parenting. Her current research is focused on family–work balance. She co-edited and contributed to *Quality and Work in a Changing Europe, Theory, Practice and Policy* (Palgrave Macmillan, 2011).

Giovanna Badalassi is member of GenderCAPP at the University of Modena and Reggio Emilia, Italy, and is a consultant expert in gender budgeting. Her recent publications include a co-authored paper on 'A Social-reproduction and Well-being Approach to Gender Budgets: Experiments at Local Government Level in Italy', which was presented to the Annual Conference of the International

Association for Feminist Economics in 2008, and *Gender Budgeting in Piedmont Region 2007–2008* (co-authored with D. Del Boca, E. Murtas and M. Zanoni) (IRES, 2009).

Loretta Baldassar is the Director of the Monash University Centre in Prato, Italy and Professor in the Department of Anthropology and Sociology at the University of Western Australia. She has published extensively on Italian migration to Australia. Her most recent publications include *Families Caring Across Borders* (with Cora Baldock and Raelene Wilding) (Palgrave, 2007) and *Intimacy and Italian Migration* (with Donna Gabaccia) (Fordham University Press, 2010). Her main fields of interest include the Australian diaspora in Italy and second-generation migrants in Italy and Australia. She is currently collaborating on projects which focus on transnational caregiving and the social uses of new technologies.

Anette Borchorst is Professor of Political Science at Aalborg University, Denmark. Among her recent publications are 'Political intersectionality: Tackling inequalities in public policies in Scandinavia', *Kvinder, Køn & Forskning*, nos 2–3 (with Mari Teigen), and 'The Multicultural Challenge to the Danish Welfare State: Tensions between Gender Equality and Diversity', in Janet Fink and Åsa Lundqvist (eds), *Changing Relations of Welfare. Family, Gender and Migration in Britain and Scandinavia* (Ashgate, 2010).

Cristina Borderías is Professor of Modern History at the University of Barcelona. She has published widely in areas relating to the history of labour, women's paid and unpaid work, and gender inequalities in Spain. Her recent publications include 'Women's work and household economic strategies in industrializing Catalonia', *Social History*, vol. 29, no. 3 (2004), pp. 373–83; *Género y políticas del trabajo en la España contemporánea* (Icaria editorial, 2007), and (with C. Sarasúa and P. Pérez-Fuentes), 'Gender inequalities in Family Consumption: Spain 1850–1930', in *Gender Inequalities, Households and the Production of Well-being in Modern Europe* (co-edited with T. Addabbo, M-P. Arrizabalaga and A. Owens) (Ashgate, 2010).

Sara Falcão Casaca is a Professor of Sociology of Work at the School of Economics and Management of the Technical University of Lisbon (ISEG-UTL) and a researcher at SOCIUS, The Research Centre in Economic and Organisational Sociology. She is a co-chair of the research network 'Gender Relations in the Labour Market and the Welfare State' of the ESA (European Sociological Association) and her main publications cover gender and labour market issues.

Francesca Corrado is a member of GenderCAPP at the University of Modena and Reggio Emilia, Italy, and is a PhD student in History of Economic Thought (University of Macerata – thesis project 'Wealth, Welfare and Well Being'). Her recent publications include *A Social-reproduction and Well-being Approach to*

Gender Budgets: Experiments at Local Government Level in Italy (co-authored with T. Addabbo, G. Badalassi and A. Picchio) (Ashgate, 2011). Her research interests include well-being gender budgets, welfare economics, and the standard of living in the history of economic thought.

Sónia Damião works for the Portuguese Institute for Employment and Vocational Training as a business investment analyst. She holds a masters degree in Economics and Social Policy from the School of Economics and Management of the Technical University of Lisbon, SEG/UTL.

Paloma de Villota is Professor of Economic Policy at the University Complutense de Madrid, Spain. Her latest publications include *El Impuesto sobre la Renta de las Personas Fisicas en Castilla y León dese la perspectiva de Género: Una propuesta a favor de las Mujeres Asalariadas* (with Ignacio Ferrari and Clara Sahagún) (Consejo Económico y Social de Castilla y León, 2008), *Estrategiaas para la integración de la perspectiva de género en los presupuestos públicos* (with Ignacio Ferrari and Yolanda Jubeto) (Ministerio de Igualdad, 2009), and a chapter (with Susana Vazquez Cupeiro) in *The Handbook of European Welfare State* (Routledge, 2009).

Florence Degavre is Senior Lecturer and Researcher at the Centre de Recherches Interdisciplinaires Travail, État et Société (CIRTES) at the Université Catholique de Louvain, Belgium. Her latest publications include 'Care as a Social Construct: The Case of Home Care Workers in Contemporary Belgium' (with M. Nyssens), in T. Addabbo et al. (eds), Gender Inequalities, Households and the Production of Well-being in Modern Europe (Ashgate, 2010), and 'La pensée "Femmes et développement"': Critique des fondements et pistes pour reconstruire un point de vue féministe croisé Nord/Sud', in I. Guérin et al. (eds), Femmes, économie et développement: Entre résistance et justice sociale (Eres/IRD, 2010).

Mónica Domínguez Serrano is Lecturer in Quantitative Methods at the Department of Economics, Quantitative Methods and Economic History and Coordinator of the masters programme on Gender and Equality, both at Pablo de Olavide University, Seville, Spain. Her most recent publications include Gender and Well-being: A New Measurement Proposal (forthcoming) and 'Work and time use by gender in European welfare systems', Feminist Economics (with Lina Gálvez and Paula Rodríguez) (forthcoming, 2011).

John Eriksen is a sociologist and Emeritus Researcher at NOVA – Norwegian Social Research Institute in Oslo, Norway, where he was formerly Research Director. With R. Richter, he edited 'Care through Cash and Public Service', European Societies, vol. 5, no. 4 (2003), pp. 342–470. He was a co-author of Eurofamcare: Supporting Family Carers of Older People in Europe (with R. Ingebretsen) (LIT Verlag, 2007), and of Livskvalitet: Forskning om det gode liv

('Quality of Life: Research about the Good Life') (with S. Næss and T. Moum) (Fagbokforlaget, 2011). He has been the editor of the Scandinavian Journal of Disability Research (Taylor & Francis) since 2008.

Lina Gálvez Muñoz is Professor of Economic History and Institutions, Vice-Rector of Graduate Studies, Director of the master's programme on Gender and Equality and the PhD programme on Development and Citizenship at Pablo de Olavide University, Seville, Spain. Her latest publications include Desiguales: Mujeres y Hombres en la crisis financiera ('Unequal: Women and Men in the Economic Crisis') (with Juan Torres López) (Icaria, 2010), and a special issue of Revista de Historia de la Economía y de la Empresa (with Francisco Comín) on De la beneficencia al estado del bienestar, pasando por los seguros ('From Charity to Welfare State, through Private Insurance')

Bernard Harris is Professor of the History of Social Policy at the University of Southampton. He has written The Origins of the British Welfare State: Social Welfare in England and Wales, 1800–1945 (Palgrave Macmillan, 2004). His is also the co-author of The Changing Body: Health, Nutrition and Human Development in the Western World (with R. Floud, R.W. Fogel and S.C. Hong) (Cambridge University Press, 2011).

Linda Lane, PhD, is Senior Lecturer at the Department of Social Work, University of Gothenburg, Sweden. Her publications include 'Conceptualizing work–life balance in the Swedish 'life puzzle' debate: Is it just about time?', in Familj, vardagsliv och modernitet (University of Gothenburg, 2010). She participated in the Sixth FP project 'Quality of Life in a Changing Europe' in 2007–2009, and was co-author of a chapter entitled 'Competing Demands: Work and Child Well-being' (with Tanja van der Lippe, S. Kabaivanov and Margareta Bäck-Wiklund), in Quality of Life and Work in Europe: Theory, Practice and Policy (Palgrave Macmillan, 2011).

Laura Merla is a National Funds for Research Postdoctoral Fellow at the Catholic University of Louvain, Belgium. Her main areas of research include the sociology of the family, gender, migration and transnational care. Recent publications include a special issue of the journal Recherches sociologiques et anthropologiques on 'Transnational Care Dynamics: Between Emotions and Rationality'. Future publications include papers in International Migration, Autrepart and the Journal of Ethnic and Migration Studies. She is currently co-editing (with Loretta Baldassar) a book on transnational families that will be submitted to Routledge (Transnationalism Series).

Anna Nikolaou is a PhD candidate at the University of Essex. Her research on 'Memory and Identity in Epirus: Ethno-cultural Affiliations, and Relationships under Reconstruction on the Greek/Albanian Border' was due to be submitted to the Sociology Department in January 2011.

Ariane Pailhé, PhD in Economics, is researcher at the Institut National d'Etudes Démographiques (INED), Paris, France. Her main fields of research are work–family conflict, gender and ethnic discrimination on the labour market, working conditions, and time allocation between spouses. She has written Entre famille et travail: Des arrangements de couple aux pratiques des employeurs (La Découverte, 2009).

Antonella Picchio is Professor of Political Economy at the Faculty of Economics of the University of Modena and Reggio Emilia. She holds a PhD in Economics from Cambridge University, has taught at the University of Rome 3 and has been a Visiting Professor at the New School of Social Research in New York. She is the author of Social Reproduction: The Political Economy of the Labour Market (Cambridge University Press, 1992; digital version 2010) and editor of Unpaid Work: A Gender Analysis of the Standards of Living (Routledge, 2003; digital version 2006). Her fields of research include: classical political economy, feminist economics, the capability approach, and gender budgets. She is currently a Fellow of the Human Development and Capability Association.

Paula Rodríguez Modroño is Lecturer in Economic History and Institutions in the Economic, Quantitative Methods and Economic History Department at Pablo de Olavide University, Seville. She teaches on the master's programmes on 'Gender and Equality' and 'Economic Development and Sustainability'. Her latest publications include a chapter on 'Welfare States, Work and Life Balance and Gender Differences in Time Use' in the book Women and the Labour Market (Fundación BBVA, 2010), and 'Work and time use by gender in European welfare systems', Feminist Economics (2011 (both with Lina Gálvez and Mónica Domínguez).

Annamaria Simonazzi is Professor of Economics at Sapienza University of Rome, President of the Scientific Committee of the Fondazione Brodolini and co-editor of Economia & Lavoro. She has published widely in the areas of macroeconomic theory and policy, the economics of the welfare state, employment and gender. Recent publications include 'Care regimes and national employment models', Cambridge Journal of Economics, vol. 33, no. 2 (March 2009), and (with Paola Villa) 'La Grande Illusion: How Italy's "American Dream" Turned Sour', in D. Anxo, G. Bosch and J. Rubery (eds), The Welfare State and Life Transitions (Edward Elgar, 2010).

Anne Solaz obtained her PhD from the University of Paris X-Nanterre in 1999. After lecturing at the University of Cergy, she took up her current post as a Research Fellow at the Institut National d'Études Démographies (INED) in September 2001.

As an economic demographer, her main research interests include the analysis of the relationship between career patterns and family events, the division of labour within couples, the evolution of family-friendly employment policies, marriage patterns and fertility.

Athina Vlachantoni is Lecturer in Gerontology at the Centre for Research on Ageing and ESRC Centre for Population Change at the University of Southampton. Her recent publications include 'The demographic and socio-economic characteristics of older carers: Evidence from the English Longitudinal Study of Ageing', Population Trends, no. 141, pp. 54–76.

Acknowledgements

This book is based on papers presented at the Symposium in Madrid in 2008 of COST Action 34 'Gender and Well-being: Work, Family and Public Policies', under the direction of Cristina Borderías (University of Barcelona). The editors would like to express their gratitude to her as well as to Bernard Harris (University of Southampton) for their scientific support in the editing process of this volume. Discussions with them as series editors have been important in shaping the focus and content of the present volume, and we are very grateful to them for their insight and their patience. Other help was provided by Conchí Villar and Mireia Singleton, successive secretaries for COST Action 34.

We held editorial meetings at Consejo Superior de Investigaciones Científicas in Madrid, at l'École des Hautes Études en Sciences Sociales in Paris and at the Université des Femmes in Brussels. We are grateful to these institutions for hosting us. Finally, we would like to thank Eleanor Rivers for copy-editing work, as well as Claire Jarvis from Ashgate for her help in preparing this manuscript and her assistance in producing the published book.

Preface

Cristina Borderías and Bernard Harris

This book is the fourth in a series of volumes under the general heading 'Gender and Well-being'. Like the first two volumes (Harris et al. 2009; Addabbo et al. 2010), it is based on a set of papers which were originally presented at a symposium funded by COST (European Cooperation in Science and Technology). The symposium was hosted by the Consejo Superior de Investigaciones Científicas in Madrid, and was organised by Paloma de Villota, Elisabetta Addis, Florence Degavre and John Eriksen.

COST is an inter-governmental framework which is designed to promote international collaboration across Europe in areas of scientific and technical research. There are currently 35 countries which are directly affiliated to COST, and 23 of these countries included participating institutions. There is also one country, Israel, which enjoys the designation of a 'co-operating state'.[1] The Madrid symposium was one of six which were funded under the auspices of COST Action 34. The Action was specifically concerned with the study of 'Gender and Well-being: Interactions between Work, Family and Public Policies'. It included individuals from 24 countries, and was co-ordinated by the University of Barcelona. The Action was chaired by Cristina Borderías, and the Vice-Chair was Antoinette Fauve-Chamoux.

The Action had two central but inter-related aims. Its first aim was to explore the impact of economic and social change on the lives of females and males using traditional indicators of well-being, such as income and wages, the allocation of household resources, access to services, and health status. The second aim was to explore the scope for the development of a new concept of well-being, and new social indicators, which would reflect the circumstances of both male and female lives. It was hoped that the development of this concept would also contribute to the emergence of a set of new criteria for evaluating the impact of social policies both now and in the future.[2]

The Madrid symposium was particularly concerned with the impact of institutions on gender and well-being. It includes 34 separate papers, focusing on a wide range of issues, ranging from the organisation of welfare in historical

---

1   See <http://www.cost.esf.org/service/faq> (accessed 8 May 2011).

2   The original prospectus for the Action is set out in the Memorandum of Understanding between the Proposer, Cristina Borderías, and COST, dated 28 April 2005. This can be downloaded from the Action website at <http://w3.cost.eu/fileadmin/domain_files/ISCH/Action_A34/mou/A34-e.pdf> (accessed 10 May 2011).

societies to discussion about contemporary equality policies, the capability approach and gender-budgeting. Several papers explored the impact of economic and demographic changes on the provision of social care. The increasing demand for care, together with the costs and benefits of delivering care, are among the most important challenges facing contemporary societies, and this focus is also reflected in the current volume.

The volume itself brings together chapters based on 11 of the papers which were originally presented in Madrid. All the chapters have been revised in the light of the discussions which took place during the symposium and conversations with the editors. As the editors point out, different kinds of institution – economic, social and cultural – influence well-being, and the gendered division of well-being, in a variety of ways. All the chapters in this volume are designed to shed new light on these questions, and by so doing, they also help to illuminate some of the ways in which families, business organisations and the state can work together to enhance the well-being of both women and men through the whole of their lives.

References

Addabbo, T., Arrizabalaga, M-P., Borderías, C. and Owens, A. (eds) (2010), *Gender Inequalities, Households and the Production of Well-being in Modern Europe*, Farnham: Ashgate.

Harris, B., Gálvez, L. and Machado, H. (eds) (2009), *Gender and Well-being in Europe: Historical and Contemporary Perspectives*, Farnham: Ashgate.

Chapter 1

Gender and Well-being:
The Role of Institutions

Elisabetta Addis, Florence Degavre, Paloma de Villota and John Eriksen

Provisioning for human basic needs is carried out in three main kinds of institutions: the familial household, the market and the institutions of the welfare state. The purpose of this book is to study the interplay among these institutions and their combined impact on people's well-being from a gender perspective. The chapters analyse some of the key policies and measures that have been implemented in European countries to sustain well-being in present and past times, and show the gendered implications of the changes that occurred.

The conceptual framework of the contributions in this book is inspired by the seminal work of Gøsta Esping-Andersen (1990) and by the comparative sociological literature he has initiated which identifies three main configurations of the institutions mentioned above: 'liberal', where the main provider is the market; 'social-democratic', where the main provider is the public sector, and 'corporatist', where family provision of care still plays the most prominent role. Some scholars have pointed out that Southern Europe constitutes a Mediterranean variation of the 'corporatist' welfare regime, characterized by low trust in the state as provider (Arts and Glissen 2002; see also Esping-Andersen 1999). The regimes also differ with respect to the main source of financing for care (private purchase, taxation, contribution), the amount and the channels of resources directed to the needy (cash transfers or transfers in kind by the state, private intra-family transfers),[1] and the arrangement of labour relations towards less commodification. However, as shown in many ways by gender theorists, this typology does not account for gender inequalities or for the way the state and the labour market intervene to reduce women's dependency on family or marital relations (Orloff 1993; Sainsbury 2000; Lewis et al. 2008). Gender stratification and its origin have thus become an increased source of questioning. Feminist literature has addressed important critiques to the usual Esping-Andersen typology before discussing new criteria to define the behaviour of European welfare states towards women (like female labour market participation, length and compensation of maternity leave),

---

1   In order to classify models, the kind of industrial relation system is also relevant, with centralised or decentralised wage-setting, and with co-operation or conflict as the prevailing wage-setting mode. We chose not to deal with these differences because they are not relevant to our theme.

and categorising them into new country clusters. In many ways, this book adds to this critical strand by developing some innovative paths both into the analysis of the interaction of institutions providing well-being and into the evaluation of their performances for women and men.

Many of the contributions in this book use renewed classifications of welfare states to study the production of well-being by institutions and its gendered aspects. In addition, they also measure social and economic inequality not only in terms of traditional welfare entitlements, but also in terms of a wider concept of well-being which is derived from the ideas of Amartya Sen and Martha Nussbaum about functioning and capabilities. In some chapters, the capability approach is applied specifically, in others it constitutes a more general orientation for the analysis of well-being. The joint usage of the sociological and economic-philosophical approaches to study the family, labour market and welfare state conundrum is one innovative characteristic of this book.

The contributions also innovate by putting policy logics alongside new and gendered indicators of well-being, analysing the latter as a dependent variable of the first. Societies are commonly classified and analysed according to the relative importance or mix of the institutions for the well-being of citizens. As mentioned above, many authors in this book use a categorisation which has become common. They see well-being in modern, capitalist societies as 'produced' by three kinds of institutions. The first are the familial households, where the first and basic levels of care, education, health provisions and comforts are provided; the second are profit and non-profit organisations selling to the households goods and services on the market that in pre-capitalist economies were produced only within the household itself, including healthcare and education-related goods and services. Third and last are the institutions of the welfare state, such as health services, mandatory schooling, retirement pensions, unemployment and other job-related insurance programmes, which either directly provide or subsidise the purchase.

It is important, however, to notice that in order to fully understand the relevance of these institutions to gender, we need to study their interplay in provisioning for human needs. These institutions determine women's labour demand (men and women are hired by the institutions of the welfare state or by market providers of care), the possibilities of consumption (earned wage can be used to buy goods and services only if such goods and services are provided by the market, or there is no need to buy them if they are provided free of charge in the family or by the public sector) and they are critical in determining the allocation of people's time, in particular women's time, between paid work and unpaid domestic production and provision of care, shaping gender relations and time use of people of both sexes. The proper balance of these institutions is a prerequisite of well-being for both: the caregivers and the care receivers, and also for satisfactory gender relations (Addis 2003).

Furthermore, this book contributes to the existing body of knowledge on gender, well-being and institutions at two levels: *empirical* and *theoretical*. Through the use of empirical material from original fieldwork or databases, various public policies and measures emanating from the local and the national level will be examined, as well as policies initiated at the level of the firm and accounts of individuals' behaviour in terms of capabilities. By doing so, the book brings together three worlds of analysis: the macro world of policies, the meso world of organisations and the micro world of individuals and households. The chapters cover several European countries with different welfare state regimes (Italy, Spain, Portugal, Greece, Germany, France, Sweden, Denmark and Great Britain), including cross-national data and comparative perspectives. The contributors have provided up-to-date data sets as well as innovative insights on the traditional welfare state's prerogatives. Some new fields are also explored, such as reconciliation policies, gender-budgeting and firms' family-friendly policies

The theoretical contribution is in line with the reflection on the development of the welfare state and its changing responsibilities in providing well-being. Three major responsibilities of today's welfare states in intervening to deliver well-being – care, economic protection and equality measures – which all affect access to resources for well-being for men and women are given special consideration. Dependency and well-being as well as the construction of care and its compensation across the life course are examined in the case of different regimes in Europe. In this context, the feminist theories used by some of the authors serve as a tool to critically assess the impact of institutional actors in providing well-being for both men and women, but most of all, to further 'engender' the various concepts used in the analysis.

The following sections of this introduction will give the reader a deeper insight into the book. The first section will explain the context in which the preparation of this book takes place. Then, since three of the important terms we use in the title are either subject to recent revision (well-being) or contested terrain in a plurality of approaches (gender and institutions), the second section will clarify the features of these concepts that are the most relevant to this book. Finally, we will introduce each of the chapters by pointing out their main contributions, and conclude by discussing the findings in the book that we consider most significant.

Context

In several ways, this book reflects the social, political and economic context of contemporary Europe. The main institutions securing the well-being of citizens, objects of our analyses, are identified for the purposes of this book as the families, the various institutions of the welfare state, and the private firms providing employment in general, and in particular those involved in the production of care services, although the institutions such as armies, parliaments and the judiciary are also involved in the production of well-being for citizens, and their activities have gendered effects. Our choice is due to the need to focus on the object of study, and also to the fact that the interplay among these institutions is fundamental to the understanding of gender roles and resource allocation between the two sexes (in terms of time and money, for example), and that their relative importance has been changing rapidly over time and space. Is it correct to say that the family might be a less important 'producer' of well-being than in earlier times, in particular in some countries? It is true that women were once the primary informal caregivers, and now the provision of care is directly affected by how care is organised or shared with the welfare state or purchased outside of the family. However, as shown, for example, in Chapter 7 by Laura Merla and Loretta Baldassar, the family role and women's primary responsibility in organising caregiving are resistant even to the strain of migration. The labour market holds a key position for women's well-being, because paid work is seen as a key route to equality and independence. However, as analysed by Sara Falcão Casaca and Sónia Damião in Chapter 9, in many countries unemployment, and particularly women's unemployment, remains at a high level. In addition, working full-time in the market puts an end to working full-time on the family, generating a conflict between the need for economic security and the need to give and receive domestic care. One solution to this conflict has been the choice of part-time work. But, often, when women take up part-time work, they enter low-paid positions or are subject to wage discrimination, affecting both their present and future incomes (pensions). The welfare state has become more important for people's well-being as more arenas of life are embraced by welfare arrangements – childcare centres, parental leave, prolonged education, healthcare, unemployment support, old age care and pension schemes. This long-term growth in publicly financed welfare provisions is subject to economic concerns, in particular in combination with high unemployment rates, increased longevity and stable age of retirement. These concerns were undoubtedly heightened by the onset of the financial crisis in 2008.

These changes in the role and place of the family, the welfare state and the labour market are accompanied – enlarged or moderated – by heavy social trends. As mentioned, increased longevity has provoked calls for pension scheme reforms which may reduce well-being, particularly for women. It has also called for more formal and informal care services for the elderly, putting pressure on families and social services that organise care. Issues associated with care have an important weight in the current volume. International migration challenges the labour market, among other things, but has also helped maintain care arrangements when fewer indigenous carers are available. Profound changes in family and household structure have several implications. More women wanting paid employment means that more jobs need to be created; at the same time, this creates a demand for care outside of their families, which in turn generates new employment in the personal services industry. This demand for more jobs is strongly supported by the female influx in higher education.

On the other hand, until the mid-1980s in OECD countries, the increase in female employment was accompanied by a decrease in fertility rate. Although this relationship has been reversed since, in the Nordic countries, with a female employment ratio almost at the same level as men's, the fertility rate still remains below the replacement level. But in other countries, the impossibility of finding employment with good salary and job security has impeded family formation, resulting in delayed births and population decline, as has occurred in Italy and Spain – especially during the 1990s, before receiving immigration influxes during the current century (de Villota 2007).

The comprehensive and women-friendly welfare states of the Nordic countries are usually seen as inspiring or as examples to be followed to achieve more gender equality. However, in Anette Borchorst's contribution in Chapter 3 as well as in Linda Lane and Margareta Bäck-Wiklund's in Chapter 11, the shortcomings of this welfare model are demonstrated: Married couples are not satisfied with their gender roles, and the welfare state has failed to integrate migrants, in particular migrant women from non-Western countries.

Conceptual Background

As mentioned at the beginning of this introduction, the three basic concepts of well-being, gender and institutions have a meaning that is controversial and subject to change, and therefore are in need of further exploration and clarification.

A Gender Perspective ...

The contributions in this book adopt a gender perspective to describe and analyse the various roles institutions play in producing well-being. Gender is the social construction prescribing for people of both sexes the proper behaviour, activities and decision power. Gender is not as fixed as sex: different notions of gender give shape, in different countries and at different times in history, to institutions. The gender perspective looks at what men and women do, and how the priorities, choices and relations of people of both sexes, which are sometimes in conflict, sometimes in co-operation, determine actual outcomes, including their well-being. It is exactly this understanding of the relations between people of different sexes – including their work, their culture, their allocation of resources and decision powers and their sexual orientations – that is the object of gender studies. Thus, by making this social construction of the individual visible and by emphasising gendered power relations, gender analysis illustrates how institutions are shaped.

Mainstream accounts treating men and women as gender-undifferentiated citizens dealing with institutions see the dynamics of other conflicting interests at play: tax payers versus users of welfare services, wage earners versus private entrepreneurs hiring them, contributors to pension funds versus pension earners, older generations versus younger generations of citizens. The gender perspective here is used, as the chapters show, to define the terms on which women's paid and unpaid work is provided and the kind of inequalities to which this division leads. In most societies it is women who, materially speaking, provide the bulk of care. But it makes a big difference if they do it as unpaid housewives, as public employees with the protection and wages of this status, or as private employees with varying degrees of job security and higher or lower wages. It makes a big difference for women's well-being as well as for the well-being of those cared for, within and outside the family. Policy proposals about taxation, contributions, pensions and labour market regulations which do not explicitly speak about gender still have an unspoken gender 'subtext'. In order to be able to make fully informed policy choices, this 'subtext' must be made explicit as it affects what men and women choose to do, their daily activities, the way they perceive themselves in the world, and therefore their well-being.

This 'subtext' has been grasped in the literature through the concept of the 'Gender Contract'. This remains very accurate, and gives an interesting insight into how the three institutions under examination interplay in shaping women and men's roles. The 'Gender Contract' is an invisible compromise at the level of social practices and representations that enrols men and women in productive and reproductive functions (Pfau-Effinger 1994). The term 'contract' here is not necessarily associated with established legal rules; it contains subtle symbolic and material terms sensitive to the relative power of men and women in society. This contract can be negotiated, however (Rantalaiho and Heiskanen 1997). In the field of care work and of the amount that is delivered, we know that women and men negotiate on an unequal basis: differences in wages, training but also social constructions of femininity or masculinity affect each gender's capability. Most of the authors in this book shed light on some of the multiple aspects of the contemporary version of the Gender Contract in European countries, while in Chapter 2, Bernard Harris, by examining the gendered nature of welfare provision before and after 1939 in England and Wales, examines the historical grounds of the contemporary contract.

... On Well-being

The gender perspective, whether applied through the macro level-related concept of Gender Contract or not, has led to a renewal of reflection on the measurement of well-being. It used to be that welfare – rather than the related concept of well-being – was traditionally measured by income per capita. From the 1960s, there was growing discontent with such a one-dimensional (economic) and often aggregate (like GNP per capita) measure to describe the complex life situation of citizens in terms of their welfare. As Nordhaus and Tobin (1973) pointed out, GNP was an index of production rather than consumption, and for this reason it could not be regarded as an appropriate measure of economic welfare. They were also very critical about the benefits and the inevitability of economic growth.[2]

It can be considered that this discontent resulted in two approaches:

1. an extended welfare concept covering many life arenas – income, employment, education, housing, health, social relations, social

---

2   On this topic, see Harris et al. (2009).

participation (level of living studies; Johansson 1979; Allardt 1975; see also Titmuss 1963);

2. an individual and self-reported well-being concept, often termed quality of life or psychological well-being (Veenhoven 1984).

Both are now established traditions, with considerable merit but lacking general acceptance as an adequate way to measure welfare and well-being. Amartya Sen's capability approach (Sen 1987) offers a more appropriate alternative. His approach is deeply rooted in philosophical notions of social justice, reflecting his perspective considering human beings as ends by themselves and the individual's ability to pursue and realise the goals he or she values. This approach supposes a rejection of the neo-classical economic model of individuals acting to maximise their own self-interest regardless of relationships and emotions, and tries to go further than the conventional analysis of economic well-being. It considers economic resources as an insufficient metric to measure quality of life. This assertion is based on two fundamental reasons: firstly, because economic resources are considered just means that have to be transformed into ends (well-being), and secondly, because many resources depend on people's life circumstances, such as friendship, family relations, informal support in case of need, which should not be described as resources with an imputable price 'even if people do make trade-offs among them' (Stiglitz et al. 2009, p. 41).

In this perspective, a person's life is as a combination of various doings and beings. The key idea of this approach is that social arrangements should aim to expand people's capabilities – their freedom to promote or achieve functionings. Functionings are defined as valuable beings and doings in an individual's life, such as a healthy body, being literate or having a decent job and so forth. Therefore, goods and services are important to the extent that they can generate capabilities.

Ingrid Robeyns notes that the development of some capabilities does not always require goods or services as an input: 'for instance being respected by your peers requires primarily respectful behavior from other people, and not necessarily any goods or services' (Robeyns 2007, p. 4).

It has to be said that freedom of choice and individual heterogeneity are included in the study of the multi-dimensional nature of welfare (Sen 1982; Sen 1987; Sen 2002; Nussbaum and Sen 1993). Sen and Nussbaum argued that in evaluating well-being, scholars and policy makers should focus on the real freedoms that people have – or don't have – to live a valuable life of their own. Therefore, they propose to consider capabilities such as being fed, healthy, educated and so on as necessary premises to undertake human activities such as being politically active or working on the labour market. Consequently, income and consumption are only means for well-being, and they appear to be very poor indicators of what really matters intrinsically – human capabilities and functionings.

Some capabilities may be considered quite elementary, such as being adequately nourished and avoiding premature mortality, while others may be more complex, such as having the literacy required to participate actively in political life. Others can be considered as instrumental capabilities –'substantive freedoms', such as the ability to engage in economic transactions, or participate in political activities. These are defined in terms of the substantive freedoms people have reason to value, instead of the concept of utility (choice, happiness) or access to resources (income, goods), and therefore represent a criticism of most standard mainstream microeconomic approaches.

Although it is important to also consider inequalities in the capability approach, it is necessary to avoid the presumption that one of them (for instance, income) will always encompass all others. On the other hand, there are certain inequalities that are very poorly understood and measured because they may have cumulative effects. For example, being poor and sick far exceeds the sum of the two separate effects, and government may act specifically to cater for those who accumulate these disadvantages.

Martha Nussbaum (2001), inspired especially by Indian women's grassroot associations, has developed a list of capabilities to try to inspire political measures to bring about a better quality of life for people. Ingrid Robeyns (2003), also inspired by the women's movement, has addressed issues that cannot be reduced to material or monetary endowments. She has emphasised the importance of reproductive health and reproductive rights, the negative effect of domestic violence, women's education and socio-economic status participation in the labour market, and time autonomy. She has deepened the understanding of how the capability approach is particularly relevant for the analysis of individual well-being in a gendered perspective. Ingrid Robeyns's list of capabilities has been designed especially for Western countries, and we believe both lists are very useful tools not only to implement adequate public policies, but to evaluate them.

To summarise, it can be said that the only way to generate capabilities out of goods and services depends on three conversion factors: social, environmental and personal. The environmental conversion factor depends on the environment (level of pollution, deforestation and so on) in which each person lives, and the personal conversion factor depends on mental (memory, imagination and so on) or physical (strength) aspects that are individually considered, which are crucial for generating different types or degree of capabilities. The relation between capabilities and functioning has also been explained very clearly by Ingrid Robeyns (2007):

> The choice of achieved functioning from a person's capability set need not be seen as an idealized choice of a purely rational agent who is detached from society; instead, the capability approach explicitly acknowledges the impact of preference formation mechanism on the preferences that people activate when they make choices, and also the potentially wide range of other social influences on decision making, such as peer pressure, social conformity, expectations from or commitments to family and friends, and so forth. In advance certain mental aspects of the person impinge on her [or his] ability to choose, for example low self-confidence, or post-traumatic anxieties. (Robeyns 2007, p. 4).

Personal and social conversion factors also affect functioning and demand careful observation, and differ among persons due to their individual circumstances, or there can also be structural social differences related to class, race, gender and so on. For example, it is quite easy to understand why it is more difficult for a woman to use her academic degree to develop self-esteem and secure economic autonomy (functionings) because social prejudices and gender discrimination in the labour market may affect her professional achievement negatively.[3]

In such a context, the task for governments is not easy to perform, as the cumulative effects of multiple disadvantages are poorly measured and inadequately understood at the individual and social levels, leading to the implementation of sub-optimal policies. For this reason, governance as legislative guarantees and the rule of law are crucial, as well as constitutional rights and rights in general, to providing people's well-being.

Access to a political voice is another fundamental dimension, together with the right to participate as full citizens in order to dissent without fear and speak up against what is perceived to be wrong. To have a say in the framing of policies is a crucial way of functioning for democratic institutions where different political groups should have opportunities for civic participation – not only for citizens, but also for immigrants (Stiglitz et al. 2009, p. 50).

The existence of universal suffrage is not the only way to evaluate the functional multi-party democracies. Popular levels of participation at different governmental levels have to be measured by indicators of political voice and governance: presence of free media, of civil organisations, trade unions and different professional bodies, and so on. The functioning of judicial systems is also a fundamental part of democratic institutions, and could be evaluated not only by considering extreme situations of corruption or political influence that really affect the roots of democratic regimes, but also by measuring the speed with which justice is delivered and the extent to which it can be accessed, both by citizens and non-citizens (residents and immigrants) (Stiglitz et al. 2009).

Before concluding, it must be pointed out that Amartya Sen's approach is an ethically or normatively individualist approach, as Ingrid Robeyns has underlined (Robeyns 2005; Robeyns 2007), but it is not ontologically or methodologically individualistic. This means that it takes into consideration the connections between people and their social relations. And this is why Sen's approach is different from ontological individualism, which only considers individuals and properties to build up societies and nothing more than the sum of them, and in the end, all social phenomena have to be explained only in relation to individuals and properties. Ethical individualism is a key issue for feminist theory, as women and children are

---

3   Conversion factors are empirically analysed by Tindara Addabbo et al. in Chapter 5 of this volume, when auditing public policies for gender-budgeting using context analysis. They point out how public employment centres can help in the conversion of the capability of working and doing business into the functionings of being employed or becoming entrepreneurs, and so on.

normally considered inside the 'box' of the family or community well-being. Only on rare occasions are the possible trade-offs between the different members of those social organisations taken into consideration. As a consequence, the lack of a perspective based on ethical individualism has hidden intra-household inequalities, as Nancy Folbre (1994), Jane Humphries ([1977] 1982) and Frances Woolley and Judith Marshall (1994) have shown for economically developed countries.

... and Institutions

The chapters in this book also contribute to an evaluation of the institutions' performance in the field of well-being for both sexes: Sara Falcão Casaca and Sónia Damião's Chapter 9 by raising the question of the need in the Mediterranean states for arrangements to improve the situation of women, in particular in relation to childbearing, and Anette Borchorst (Chapter 3) and Linda Lane and Margareta Bäck-Wiklund (Chapter 11) by demonstrating that the welfare state is not particularly gender-sensitive.

The concept of 'institution' can be used in various and sometimes confusing ways by people working in different fields and cultural traditions. In sociology, institutions are usually defined as 'social facts', stable in time (Dubet 2006, p. 635). Family, church, school and the state are considered as main institutions, but so are moral codes, norms and laws. Everett Hugues (1996) speaks about institutions as organisations that are able to distribute norms and goods, while François Dubet gives them a more political sense: apparels, laws, representations and activities which operate the transmutation from 'nature' into 'society' (Dubet 2006, p. 634). In other words, institutions are actors that organise, regulate and legitimise the rules and norms that are relevant in public and private spaces. This is not only true in the political field. Institutions proceeding from the state have also been studied by socio-economists in terms of their regulating role in the market. Economics builds on one central metaphor – the equilibrium of demand and supply – to describe and understand one particular institution – the market. and then tries to extend the methodology to understand the market to a number of other institutions, notably the family, but also bureaucracies, performing arts and other social phenomena, in an expansion labelled by critics as 'economics imperialism'. Polanyi, for example, insisted on the important role of institutionalised solidarity bonds in order to 'embed' the market principle and selfish interests (Polanyi [1944] 1983, p. 237). To him, an economy is an 'institutionalised process' characterised by its tendency towards disembeddedness. Institutions, in this context, supervise and regulate the market. In a less heterodox approach to economics, Ronald Coase (1937), and after him Oliver Williamson (1975), explained why contracts – considered as institutions – were necessary in order to achieve efficiency in a capitalist economy. The conceptions of these precursors of the neo-institutionalist stream are considered as breaking with the neo-classical tradition in economics which generally denies the existence of any institutions, concentrating on the atomistic individual. Neo-institutional economics also favours the analysis of market, contracts and organisations (that is, firms) in terms of institutions, considering the two latter as complementary to the first, and palliating its failures. In this important economic stream, institutions are considered as a set of crystallised human relations answering the market's insufficiencies (Lemaître 2009).

Institutions like the educational system or public administration can be seen as means of achieving justice and equality, or can also be seen as reproducing class inequalities; both interpretations may be true at the same time (Erikson and Goldthorpe 1992; Shavit and Blossfeldt 1993; Breen 2004; Sørensen 2006). It has also been demonstrated how gender and ethnic discriminations have been present in public and private institutions. On this last point, feminist studies have made decisive contributions. The long-running patriarchal functioning of the family, the workplace and social movements emerged from remarkable studies in women's history, while feminist sociology revealed contemporary aspects of this functioning. In the double emancipation process of women – from biology and the patriarchal functioning of society – institutions play an important role, however. If gender plays a role in shaping institutions, institutions determine gender outcomes as well. Synthetically and roughly speaking, one could say that an important part of feminist research can be considered an attempt to deconstruct the internal functioning of institutions and to reveal their sexism, while another important part is concerned with the impact of (gendered) institutions on the global functioning of societies, and on shaping women's lives in particular.

Contents of the Book

The book is organised into three parts. The chapters in Part I are more theoretical in nature. The framework of analysis is such that these chapters lay down the grounds for the debate. Although each of them is a case study, it is a case study that applies more general categorisations to the field of analysis, making it intelligible. They provide the keynote to the entire volume. They do so for the historical dimension (Bernard Harris, Chapter 2), for the central concern of the allocation of time to paid and unpaid care (Lina Gálvez Muñoz, Paula Rodríguez and Mónica Domínguez Serrano), for the problems related to public policy and policy evaluation (Tindara Addabbo, Giovanna Badalassi, Francesca Corrado and Antonella Picchio, Chapter 5), and for the general debate on the evaluation of welfare regimes (Anette Borchorst, Chapter 3).

Part II deals with the interplay between family-provided care and institutionally provided care. Care is seen here both as a need (making human interdependency visible) and a right (the right to be cared for and to care for). Care for the elderly is a paradigmatic locus of this interaction in all the chapters. Care is also connected to gender and migration through the analysis of the traditional role of women as caregivers (Annamaria Simonazzi, Chapter 6), but also through more unknown aspects, like the caring of migrants for their parents left behind in their home countries (Laura Merla and Loretta Baldassar, Chapter 7). The production of entitlements in the welfare system connected to family care provision via the recognition of pension credits is discussed by Athina Vlachantoni in Chapter 8.

Part III deals with the interplay between family-provided care and women's presence in the paid labour market. It explores the important issue of how the burden of care affects women's position in the paid labour market, interfering with the well-being both of women and of those cared for. This conflict between women's roles is particularly strong in Mediterranean welfare regimes, as shown by Sara Falcão Casaca and Sónia Damião in Chapter 9. 'Reconciliation policies' (Laura Alipranti-Maratou and Anna Nikolaou, Chapter 10) tries to overcome the problem, with mixed results. Labour market participation by itself also affects people's well-being, as shown by the analysis of Ariane Pailhé and Anne Solaz of the French case in Chapter 12, while Linda Lane and Margareta Bäck-Wiklund debate the Scandinavian model of work–life balance in Chapter 11.

The common core of the chapters in Part I, 'Gender and Welfare Regimes: Historical and Theoretical Perspectives', is the functioning of the welfare state in different contexts. Central topics are the division between paid and unpaid labour, the subsequent time-autonomy, active intervention in institutions like the family or the market, or changes in citizens' rights, including rights of the two sexes. This first part also shows how women have been secondary for welfare policies and in gaining full citizen rights in England and Wales, and how they still are in welfare states of the Mediterranean type, but also, to some extent, in the comprehensive welfare states of the Nordic type with a long history of aiming for full gender equality. One of the proposed tools to improve substantive gender equality is a strategy to make public budgets more sensitive to the needs of women by means of gender-budgeting.

Chapter 1 by Bernard Harris is an explicitly historical chapter where the roots of gender inequality in England and Wales are traced in the long term. This chapter draws on Marshall's distinction between the civil, social and political rights of citizenship to provide a new account of the relationship between gender and welfare provision in Britain during the nineteenth and twentieth centuries (Marshall 1965). Marshall argued that these rights had become separated during the course of the eighteenth and nineteenth centuries, and were only re-integrated during the first half of the twentieth century. During the nineteenth century, when social rights were divorced from political rights, the majority of welfare recipients were female and the receipt of poor relief was associated with dependent status. During the twentieth century, a new set of welfare provisions was introduced and restrictions on the exercise of political rights were removed. These changes enabled a new generation of men to exercise their social rights without surrendering their political rights, but they also generated new forms of inequality within the welfare system. The impact of these inequalities on the welfare entitlements of men and women is still apparent today.

In Chapter 2, Anette Borchorst presents a critical analysis of the Scandinavian welfare states and their experiences in generating gender equality. In these countries, equality was and still is high on the political agenda. Income inequality is relatively low, and the commitment to gender equality is high. Women participate in paid work almost as often as men, and both men and women occupy high offices in political life. The dominant measure implemented by the welfare state is the dual-breadwinner model, supported by the availability of childcare facilities for pre-school children and long, paid parental leaves. This is accompanied by birth rates that stay below the replacement rate but are comparatively higher than average European standards. This pattern is contrary to many other countries in Europe, as demonstrated in other chapters in this book (see Chapters 4, 8, 9 and 10).

However, as Anette Borchorst notices, different authors make different evaluations of the outcomes in the Scandinavian countries. While Helga Hernes (1987) has termed the Scandinavian welfare state 'women-friendly', Yvonne Hirdman (1996) has concluded (from Swedish data) that the traditional gender system has remained intact due to gender segregation and a hierarchy based on the male norm. One reason for these different evaluations could be that while Helga Hernes focused on the welfare state, Yvonne Hirdman focused on the labour market. Anette Borchorst supplements this evaluation of the Scandinavian welfare states and their gender equality efforts by pointing to some paradoxes. Referring to Marshall's distinction between civil, political and social rights, the author notices that Scandinavian women obtained political rights quite early on and have had high levels of political representation, but are no longer in the lead in comparison with other European countries. Further, in Scandinavia, the labour markets are highly gender-segregated, and the high birth rates and long parental leaves enjoyed by Scandinavian mothers are accompanied by 'a child penalty' – loss of pay, career and pensions. It is also noteworthy that the Scandinavian welfare states have failed to integrate non-Western immigrant women. Anette Borchorst concludes that the Scandinavian experience demonstrates that the universal breadwinner vision has obvious shortcomings: it is driven by a narrow utilitarian policy logic that restricts women's options and makes gainful employment imperative. It does not generate gender equality unless men participate on an equal level in care work.

Chapter 3 by Lina Gálvez Muñoz Paula Rodríguez and Mónica Domínguez analyses the experience of the Mediterranean countries, which can be characterised in gender terms as having low female market participation rates and low fertility rates. This demonstrates that these societies are not only highly unequal, but also non-sustainable, since the fertility rate is well below the level needed for the population to reproduce itself. Considering this point, it must be underlined that since the mid-1980s onward important demographic changes have been observed in some OECD countries which show a positive correlation between fertility rates and women's employment. On the one hand, Namkee Ahn and Pedro Mira (1999) have considered the incidence of the high level of youth unemployment during the 1980s and 1990s in Italy and Spain as an important factor in explaining the dramatic decline in fertility rates during those decades. On the other hand, Alicia Adsera (2004) has stressed that during the last two decades a silent demographic transformation with important economic and political consequences has occurred, in which the correlation between fertility and female labour participation rates across OECD countries has become positive. She extols the virtue of what occurs in Northern European countries, where income tax and dependent children benefits encourage fertility and a commitment to a life-long labour market career for women, as noted also in de Villota (2007).

Besides, it is not highlighted enough that the Mediterranean countries also show a more unequal distribution of unpaid domestic and care work, together with some Eastern European countries. The study presents an international time-use study based on the Eurostat Time Use Survey 2003 (covering 15 European countries), paying special attention to paid–unpaid work dynamics and to free time differences by gender, with particular reference to the Southern European welfare model. Time-use data allow the authors to show how housework and care work that take place outside the market represent an essential and distinctive part of the economy. Although Anette Borchorst in Chapter 2 highlighted some of the limitations of the Nordic welfare states, this chapter argues that institutional developments and public policies in Mediterranean countries have evolved in a less female-friendly environment than in other welfare regime types, such as the Nordic ones, which still appear to possess a more even distribution of total work by gender.

Finally, in the concluding chapter of this part, Tindara Addabbo, Giovanna Badalassi, Francesca Corrado and Antonella Picchio illustrate a new approach to the analysis of the budget of public entities from the gender viewpoint, based on Sen and Nussbaum's capability approach as it has been experimented with in Italy at local government level. The authors consider this approach the most adequate to deal with gender inequalities because it includes unpaid work as a major component of the total work of women and men and it also includes in the analyses the process of social reproduction. This approach has been applied at various levels of local governments in Italy. Well-Being Gender Budgets (WBGBs) can also be applied to other countries and at different levels of government. WBGBs have the potential to become the key to greater co-ordination of policies and to serve as a basis for social participation and for public debate because of their effectiveness in capturing women's and men's well-being in a given territory.

Part II of the book deals with gender, the provision of care (in the family and in the household), and the policy choices associated with this. It considers how the welfare state can organise care to meet the needs both of women as main caregivers and of those in need of care. Long-term care responsibility towards elderly people is one of the greatest challenges for European societies, where demographers predict that the number of older dependent people in Europe will approximately double between the present day and 2060 (EU-27) (ECFIN 2009, p. 150). One can ask how European societies will respond to this challenge at a time when demand for care is supposed to increase (ECFIN 2009, p. 145), long and heavy unpaid commitments by women can no longer be expected (if they ever really could), and flexible labour markets are putting pressure on life–work balance. States are opting for various degrees of marketization (giving to the market care provisions mediated by the family) and de-institutionalisation (people receiving care in their own homes). Therefore, the question 'Who is caring today?' is indeed an important one, and it must be examined both at the level of the state and at the level of individuals, as public provisions have important incentive effects on individual behaviour. Elderly care in particular could be monetised, and a family member might substitute for a public institution, or be in charge of translating a monetary subsidy in a market purchase. The family – and women in it – react to public policy choices, and a configuration of care is created.

In a comparative analysis of care policies in European societies, Anna-Maria Simonazzi asks whether care regimes are converging towards a common European model with more home-based care, which depends on women both in the formal and informal care markets. Originally, care regimes referred to resources dedicated to lone mothers in different European Welfare States (Lewis and Hobson 1997). Two ideal-type came out of this study: the 'caregiver social wage' model and the 'parent/worker' model. The concept of care regime has become more complex, however, and nowadays tends to integrate elements other than lone mothers' rights and their role in care work. The care regimes present a strong formal dimension in the sense that they integrate measures that states put at the disposal of people who provide or receive care: types of cash benefits which might be provided (unconditional versus tied cash benefits), labour market regulations, special leaves, social insurance, or foster care for elderly or frail adults. But the concept has roots in the informal arrangements, remunerated or unremunerated, that are developed by individuals to fulfil their own care needs: payments to individual carers within families and households versus the public provision of institutionalised services, the role of undocumented workers or any other informal and remunerated solutions. Care regimes express the strategies *vis-à-vis* care as they are pursued by the different states. Annamaria Simonazzi uses the type of public intervention in response to new needs in long-term care ('in cash' or 'in kind') to establish a new distinction among care regimes, and draws a link with the new care market that these interventions have created.

The concept of care regimes is a useful tool to analyse political strategies towards care. However, at this stage in the development of care regime theory, one important question is left aside: the role of individual preferences in the choice of care organisation. The identification of care regimes does not in itself say much about how 'real people' cope with the different possibilities that are offered in terms of care, how they make use of the set of possibilities that are put at their disposal, and how they 'invent' their own arrangements. The issue of individual care arrangements is taken up in Chapter 7 by Laura Merla and Loretta Baldassar, who investigate transnational family caregiving in a comparison between Australia, EU and Latin America. They apply the capabilities approach to examine transnational family practices and the exchange of care between adult migrant children and their ageing parents living at a distance. One aim of the chapter is to raise awareness about the importance of transnational familial caregiving for migrant well-being. Using qualitative oral history data, they highlight the role of the state in facilitating caregiving across distance between the countries where the parents are living, in this case El Salvador and Italy, and the country where the children reside, in this case Australia. The ability to practise transnational caregiving is defined as a 'capability' that is influenced by a further set of 'capabilities', including mobility, social relations, time-autonomy, education and knowledge, paid work and communication. Access to, and use of, these capabilities is strongly influenced by both the home and host countries' formal institutional and informal policies. The family, considered here as a social institution, plays a key role in mediating the access of both migrants and parents to transnational caregiving-related capabilities.

In Chapter 8, Athina Vlachantoni discusses the paradox of some welfare arrangements that are intended to improve the well-being of women, but in practice may have the opposite effect. Her example is the system of credit rights (future pension) for unpaid care work in the home for own family members (own children, spouses, elderly parents) introduced in many European countries.

The background for introducing such care credits is pension systems. Even though they were originally introduced to help people on low incomes, mostly female (at least this was the case for non-contributory schemes; see Chapter 2), present-day pension schemes favour the full-time and long-term employed – men – thus they fail to address the division between paid and unpaid labour – that is, much of women's traditional work. Following demographic changes, pension systems have been reformed across Europe, and credits for caring for own family members have been included. Such credits are included in the carer's working record as if the carer were employed in the labour market.

Care credits acknowledge and compensate carers for time spent outside paid work, and in this sense care credits contribute to the well-being of women. They recognise individual rights to make choices, they ensure valorisation of unpaid care work in practice, and they promote gender equality in terms of pension accumulation. On the other hand, care credits tend to preserve women's and men's traditional roles, since – under the present wage structure – the family will suffer least income loss if women take on care duties and give up their jobs, fully or partly. Care credits can be seen as the primary compensatory mechanism for persons devoted to caring for dependent household members. But the arrangement needs reorganisation to support gender equality: it must be incorporated into a wider social policy framework, extended to cover care for the elderly (in countries where it does not do so), and not least, compensation must be increased to a level that allows real choice between work and care for both men and women. The convergence towards a common caregiving model, as described by Annamaria Simonazzi, hardly seems to improve the independence and well-being of women. Modern care systems (increasingly home-based) still depend on women, and various measures implemented to alleviate – or improve – the well-being of caring women are insufficient. Care credits and payment-for-care schemes are insufficient or compensatory at best, and in any case, they tend to reinforce traditional gender roles. Modern care systems are in many countries dependent on immigrant labour, often women, often undeclared, and paid at low rates in the informal market. This creates a care scarcity in the migrants' home countries and maintains the imbalance in gender roles in the host countries, rather than bringing men into care. Modern care systems are also closely linked with low birth rates. In particular in countries with extensive family care and little public care, birth rates are low and remain low, far below replacement level.

Thus, Part II demonstrates that while politicians in many countries prefer care to be a private or family responsibility supported by welfare arrangements (as cash or rights), such policies may result in negative arrangements for most women, and will affect the sustainability of both the migrants' home societies and the societies to which they migrate.

Part III is primarily concerned with the attempt to reconcile the demands of the labour market with those of family life. It explores inequalities between men and women in this domain, and examines the extent to which public policy has been able to deal with the conflicts that arise when individuals are called upon to combine participation in the labour market with family responsibilities. It also emphasises the importance of employers' policies in helping people to address these issues.

In Chapter 9, Sara Falcão Casaca and Sónia Damião study how Southern European welfare states are slowly evolving towards dual-breadwinner models, with growing concern for work–life reconciliation in public policies – far from enough, though. In fact, during recent years globalisation has imposed pressure to increase business productivity and competition, making it very difficult for women to combine family or personal life with the increasing demands of the labour market. Casaca and Damião discuss the role of the welfare state in the modernisation of gender roles in Portugal, Spain, Italy and Greece. According to their work, standard classifications of welfare regimes are not gender-sensitive and do not account for the specific gender regimes of Southern Europe. In addition, care regimes are evolving at different rates. The weakening of the male breadwinner model is most noticeable in Portugal, but is also apparent in Spain. They argue from the Mediterranean experience that gender equality cannot be achieved in the Southern European countries unless radically improved parental leave and affordable and high-quality daycare are provided.

In Chapter 10, Laura Alipranti-Maratou and Anna Nikolaou focus on reconciliation policies in Greece, and examine critically how the problem is formulated in policy frames and public discourse. They start by noticing that socio-economic developments in the countries of the EU have enhanced the social and productive role of women by raising educational standards and increasing their participation in the labour market. As a result, women are called on to combine work and caring responsibilities. Reconciliation, equal opportunities and family policy in Greece constitute fields that have been closely connected, with a commitment to promoting women's access to employment. They present a brief overview of the measures regarding reconciliation of work and family, and the public debate about gender equality. They also introduce some of the findings of MAGEEQ, a large-scale European collaborative study including Austria, Greece, Hungary, the Netherlands, Slovenia and Spain. The study involved the analysis of public documents with respect to gender equality in three policy fields – politics, family policy and domestic violence – and showed that the policy framing had an important effect on the policies enacted.

Part III ends with two important national case studies. Chapter 11 provides the second evaluation (in addition to Chapter 3) of the merits of the Scandinavian welfare regime for achieving gender equality. Here, Linda Lane and Margareta Bäck-Wiklund examine work–life conflicts among Swedish dual-breadwinner families. According to comparative data, they find – maybe somewhat unexpectedly – that Swedish dual-breadwinners families are experiencing more work–life conflicts than dual-breadwinner families in other countries. This dissatisfaction with current gender roles in Sweden (and other Nordic countries), when it comes to combining work and family life, may partly reflect high ambitions and the long-term pursuit of full gender equality. While women and men have reported similar levels of perceived work–life conflict, gendered expectations have played an important role in perceived work–life conflict when the household domain is included. For women, household disagreements have reflected the link between work–life conflicts and the double burden of paid and unpaid work. Men have found it difficult to live up to Swedish equality goals and perform their fair share of household work. In other words, in a country known for its long-term quest for full gender equality and for comprehensive welfare arrangements to achieve this goal, work–life conflict has not been overcome. Rather, this conflict is an integral part of Swedish dual-breadwinner families' lives, the authors observe. How can this be? The key element is time shortage. Time spent on work necessarily restricts the amount of time available for other demands, such as caring and housework. In Sweden, where labour market participation is high both from men and women, and the welfare state provides economic and social support that enables both to combine the multiple roles of work and family life, there is still considerable dissatisfaction in everyday life. While the patterns of paid work have changed considerably, the patterns of unpaid work have not. Women contribute substantially to household income through their work in the labour market, *and* they continue to perform the bulk of unpaid household work. This is because the way in which partners in dual-breadwinner families share work and household demands will depend on the gender ideology they hold and the power each partner can wield to demand a fair share of work from the other. In the end, the unequal distribution of unpaid work results in time shortages, in particular for women, and diminishes their opportunities to develop all their capacities. This scarcity of time for women constitutes a situation that can be observed in all the European countries considered in this book.

In Chapter 12, Ariane Pailhé and Anne Solaz, standing in the framework of the economic literature on self-perceived job satisfaction, present interesting results for France, where firms' family-friendly policies have long been noted. They study the determinants of individual satisfaction concerning the balance between work and family. The literature on work satisfaction is a branch of a larger field that may be labelled 'sociology and economics of happiness'. It is a field of research that developed starting with the findings known as 'the Easterlin Paradox': there is very little correlation between income growth and perceived satisfaction and/ or perceived happiness in developed countries. After a sufficient level of income is achieved, the ability to transform income into happiness ceases. Other factors, such as health, social relationships and job satisfaction, become more important than income levels. One important fact that emerged from this literature is that women, controlling for levels of income, job satisfaction and other known variables affecting happiness, are happier than men almost everywhere.[4]

The findings in this chapter confirm how in France as a whole, people are satisfied with their balance between family and work, and women are even a little more satisfied than men. At the same time, French fertility remains at a relatively high level within Europe. One explanation advanced is the family-friendly environment which allows mothers – even those with young children – to continue to work without feeling upset. Family-friendly environments may have different mediums – public policies, social and cultural norms and the workplace – topics that are under-researched. Firms may be involved in the balance between family and work through schedule flexibility, in-kind benefits and financial benefits.

The merit of the econometric approach taken in this chapter is the mix of individual determinants, household determinants and company determinants, enabled by the survey linking individuals and their workplaces. The data set used in this chapter comes from the Families and Employers Survey conducted by the Institut National d'Études Démographiques (France) in 2004–2005. It is presented in two steps. First, using factor analysis, the authors present a typology of companies according to the degree of 'family-friendly policies' they have set up. Secondly, those groups formed by the cluster analysis are seen as explanatory variables of an ordered probit analysis of employees' satisfaction with work– family balance, controlled for socio-demographic covariates. The results show that employers' policies and practices are only partially determinant; individual working conditions are the most important determinants. The companies' practices, especially their flexible schedules, have a strong impact on mothers' satisfaction, whereas fathers' satisfaction depends more on working atmosphere and family-friendly acceptance of peers and supervisors.

Important Lessons

We noted at the beginning of this introductory chapter that the most important objects of our inquiry are all in a state of flux, either as a subject under deep revision (well-being) or as particularly complex to deal with (gender and institutions). This introduction does not aim to provide a synthesis or policy prescription, but to draw a line between the different contributions showing how rich and full a

---

4   Some of these issues have been discussed in a recent review of the literature on 'subjective well-being' for the UK Treasury – see Lepper and McAndrew (2008).

gendered view of institutions and institutional change can be, and how important it is for the production and evaluation of people's well-being. However, we have tried here to grasp and convey to the reader the most recent approaches in these fields. In conclusion, we will summarise the most important findings that emerge from the work as a whole.

The Need for an Integrated Approach

The main characteristic emerging from the studies contained in this volume is the close interdependence between social and labour market policies in the context of fundamental changes in both working patterns (the increase in female labour force participation rates) and social needs (including population ageing). Therefore, one lesson which might follow from the research contained in this book is the need for a more integrated approach both to welfare analysis and to welfare policy, which takes account not only of basic welfare entitlements, but also the need for supportive forms of service provision and the details of employment regulation. One related point that recurs throughout the book is that this interdependence requires scholars to develop new and more powerful integrated indicators which are capable of evaluating and giving orientation to social and economic intervention, and which incorporate the new findings of moral philosophy, as Sen and Nussbaum have only begun to show.

Applied Use of a New Theoretical Approach

Another lesson that emerges from the book is the possibility of applying the capabilities approach as a methodological tool for the applied purpose of gender-budgeting. This possibility is quite innovative, and can help to improve public policies. It should be pointed out that the discussion on gender-budgeting, compared to other contemporary debates over public policies, has incorporated feminist reflections on theories of justice, and especially criticisms about the liberal distributive concept of equal opportunities as reformulated by means of John Rawls's (1973) and Ronald Dworkin's (2000) theories. In this sense, the gender-budgeting debate triggers essential questions for feminist theory: What do we understand by justice, by equality, by rights? Do our notions of justice, equality and rights include women, or is it necessary to approach them from a different perspective in order to incorporate women's needs? On the other hand, in relation to the budget field, 'well-being' that includes women requires not only the approach of traditional distributive budgets, but reformulation of the analysis, and in this sense, a recognition of women in public policies. This places discussions on gender-budgeting in a different frame: the well-being frame. The implication of these changes is developed in Chapter 5 by Tindara Addabbo, Giovanna Badalassi, Francesca Corrado and Antonella Picchio, which shows how gender budgets based on the well-being approach can allow us to see women as a multiple subject, and not as a category. Their analysis of the importance of gender-budgeting at the local level is very relevant because they connect the problem of who decides and how with the possibility that local governments offer a more democratic space for the determination of the definition of well-being. In fact, as they say:

> well-being gender budgets ... can also be applied to other countries and at different levels of government. They could in fact become a key to a greater coordination of policies and a basis for social participation in public debate on both the concept and the actual experience of women's and men's well-being in a given territory. (see Chapter 5 in this volume)

Centrality of the Issue of Time Allocation

Many of the chapters insist on the use of time as a major indicator of well-being, because gender inequality is particularly present in time use. According to the list of capabilities elaborated by Ingrid Robeyns (2003, p. 75), 'gender inequality includes inequality in time allocation, leisure time, time related stress, and so forth. This is an important social issue in some Western societies.' For example, in Chapter 11, Linda Lane and Margareta Bäck-Wiklund explain dissatisfaction with present gender roles in Sweden in terms of time use and time squeeze. In Sweden, as elsewhere, women still take on the double burden of paid and unpaid work, and thus feel the pressure of work demands more than men. This is seen by many women as an unfair distribution of household work that can be expressed in the number of hours that men and women devote to it. As the authors point out and the survey shows, there still exists a partner disagreement over what needs to be done and who should do what. This could be considered a significant indicator of work–life conflict. Equality and equity between the sexes are official goals, but gender inequality can be seen in the unfair distribution of unpaid work that still exists. The Mediterranean countries present an even more uneven gender distribution of total work, demonstrating how institutional developments and public policies have evolved in a 'less female-friendly environment than in other welfare regimes', as Lina Gálvez Muñoz, Paula Rodríguez Modroño and Mónica Domínguez Serrano pointed out in Chapter 5. Autonomy in the use of time – the ability to decide freely how to best spend one's time for different purposes – is fundamental for achieving well-being and for evaluating welfare regimes.

Large Potential for New Research

Finally, this book shows that we need 'gendering' – accounting for the process of social construction of men and women and for their relative positions in society, to fully describe institutions and understand their functioning. The contributions show how large the potential of research is in the area of institutions producing well-being in a gender perspective. Most chapters use a theoretical structure applied to a single case study. These structures could be most fruitfully applied to other national or transnational examples, to render these new approaches systematic.

Since national cases were investigated and described in terms of their specific features and merits, the policy suggestions may or may not be relevant for policy reforms in for other countries – and it would be worthwhile to investigate this issue. Other chapters are comparative, and demonstrate differences and similarities between European welfare states. The main policy contribution, Tindara Addabbo, Giovanna Badalassi, Francesca Corrado and Antonella Picchio's Chapter 5 on gender-budgeting, is methodological, and the central idea of writing down gender accounts of public spending can be applied to all countries at different levels – central or local – of an individual institution. The application of gender-budgeting techniques to the study of public finances is considered one of the most promising new research avenues. We expect that much of the research presented in this book will have follow-ups, and that the cross-fertilisation of themes and approaches that went on in the Madrid symposium and in the other meetings of Cost Action 34 (see Preface) will result in the further findings and in the advancement of gender-conscious policy making at the national as well as at the European level.

References

Addabbo, T. and Picchio A. (2009), 'Living and Working Conditions: Perspectives, Concepts and Measures', in B. Harris, L. Gálvez and H. Machado (eds), *Gender and Well-being in Europe*, Farnham: Ashgate.

Addis, E. (2003), 'Unpaid and Paid Caring Work in the Reform of Welfare States', in A. Picchio (ed.), *Unpaid Work and the Economy*, New York: Routledge, pp. 189–223.

Adsera, A. (2004), 'Changing fertility rate in developed countries: The impact of labour market institutions', *Journal of Population Economics*, vol. 17, pp. 17–43, <http://www.jordipujol.cat/files/adsera_04.pdf> (accessed 8 May 2011).

Ahn, N. and Mira, P. (1999), *A Note on the Changing Relationship between Fertility and Female Employment Rates in Developed Countries*, Madrid: Fundación de Economía Aplicada, Working Paper no. 3, February, <ftp://ftp.cemfi.es/wp/99/9903.pdf> (accessed 8 May 2011).

Allardt, E. (1975), *Att ha, att älska, att vara: Om välfärd i Norden*, Lund: Argos.

Arts, W. and Gilissen, J. (2002), 'Three worlds of welfare capitalism or more? A state of the art report', *Journal of European Social Policy*, vol. 12, no. 2, pp. 137–58.

Bettio, F. and Plantenga, J. (2004), 'Comparing care regimes in Europe', *Feminist Economics*, vol. 10, no. 1, pp. 85–113.

Bourdieu, P. and Passeron, J.C. (1970), *La reproduction: Eléments pour une théorie du système d'enseignement*, Paris: Editions de Minuit.

Breen, R. (ed.) (2004), *Social Mobility in Europe*, Oxford: Oxford University Press.

Carrasco, C. (2009), 'Beyond Equality: Towards a System of Non-androcentric Indicators', in B. Harris, L. Gálvez and H. Machado (eds), *Gender and Well-being in Europe*, Farnham: Ashgate.

Castles, F.G. (1993), *Families of Nations: Patterns of Public Policy in Western Democracies*, Aldershot: Dartmouth.

Coase, R. (1937), 'The nature of the firm', *Economica*, no. 4, pp. 386–405.

De Villota, P. (2006), 'Birth Rate and Women's Rights in Europe', in H. Widdows, I.A. Idiakez and A.E. Cirión, *Women's Reproductive Rights*, Basingstoke: Palgrave Macmillan, pp. 50–70.

Delphy, C. (1998), *L'ennemi principal: Économie politique du patriarcat*, Collection Nouvelles Questions Feminists, Paris: Syllepse.

—— (2001), *L'Ennemi principal: Penser le genre*, Collection Nouvelles Questions Feminists, Paris: Syllepse.

Dubet, F. (2006), *Injustices*, Paris: Seuil.

Dworkin, R. (2000), *Sovereign Virtue: The Theory and Practice of Equality*, Cambridge, MA: Harvard University Press.

ECFIN (2009), 'The 2009 Ageing Report: Economic and budgetary projections for the EU-27 member states (2008–2060)', *European Economy*, 2/2009.

Erikson, R. and Goldthorpe, J. (1992), *The Constant Flux: A Study of Class Mobility in Industrial Societies*, Oxford: Clarendon Press.

Esping-Andersen, G. (1990), *The Three Worlds of Welfare Capitalism*, Cambridge: Polity Press, and Princeton, NJ: Princeton University Press.

Esping-Andersen, G. (1999). Social Foundations of Postindustrial Economies. Oxford: Oxford University Press.

Folbre, N. (1994), 'Children as public goods', *American Economic Review*, vol. 84, no. 2, pp. 86–90.

Goffman, E. (1979), *Asiles: Études sur la condition sociale des malades mentaux et autres reclus*, Collection 'Le Sens Commun', Paris: Editions de Minuit.

Harris, B., Gálvez, L. and Machado, H. (2009), 'Gender and Well-being from the Historical and Contemporary Perspective', in B. Harris, L. Gálvez and H. Machado (eds), *Gender and Well-being in Europe: Historical and Contemporary Perspectives*, Farnham: Ashgate, pp. 1–20.

Hernes, H.M. (1987), *Welfare State and Women Power. Essays in State Feminism*, Oslo: Norwegian University Press.

Hirdman, Y. (1990), 'Genussystemet', in *Demokrati och Makt i Sverige*, Maktutredningens huvudrapport, SOU 1990:44, pp. 73–114.

—— (1996), *Key Concepts in Feminist Theory: Analyzing Gender and Welfare*, Aalborg: Aalborg University, FREIA Paper 34.

Hugues, E.C. (1996), *Le regard sociologique*, ed. J.M. Chapoulie, Paris: Editions de l'EHESS.

Humphries, J. ([1977] 1982), 'The working-class family, women's liberation and class struggle: The case of nineteenth century British history', *Review of Radical Political Economics*, vol. 9, no. 3 (Fall 1977), pp. 25–41; revised version in Spanish translation, in *Debate Sobre la Mujer en America Latina y el Caribe: Discussions Acerca de la Unidad Production Reproduction*, ed. Magdalena Leon del Leal (1982).

Johansson, S. (1979), *Mot en teori för social rapportering*, Stockholm: Institutet för Social Forskning.

Klasen, S. (2008), 'Gender and Well-being: What Does the Capability Approach Have to Offer?', lecture given at the COST Action 34 Madrid symposium, 26–28 June.

Lemaître, A. (2009), *Organisations d'économie sociale et solidaire: Lectures de réalités Nord et Sud*, Louvain-la-Neuve: Presses Universitaires de Louvain.

Lepper, J. and McAndrew, S. (2008), *Developments in the Economics of Well-being*, Treasury Economic Working Paper no. 4, <http://www.hm-treasury.gov.uk/treasury_economic_workingpaper4.htm> (accessed 8 May 2011).

Lewis, J. (2003), 'Erwerbstätigkeit versus betreuungsarbeit', in U. Gerhard, T. Knijn and A. Weckwert (eds), *Erwebstätige Mütter: Ein europäischer Vergleich*, Munich: Beck.

—— and Hobson, B. (1997), 'Introduction', in J. Lewis (ed.), *Lone Mothers in European Welfare Regimes: Shifting Policy Logics*, London: Jessica Kingsley, pp. 1–20.

——, Campbell, M. and Huerta, C. (2008), 'Patterns of paid and unpaid work in Western Europe: Gender, commodification, preferences and the implications for policy', *Journal of European Social Policy*, vol. 18, no. 1, pp. 21–37.

Marshall, T.H. (1965), *Class, Citizenship and Social Development*, New York: Anchor Books.

Mesure, S. and Savidan, P. (2006), *Dictionnaire des sciences humaines*, Paris: Presses Universitaires de France.

Nordhaus, W and Tobin, J. (1973), 'Is Growth Obsolete?', in M. Moss (ed.), *Measurement of Economic and Social Performance*, New York: National Bureau of Economic Research, pp. 509–64.

Nussbaum, M.C. (2001), *Women and Human Development: The Capabilities Approach*, Cambridge: Cambridge University Press.

—— and Sen, A. (1993), *The Quality of Life*, Oxford: Clarendon Press.

OECD (1999), *A Caring World: The New Social Policy Agenda*, Paris: OECD.

Orloff, A.S. (1993), 'Gender and the social rights of citizenship: The comparative analysis of gender relations and welfare states', *American sociological Review*, no. 58, pp. 303–28.

Pfau-Effinger, B. (1994), 'The gender contract and part-time paid work by women: Finland and Germany compared', *Environment and Planning*, vol. 26, no. 9, pp. 1,355–76.

Picchio, A. (2008), 'Capability Approach and Classical Political Economy', paper presented at the COST Action 34 Madrid symposium, 26–28 June 2008.

Polanyi, K. ([1944] 1983), *La grande transformation: Aux origines politiques et économiques de notre temps*, Paris: NRF, Gallimard.

—— (1975), 'L'économie en tant que procès institutionnalisé', in K. Polanyi, C. Arensberg, and H. Pearson, *Les systèmes économiques dans l'histoire et la théorie*, Paris: Larousse, pp. 39–260.

Rantalaiho, L. and Heiskanen, T. (eds) (1997), *Gendered Practices in Working Life*, London: Macmillan.

Rawls, J. (1973), *A Theory of Justice*, Oxford: Oxford University Press.

Robeyns, I. (2002), 'Gender Inequality. A Capability Perspective', PhD thesis, Cambridge University.

—— (2003), 'Sen's capability approach and gender inequality: Selecting relevant capabilities', *Feminist Economics*, vol. 9, nos 2–3, pp. 61–92.

—— (2005), 'The capability approach: A theoretical survey', *Journal of Human Development*, vol. 6, no. 1, pp. 93–114.

—— (2007), 'Social Justice and the Gendered Division of Labour: Possibilities and Limits of the Capability Approach', paper prepared for presentation at the Cost Action 34 Conference, Barcelona, 25–27 June 2007.

Sainsbury, D. (2000), *Gendering Welfare States*, London: Sage Publications.

Sen, A. (1980), 'Equality of What?', in S. McMurrin (ed.) *The Tanner Lectures on Human Values*, vol. 1, Cambridge: Cambridge University Press.

—— (1982), *Choice, Welfare and Measurement*, Oxford, Blackwell.

—— (1987), *The Standard of Living*, Cambridge: Cambridge University Press.

—— (1990), 'Gender and Co-operative Conflict', in I. Tinker (ed.), *Persistent Inequalities*, New York: Oxford University Press, pp. 123–49.

—— (2002), *Rationality and Freedom*, Cambridge, MA: Belknap Press.

Shavit, Y. and Blossfeldt, P. (1993), *Persistent Inequality: Changing Educational Attainment in Thirteen Countries*, Boulder, CO: Westview Press.

Siim, B. (2000), *Gender and Citizenship: Politics and Agency in France, Britain and Denmark*, Cambridge: Cambridge University Press.

Sørensen, A. (2006), 'Welfare states, family inequality, and equal of opportunity', *Research in Stratification and Mobility*, vol. 24, pp. 367–75.

Stiglitz, E., Sen, A. and Fitoussi, J.P. (2009), *Report by the Commission on the Measurement of Economic Performance and Social Progress*, <http://www.stiglitz-sen-fitoussi.fr/documents/rapport_anglais.pdf> (accessed 8 May 2011).

Titmuss, R.M. (1963), *Essays on the Welfare State*, London: George Allen & Unwin.

Veenhoven, R. (1984), *Conditions of Happiness*, Dordrecht: Kluwer Academic.

Wall, R. (2009), 'Gender-based Economic Inequalities and Women's Perception of Well-being in Historical Populations', in B. Harris, L. Gálvez and H. Machado (eds), *Gender and Well-being in Europe*, Farnham: Ashgate, pp. 23–58.

Williamson, O.E. (1975), *Markets and Hierarchies, Analysis and Antitrust Implications: A Study in the Economics of Internal Organization*, New York: Free Press.

Woolley, F. and Marshall, J. (1994), 'Measuring inequality within the household', *Review of Income and Wealth*, vol. 40, no. 4, pp. 415–31.

PART I
Gender and Welfare Regimes: Historical and Theoretical Perspectives

Chapter 2

Gender and Social Citizenship in Historical Perspective: The Development of Welfare Policy in England and Wales from the Poor Law to Beveridge

Bernard Harris

As Peter Breiner (2006, p. 1) has recently pointed out, 'almost all examinations of modern citizenship are compelled at a minimum to pay lip-service to T.H. Marshall's renowned essay, "Citizenship and Social Class"'. In that essay, Marshall (1950, pp. 10–14) drew an important distinction between what he described as the civil, political and social rights associated with citizenship in England and Wales from the Middle Ages onwards. Marshall's account of the development of these rights has often been seen as a causal account in which civil rights provided the foundation for the acquisition of political rights which led, in turn, to the acquisition of social rights (see, for example, Pierson 1998, pp. 20–22; Lister 2003, p. 70), but this may not be an entirely accurate summary of its author's intentions.

Although Marshall thought that social rights were radically curtailed during the course of the nineteenth century, he did not argue that they were eliminated altogether, and even though he thought that the acquisition of political rights (by men) had contributed to the expansion of social rights, he did not regard this as being either a necessary or a sufficient condition for their development (Marshall 1950, pp. 21–46). Instead, one of the main aims of his paper was to examine the way in which the possession of one set of rights had become separated from the possession of a different set of rights, and the way in which the process of welfare reform in the first half of the twentieth century enabled the three types of rights to be brought back together. In this sense, his paper was not designed to explain the 'evolution' of Britain's welfare state, but rather to identify the particular meaning of that welfare state.

This chapter seeks to explore the implications of this argument for our understanding of the relationship between gender and the history of British social policy since the introduction of the New Poor Law in 1834. During the nineteenth century, as Marshall (1950, p. 24) explained, it was often assumed that the possession of social rights was incompatible with the full exercise of either civil or political rights, and this was reflected in the organisation and distribution of poor relief. After 1906, the Liberal governments of Henry Campbell-Bannerman and Herbert Asquith introduced a series of reforms which removed some of the constraints on the exercise of welfare rights and allowed a new generation of men to receive social benefits. Forty years later, Clement Attlee's Labour government sought to extend the scope of the Liberal reforms to the entire population, so that many women and children became eligible for benefits which had previously been restricted to male breadwinners. However, as many commentators have recognised, the new benefits did not introduce an era of gender equality because many of the benefits extended to the female population continued to depend on their relationship to a male partner (see, for example, Pedersen 1990, pp. 983–4; Pedersen 1993, pp. 1–21).

Although other commentators have also explored the relationship between gender and entitlement in the history of British welfare provision, they have tended to approach the issue in a rather different way. Several authors have examined the ways in which 'women's agency' contributed to the development of Britain's welfare state (see, for example, Thane 1991; Lewis 1994), and both Pat Thane (1978b) and Mary Daly (1998) have emphasised the essential continuity between the ways in which the poor law and its successors dealt with women's claims for income maintenance. In contrast, the main aim of this chapter is to show how the changing relationship between social and political rights affected the welfare entitlements of both men and women between the introduction of the New Poor Law and the creation of the 'classic' welfare state after 1945.

Gender and Welfare under the New Poor Law

The foundations of the English system of poor relief were laid by a series of Acts passed during the late fifteenth and sixteenth centuries, culminating in the Elizabethan Poor Law Acts of 1597 and 1601 (Slack 1995, pp. 1–13). These Acts gave the churchwardens and overseers of each parish the right to levy a tax, or poor rate, on every inhabitant or occupier of land, and made them responsible for 'setting the poor on work', maintaining those who were unable to work, and making arrangements for pauper children to become apprentices. Although several additional Acts were passed throughout the seventeenth and eighteenth centuries, the basic framework of poor law provision remained intact until the passage of the Poor Law Amendment Act in 1834. This Act broke new ground by establishing a central government body, known as the Poor Law Commission, and giving it the power 'to make and issue ... rules, orders and regulations for the management of the poor' in England and Wales. It also gave the Commissioners the power to combine individual poor law parishes into Unions 'for the administration of the laws for the relief of the poor', and enabled them to order the construction of workhouses if there was sufficient support from local ratepayers (Harris 2004, pp. 40–49).

Although the Act was primarily an administrative measure, its underlying aim was to reduce the 'burden' of poor relief by making it much more difficult for able-bodied men, in particular, to claim relief (Parliamentary Papers 1840, p. 5). During the early years of the New Poor Law, the Commissioners sought to achieve this aim by insisting that relief should only be given to able-bodied men (and their families) if they were prepared to enter a workhouse, but they were subsequently obliged to relax this policy and allow Boards of Guardians to distribute outdoor relief to able-bodied men who were willing to perform an 'outdoor labour test' (Harris 2004, pp. 49–50). However, despite this, the number of able-bodied men who received poor relief remained very low, as Table 2.1 demonstrates. On 1 January 1859, the total number of able-bodied men in receipt of poor relief was 32,363, of whom 6,245 were being relieved inside a workhouse. The majority of those who received outdoor relief were being relieved as a result of their own sickness or that of another family member. Only 85 were receiving relief as a result of 'sudden or urgent necessity', and only 2,459 were being relieved 'on account of want of work or other causes'.

Although the architects of the New Poor Law were particularly concerned to restrict the relief entitlements of able-bodied men, these restrictions had a direct impact on the welfare of the women and children whose husbands and fathers were denied poor relief. The significance of this is underlined by evidence from other sources which demonstrates that women and children tended to bear the brunt of poverty in poor households (Thane 1978b, pp. 33–5; Harris 1998, p. 418; Harris 2008, p. 194). However, many women also faced particular difficulties when applying for relief independently, as Pat Thane (1978b) has demonstrated. Married women only retained a right to relief in the parish or Union of their husbands' birth, and this meant that many widows and deserted wives were transported back to their husbands' birth-parishes in order to seek relief. Many poor law authorities were also reluctant to give outdoor relief to widowed or separated mothers, on the grounds that the workhouse would provide a more suitable environment for the upbringing of their children, and they stigmatised unmarried mothers inside the workhouse by requiring them to perform the most onerous tasks. During the 1870s, the central authority launched a 'crusade' against outdoor relief, and this led to a further reduction in the number of women who received assistance outside the workhouse. For the first time, women could be asked to perform an 'outdoor labour test' in order to demonstrate their need for relief, and new restrictions were placed on the welfare rights of deserted mothers (Thane 1978b; Harris 2004, pp. 54–6).

However, despite these difficulties, women continued to form a majority of the adult recipients of poor relief throughout the period 1834–1914, although there were important differences in respect of the numbers of men and women who were relieved inside and outside the workhouse, and in the numbers of male and female paupers who were described as being either able-bodied or non-able-bodied. The statistics for indoor pauperism are summarised in Table 2.A.1 (see Appendix). This table shows that, during the 1850s, the numbers of men and women who received indoor relief were roughly equal, but the proportion of female inmates who were able-bodied was consistently greater. This continued to be the case during the following decades, but the overall number of male inmates

           Gender and Well-Being

Table 2.1   **Able-bodied men in receipt of poor relief, 1849–59**

	Indoor relief		Outdoor relief				
	Married	Others	Relieved in cases of sudden and urgent necessity	Relieved in cases of their own sickness, accident or infirmity	Relieved on account of sickness, accident or infirmity of any of the family, or of a funeral	Relieved on account of want of work, or other causes	Total
1 Jan. 1849	2,389	8,695	708	25,506	10,996	17,427	65,721
1 July 1849	802	3,948	506	22,257	8,815	8,719	45,047
1 Jan. 1850	1,690	8,160	308	22,650	9,071	9,314	51,193
1 July 1850	512	3,085	201	18,604	6,790	4,440	33,632
1 Jan. 1851	1,396	6,958	200	19,799	7,489	5,347	41,189
1 July 1851	432	2,857	190	17,147	6,539	4,356	31,521
1 Jan. 1852	1,001	5,681	220	17,650	6,801	4,108	35,461
1 July 1852	430	2,956	102	17,049	6,442	2,677	29,656
1 Jan. 1853	749	4,630	125	17,179	6,476	1,611	30,770
1 July 1853	151	2,124	81	14,392	5,394	1,084	23,226
1 Jan. 1854	1,192	6,307	225	17,606	7,431	3,216	35,977
1 July 1854	446	3,156	133	15,967	6,849	2,246	28,797
1 Jan. 1855	1,052	5,331	116	17,781	7,587	4,245	36,112
1 July 1855	430	3,349	97	16,877	6,644	2,498	29,895
1 Jan. 1856	998	5,495	164	18,526	7,579	4,967	37,729
1 July 1856	259	2,842	78	15,556	6,001	1,479	26,215
1 Jan. 1857	842	5,052	88	17,210	6,835	3,784	33,811
1 July 1857	249	3,099	117	15,402	6,053	1,575	26,495
1 Jan. 1858	957	6,505	141	19,146	7,820	12,155	46,724
1 July 1858	217	3,195	78	15,544	5,698	2,402	27,134
1 Jan. 1859	552	5,693	85	17,239	6,335	2,459	32,363

Source: Parliamentary Papers (1859), pp. 196–9.

began to outstrip the number of female inmates at the end of the 1860s, and by 1913 more than three-fifths of all adult inmates were male, with more than 64 per cent of all adult male paupers receiving relief inside a workhouse (see also Table 2.A.2 in the Appendix).

Even though the number of adult males inside the workhouse ultimately outstripped the number of adult females, the majority of paupers were supported outside the workhouse, and the majority of outdoor paupers were female. This included both able-bodied and non-able-bodied paupers, as Table 2.A.2 demonstrates. During the 1850s, the number of able-bodied women who received outdoor relief exceeded the number of able-bodied men because, in addition to the wives of able-bodied men, relief was also granted to single women without children, unmarried mothers, widows and the wives of prisoners, members of the armed forces and other non-resident males. The central authority did not publish the same amount of information for later decades, but it is reasonable to assume that the broad pattern did not change. These statistics reflect the fact that women faced a much greater risk of poverty as a result of lower wages and more limited labour market opportunities, as well as greater longevity (Thane 1978b, pp. 33–5). However, they also reflect the way in which considerations of gender influenced the development and application of poor law policies. As Lynn Lees (1998, p. 179) has argued, even though the amounts of relief provided by the poor law authorities were often meagre at best, poor law officials were more willing to offer relief to women, children and the elderly than to Irish immigrants or healthy adult males.[1]

Pauper Disenfranchisement and Welfare Reform

Although tests such as the workhouse test and the outdoor labour test played an important part in deterring able-bodied men from seeking poor relief, they were not the only factors which discouraged people from becoming paupers. After 1832, the recipients of poor relief were legally prevented from voting in parliamentary elections, and although this made little difference to women, who were prevented from voting until 1918, it became increasingly important for men who might otherwise have been able to exercise their own voting rights. The significance of this was underlined by changes in franchise law and by the gradual expansion of poor law services.

As is well known, the basis of voting rights in the mid-nineteenth century was laid down by the Representation of the People Act of 1832. The Act granted voting rights to the freeholders of property worth more than £10 a year and to the tenants of properties worth more than £50 a year in County areas (2 William IV C. 45, sections 18–20). It enfranchised approximately 717,000 men, or roughly one-fifth of the adult male population (Pugh 1999, p. 49). Voting rights were extended more dramatically by the Acts of 1867 and 1884. The 1867 Act gave the vote to householders and lodgers in borough districts (30 & 31 Vict. C. 102, sections 3–6), and the 1884 Act established uniform rights for householders and lodgers throughout the country (48 Vict. C. 3, sections 2–3). As a result of these changes,

---

1   This point has also been made by Goose (2005), p. 357.

more than 60 per cent of adult males enjoyed the right to vote in parliamentary elections by the end of the century (Pugh 1999, p. 106).

However, there was also a long-standing tradition that political rights should be denied to individuals in receipt of poor relief. In 1795, Charles James Fox pointed out that, with very few exceptions, 'all those ... who had at any time received relief from the parish' were excluded from voting in parliamentary elections (Parliamentary History of England 1795, col. 702), and this tradition was reinforced by the Reform Acts of 1832 and 1867. The 1832 Act excluded anyone 'who shall within twelve calendar months next previous to the last day of July in such year have received parochial relief' from voting in cities or boroughs (2 William IV C. 45, section 36), and the 1867 Act extended this prohibition to voters in County areas (30 & 31 Vict. C. 102, section 40). The Divided Parishes and Poor Law Amendment Act of 1876 prevented anyone 'who shall be in receipt of relief given to himself or his wife or child, or who shall have been in receipt of such relief on any day during the year last' from voting in any local elections, including the election of members of Boards of Guardians (39 & 40 Vict. C. 61, section 14).

Although parliament denied the vote to those who had been in receipt of poor relief, voting rights were extended to the recipients of other forms of public welfare provision, including both public vaccination and the payment of school fees by School Boards. The Vaccination Act of 1867 stated that even though the poor law authorities were responsible for the administration of the public vaccination service, vaccination against smallpox 'shall not be considered to be parochial relief', and neither the recipients of vaccination nor their parents should suffer any disabilities or disqualifications as a result of this service (30 & 31 Vict. C. 84, section 26). The Elementary Education Act of 1870 allowed School Boards to remit the fees of any child whose parents were unable to pay them, but such remission 'shall not be deemed to be parochial relief ... to such parent' (33 & 34 Vict. C. 75, section 17). However, the inclusion of these clauses only served to underline the fact that the recipients of benefits which were regarded as poor relief continued to be disqualified from exercising the right to vote.

These developments highlighted a growing tension associated with the expansion of public welfare services during the course of the nineteenth century. On the one hand, parliament was anxious to maintain the deterrent aspects of the poor law, and these were reinforced during the 'crusade against outdoor relief' of the 1870s, but it also recognised that there might be circumstances in which it was in the interests of the public as a whole for individuals to avail themselves of the services which the state provided. These tensions came to a head over the development of poor law medical services in the 1870s and 1880s. Even though parliament wanted to discourage individuals from making themselves dependent on the receipt of poor relief, it also wanted to encourage people to take fuller advantage of some of the services which the poor law provided. It was also becoming increasingly aware of the demand for exemptions from some of the disabilities associated with pauper status on grounds of both political and social justice.

During the 1860s and 1870s, medical authorities were becoming increasingly aware of the role played by infected individuals in the transmission of infectious and contagious diseases, and this highlighted the need to ensure that individuals who might be suffering from these conditions should seek medical attention at the earliest opportunity (Harris 2004, p. 97). This was made more difficult if the same individuals were discouraged from seeking medical assistance under the poor law by the imposition of pauper disabilities. As a result of this, the Liberal MP for Liverpool, William Rathbone, made two unsuccessful attempts to introduce legislation which would have ensured that no person should be disqualified from voting in a parliamentary election because:

> he, or any member of his family, has ... received medical treatment or relief for any infectious or contagious disease as an in-patient or out-patient of any hospital, infirmary or dispensary established or maintained by any sanitary ... or poor law authority. (Parliamentary Papers 1878a; Parliamentary Papers 1878b)

The issue resurfaced during the debates on the Representation of the People Bill in 1884 and on the Registration (Occupation Voters) Bill in 1885. On 12 May 1885, the Liberal MP for Christchurch, Horace Davey, proposed an amendment to the Registration Bill which would have meant that 'medical and surgical relief and the giving of medicine shall not be deemed to constitute parochial relief within the meaning of the Representation of the People Acts' (Parliamentary Debates 1884, cols 859–66; Parliamentary Debates 1885a, cols 1,802–10; Parliamentary Debates 1885b, cols 387–91, 958–70).

Although Davey's amendment was rejected, it paved the way for two further bills, introduced over the course of the following two months, which were both designed to dissociate the receipt of medical relief from the disabilities which were associated with the receipt of other poor law services. In June, the Liberal MP for Ipswich, Jesse Collings, introduced a Private Member's Bill which proposed that:

> no person shall be disqualified from being registered as a voter or from voting under any Act relating to the Representation of the People by reason of the receipt ... of parochial or poor law relief in the form of medical or surgical assistance or medicine. (Parliamentary Papers 1884a)

In July, the government introduced a bill of its own, which allowed the recipients of medical relief to vote in all elections other than the election of Boards of Guardians (Parliamentary Papers 1884b). This bill became law on 30 July (48 & 49 Vict. C. 46) and provided a template for further attempts to extend voting rights to other recipients of poor relief and related services over the next two decades (see, for example, Parliamentary Debates 1906, col. 1585).

The debates over these bills reflect the changing nature of the debate over pauper disabilities. In 1884, when the Irish MP Andrew Commins sought to extend voting rights to the recipients of medical relief in the Representation of the People

Bill, his arguments were largely related to the control of infectious diseases. He pointed out that the Public Health Act of 1875 gave magistrates the power to order people who were suffering from infectious diseases to be admitted to a public hospital, and he argued that they should not be disenfranchised as a result of an obligation imposed upon them for the public good (Parliamentary Debates 1884, cols 859–66). However, when MPs agreed to support the government's Medical Relief (Disqualifications Removal) Bill in 1885, they did so on the basis that no form of medical relief should disqualify a man from exercising his right to vote, and that there was a fundamental difference between the receipt of medical assistance and other forms of poor relief. As the Conservative MP for Hertfordshire, Frederick Halsey, explained, 'in the majority of cases illness came upon people suddenly, often at most difficult times', and this meant 'that medical relief stood on a totally different footing to any other form of relief' (Parliamentary Debates 1885c, col. 1,434).

Although MPs such as Halsey accepted the idea that voting rights should be granted to the recipients of medical relief, they continued to argue that men who received other forms of poor relief should be excluded from the rights of political citizenship, and this principle was reaffirmed on a number of occasions during the 1890s and early 1900s. In 1892, Sir Wilfred Lawson argued that men who were employed by Boards of Guardians on public works schemes should be allowed to retain the right to vote in all parliamentary and local elections (Parliamentary Papers 1892), and Sir Theodore Fry introduced a very similar bill in 1895 (Parliamentary Papers 1895a), but both measures were defeated. However, when parliament passed the Unemployed Workmen Act in 1905, it did agree that 'the provision of temporary work or other assistance for any person under this Act shall not disentitle him to be registered or to vote in a Parliamentary, county or parochial election, or as a burgess' (5 Edw. VII C. 18, section 1.7).

These were not the only attempts to either modify or remove the restrictions placed on the voting rights of poor relief recipients in this period. In 1895, Samuel Hoare proposed that paupers should not be disqualified from exercising the right to vote if they received poor relief in an area which had been formally identified as a 'distressed district' (Parliamentary Papers 1895b), and three separate attempts were made to protect the voting rights of members of friendly societies who received poor relief in 1900, 1901 and 1902 respectively (Parliamentary Papers 1900; Parliamentary Papers 1901; Parliamentary Papers 1902). In 1905 and 1906, the Liberal MP for Manchester, Charles Schwann, tried to abolish the pauper disqualification clauses altogether, and his colleague, Patrick Marnham, attempted to extend the protection provided by the Unemployed Workmen Act to individuals employed in poor law labour yards in 1906 and 1908 (Parliamentary Papers 1905; Parliamentary Papers 1906a; Parliamentary Papers 1906b; Parliamentary Papers 1908). However, despite these efforts, many MPs continue to argue that men who exercised their right to claim poor relief forfeited their right to be treated as political citizens. As the Conservative MP for Wigan, Sir Francis Powell, explained, when outlining his objections to Marnham's bill in 1906:

although [the] Bill discriminated in the preamble by using the word 'deserving', there was no such discrimination in [its] enacting clauses .... How could they treat a person who was little more than a tramp or a vagrant in the same way as they treated the deserving persons to whom reference had been made by preceding speakers? (Parliamentary Debates 1906, col. 1,588)

Extending the Boundaries of Welfare Provision

By the end of the nineteenth century, there was a growing recognition of the need for some form of welfare reform. This was encouraged by the publication of new studies of poverty in London and York by Charles Booth and Seebohm Rowntree and by mounting fears about 'physical deterioration', and it reflected widespread concerns on the part of the political élite about the rise of the new Labour Party and the 'quest' for national efficiency (Harris 2004, pp. 151–7). In 1905, the outgoing Conservative government appointed a Royal Commission to investigate the operation of the poor laws, and this led to the publication of both majority and minority reports in 1909. However, instead of either reforming or abolishing the Poor Law, the Liberal government of 1906–14 decided to follow an alternative approach, based on the development of new forms of welfare provision to run alongside it. This approach enabled the government to introduce a new range of welfare benefits which could be claimed by 'respectable' workers without incurring the disabilities associated with the receipt of poor relief. This was particularly important for adult men, who were now able to claim welfare benefits for themselves and their families without surrendering their rights as political citizens (Harris 2004, pp. 57–8, 165).

The government's approach was reflected, initially, in the introduction of the Education (Provision of Meals) Act of 1906. This Act was based on a private member's bill which had been introduced by a Labour MP, W.T. Wilson, earlier in the year. Its primary aim was to enable local authorities to cooperate with voluntary agencies to provide school meals to children whose parents could afford to pay for them, but it also allowed the authorities to give free meals to children who were 'unable by reason of lack of food to profit from the education provided for them', and by 1914 it had been adopted by more than 130 local education authorities (Harris 1995b, p. 77; Harris 2004, pp. 157–8). Although this was in many ways a rather minor measure, it represented a major extension of the scope of public welfare provision outside the poor law, as many contemporary observers recognised. In 1914, the conservative constitutional theorist Alfred Venn Dicey summarised its significance in the following terms:

No one can deny that a starving boy will hardly profit from the attempt to teach him the rules of arithmetic. But it does not necessarily follow that a local authority must therefore provide every hungry child at school with a meal ... [or] that a father who first lets his child starve, and then fails to pay the price legally due from him for a meal ... should ... retain the right of voting for a Member of Parliament. Why a man who first neglects his duty as a father and then defrauds the state should retain his full political rights is a question easier to ask than to answer. (Dicey 1962, p. l)

The next major reform to raise significant questions about the relationship between the social and political rights of citizenship was the Old Age Pensions Act of 1908. As John Macnicol (1998, pp. 60–84) has shown, the earliest proposals for the establishment of old age pensions were designed to encourage young people to behave in a more sober and thrifty way by saving money for their own old age, but there was also growing evidence that many older people were experiencing considerable poverty. In 1895, the Royal Commission on the Aged Poor highlighted the fact that many elderly people were living in poverty because they were not prepared to apply for poor relief, and Seebohm Rowntree claimed that as much as 10 per cent of the household poverty in York in 1899 was attributable to the illness or old age of the principal wage-earner (Harris 2004, p. 57). These revelations reinforced the growing demand for a non-contributory pension scheme, and this culminated in the 1908 Act. The Act provided a means-tested benefit of up to 5s. a week for men and women over the age of 70 with an annual income of less than £31 10s.[2] However, it was not supposed to be paid to people who had recently received poor relief, and it was conditional on tests of behaviour and good character (Macnicol 1998, pp. 155–63; Harris 2004, p. 159).

The introduction of old age pensions represented a significant moment in the history (or pre-history) of the British welfare state for a number of reasons. In the first place, it is important to recognise that one of the main arguments in favour of the introduction of a non-contributory scheme was an acknowledgement of the fact that it would be very difficult for low income-earners in general, and women in particular, to afford the level of contributions needed over the course of their working lives to finance their own pension arrangements (Thane 1978a). Second, it is also necessary to recognise that the circumstances of both economics and demography meant that the majority of those who received old age pensions after 1908 were likely to be female, as Table 2.2 demonstrates. However, the introduction of old age pensions also possessed a major symbolic importance for elderly men because it meant, for the first time, that they were able to claim a cash benefit from the state without surrendering their rights as political citizens.

---

2   Before 1971, the main units of currency in the United Kingdom were pounds, shillings and pence (£. s. d.). Each £1 contained 20s., and each 1s. contained 12d. In 1901, Seebohm Rowntree estimated that the sum needed to maintain a family of two adults and three children in a state of 'merely physical efficiency' was 21s. 8d. a week, including rent (see Harris 2000, pp. 78–80).

Table 2.2   **Number of pensions payable in England and Wales, and in the United Kingdom, 1909–14**

	England and Wales			United Kingdom		
	Male	Female	Total	Male	Female	Total
26 Mar. 1909	—	—	393,700	—	—	647,494
31 Mar. 1910	—	—	441,489	—	—	699,352
31 Mar. 1911	—	—	613,873	—	—	907,461
29 Mar. 1912	—	—	642,524	351,397	590,763	942,160
28 Mar. 1913	245,418	423,228	668,646	363,811	604,110	967,921
27 Mar. 1914	251,126	433,509	684,635	369,365	614,766	984,131

Sources: Annual Reports of the Local Government Board, 1908–14.

The significance of these changes was underlined by the National Insurance Act of 1911. Part I of this Act introduced a national health insurance scheme which, at the time of its inception, covered approximately 13 million workers engaged in manual occupations earning less than £160 a year. Under the scheme, female employees paid 3d. a week and male employees 4d. a week, and their contributions were supplemented by additional contributions from their employers (3d. a week) and the state (2d. a week). If they were unable to attend work as a result of ill health, insured women were able to claim a weekly benefit of 7s. 6d. for the first 26 weeks of their illness and insured men were able to claim a weekly benefit of 10s.; both men and women were eligible for a disablement benefit of 5s. a week if they remained off work for more than 26 weeks. The scheme also provided insured workers with a range of other benefits, including access to a general practitioner, free accommodation in a tuberculosis sanatorium for themselves and their dependants, and a maternity allowance of 30s. for insured women and the wives of insured men (Harris 2004, pp. 162–3).

The second part of the Act was designed to provide compensation for loss of earnings as a result of unemployment. Under this scheme, both employees and employers contributed 2½d. a week and the state contributed the equivalent of 1.67d. per week. In return for their contributions, insured workers were entitled to claim an unemployment benefit of 5s. a week for up to 15 weeks in each 52–week period. When the scheme was first introduced, it was confined to approximately 2.25 million workers in a small number of clearly defined occupations, but both the extent and the coverage of the scheme expanded dramatically after 1918. By the end of 1921, the scheme covered the vast majority of manual workers and non-manual workers earning less than £250 a year, and provided insurance against both short- and long-term periods of unemployment. The financial value of the benefits was greatly enhanced by the addition of separate allowances for the dependants of insured workers from November 1921 onwards (Harris 2004, pp. 163, 204–5).

Although the National Insurance Act has often been depicted as a major extension of public welfare provision, it also represented a major change in the relationship between social and political citizenship. During the nineteenth century, it was widely accepted that a man who applied for poor relief during periods of financial hardship forfeited his rights as a political citizen, but the introduction of both the health and unemployment insurance schemes enabled working men to obtain statutory welfare benefits without surrendering their rights as political citizens. This was also reflected, if only implicitly, in many of the arguments used by the supporters of national insurance when they claimed (as Winston Churchill did) that the introduction of these schemes would help to 'increase the stability of our institutions by giving the mass of industrial workers a direct interest in maintaining them' (see Harris 2004, p. 155).

However, the introduction of national insurance also had a profound impact on the gendered nature of welfare entitlements in Britain between 1911 and 1939. As we have already seen, the main role of the poor law was to provide welfare support to those who were on the margins of the regular labour force, and the majority of these individuals were either children, adult women, or the elderly. By contrast, the unemployment and health insurance schemes were designed to offer statutory welfare benefits to those who were normally in paid employment, and the majority of these workers were adult men. These differences were reflected in the statistics of both unemployment and health insurance (see Tables 2.3 and 2.4). In 1936, only 22 per cent of women between the ages of 16 and 64 were eligible for unemployment insurance, but 64 per cent of men aged 16–64 were covered by the scheme, and in 1938 63 per cent of the entire male population was eligible for health insurance, but the equivalent proportion of the female population was less than 30 per cent.

In addition to the expansion of the unemployment and health insurance schemes, the inter-war period also witnessed a major change in pension provision, with the introduction of the Widows', Orphans' and Old Age Contributory Pensions Act of 1925. This Act was grafted onto the existing health insurance scheme and established a basic pension of 10s. a week for insured workers between the ages of 65 and 70, the wives of insured men (where the man was over the age of 65 and the woman was aged between 65 and 70) and the widows of insured men, with additional allowances for the widows' children and for orphans. In 1929, a second Act was passed, granting pension rights to the widows of men who had died before the 1925 Act came into operation, and a third Act was passed in 1936.

Table 2.3   Number of workers eligible for unemployment insurance benefits in Great Britain, 1922–36 (See facing page)

Note to Table 2.3: Figures for the employed population and total population aged 16 and over and 16–64 have been estimated from the census returns for 1921 and 1931.

Source: Parliamentary Papers (1937), pp. 2, 3, 14.

| | Insured population ≥16 | | Employed population ≥16 | | Total population ≥16 | | Total population 16-64 | | Insured population as % of | | | |
| | | | | | | | | | Employed population ≥16 | | Total population ≥16 | |
	Male	Female	Male	Female	Male	Female	Male	Female	Male	Female	Male	Female
1922	8,189,290	2,991,660	13,205,294	5,366,713	14,165,329	16,169,339	13,029,898	14,648,413	62.02	55.74	57.81	18.50
1923	8,335,200	2,896,780	13,331,214	5,426,970	14,327,803	16,330,247	13,160,219	14,768,129	62.52	53.38	58.18	17.74
1924	8,390,000	2,977,510	13,457,135	5,487,228	14,490,276	16,491,155	13,290,540	14,887,846	62.35	54.26	57.90	18.06
1925	8,553,790	3,069,430	13,583,055	5,547,486	14,652,750	16,652,063	13,420,861	15,007,562	62.97	55.33	58.38	18.43
1926	8,680,970	3,092,730	13,708,976	5,607,744	14,815,224	16,812,971	13,551,183	15,127,279	63.32	55.15	58.59	18.39
1927	8,745,500	3,130,100	13,834,897	5,668,001	14,977,698	16,973,878	13,681,504	15,246,996	63.21	55.22	58.39	18.44

| | Insured population ≥16 | | Employed population 16-64 | | Total population ≥16 | | Total population 16-64 | | Insured population as % of | | | |
| | | | | | | | | | Employed population 16-64 | | Total population 16-64 | |
	Male	Female	Male	Female	Male	Female	Male	Female	Male	Female	Male	Female
1928	8,469,700	3,159,300	13,287,782	5,575,194	15,140,172	17,134,786	13,811,825	15,366,712	63.74	56.67	61.32	20.56
1929	8,597,300	3,236,700	13,410,463	5,634,756	15,302,645	17,295,694	13,942,146	15,486,429	64.11	57.44	61.66	20.90
1930	8,769,000	3,369,000	13,533,144	5,694,319	15,465,119	17,456,602	14,072,467	15,606,145	64.80	59.16	62.31	21.59
1931	9,021,000	3,479,000	13,655,825	5,753,881	15,627,593	17,617,510	14,202,788	15,725,862	66.06	60.46	63.52	22.12
1932	9,139,300	3,403,700	13,778,506	5,813,443	15,790,067	17,778,418	14,333,109	15,845,579	66.33	58.55	63.76	21.48
1933	9,181,400	3,438,600	13,901,187	5,873,006	15,952,541	17,939,326	14,463,430	15,965,295	66.05	58.55	63.48	21.54
1934	9,266,600	3,423,400	14,023,868	5,932,568	16,115,014	18,100,234	14,593,751	16,085,012	66.08	57.71	63.50	21.28
1935	9,356,000	3,424,000	14,146,549	5,992,130	16,277,488	18,261,142	14,724,072	16,204,728	66.14	57.14	63.54	21.13
1936	9,538,000	3,512,000	14,269,230	6,051,693	16,439,962	18,422,050	14,854,394	16,324,445	66.84	58.03	64.21	21.51

Table 2.4   **Number of workers eligible for statutory health insurance benefits in the United Kingdom, 1914–38**

	No. of persons eligible for health insurance benefits (1,000s)		Population (1,000s)		Eligible persons as % of population	
	Men	Women	Men	Women	Men	Women
1914[a, b, c]	9,667	4,020	20,187	21,527	47.89	18.67
1915[b, c, d]	9,947	4,146	18,311	21,744	54.32	19.07
1916[b, c, d]	10,316	4,532	17,536	21,901	58.83	20.69
1917[b, c, d]	10,514	4,853	16,977	22,030	61.93	22.03
1918[b, c, d]	10,705	5,183	16,742	22,094	63.94	23.46
1919[b, c, d]	10,308	5,139	18,173	22,074	56.72	23.28
1920[b, c, d]	10,215	5,064	19,920	22,192	51.28	22.82
1921[b, c]	10,245	4,905	20,446	22,369	50.11	21.93
1922[c]	10,429	5,043	21,226	23,146	49.13	21.79
1923	10,687	5,214	21,328	23,269	50.11	22.41
1924	10,946	5,415	21,508	23,407	50.89	23.14
1925	11,110	5,513	21,567	23,492	51.51	23.47
1926	11,427	5,640	21,662	23,570	52.75	23.93
1927	11,607	5,747	21,733	23,656	53.41	24.29
1928[e]	11,901	5,985	21,823	24,024	54.54	24.91
1929	12,064	6,097	21,877	23,796	55.14	25.62
1930	12,326	6,199	21,986	23,880	56.06	25.96
1931	12,469	6,239	22,087	23,987	56.46	26.01
1932	12,566	6,258	22,235	24,100	56.52	25.97
1933	12,463	6,228	22,332	24,189	55.81	25.75
1934	12,522	6,273	22,403	24,263	55.89	25.85
1935	12,705	6,347	22,504	24,364	56.46	26.05
1936	13,246	6,573	22,605	24,476	58.60	26.85
1937	13,546	6,735	22,726	24,563	59.60	27.42
1938[f]	14,303	7,285	22,822	24,672	62.67	29.53

Notes:

[a] The figures for 1914 are for the period 12 January 1914–31 December 1914; all other figures are for calendar years.

[b] The figures for the years 1914–21 are for Great Britain only (excluding Ireland).

Notes continued and Source line for Table 2.4:

ᶜ The figures for the years 1914–22 include older members (aged 70 and over) who qualified for medical benefit in Scotland, Wales and (in 1922 only) Northern Ireland, but they do not include equivalent individuals in England. The English members are included from 1923 onwards.

ᵈ Population figures for 1915–20 are for civilians only.

ᵉ Individuals aged 65–70 ceased to be eligible for sickness and disablement benefits from 2 January 1928 onwards, but they continued to be eligible for medical benefit.

ᶠ Under the terms of the National Health Insurance (Juvenile Contributors and Young Persons) Act, 1937, boys and girls aged 14–16 became eligible for medical benefits from 4 April 1938.

Source: Harris (2004), p. 224.

In 1937, the scheme was extended to enable women with an annual income of less than £250 and men with an annual income of less than £400 to insure themselves voluntarily (Harris 2004, p. 216).

Although the Acts represented a substantial increase in the extent of state support for widows, orphans and older people of both sexes, many contemporaries complained about the method by which they were financed and the level at which benefits were paid. In 1937, the contemporary research organisation Political and Economic Planning pointed out that even though the majority of women married men who were older than themselves, they still had to wait until their husbands had reached the age of 65 before they themselves could benefit, and this was reflected in the smaller number of women in the 65–70 age bracket who received contributory pensions (see Table 2.5). The development of the scheme also reflected the way in which the entitlements of female claimants depended on the status and contributions of a male breadwinner or pensioner. It therefore provided a further illustration of the gendered nature of welfare provision before 1939 (Harris 2004, p. 216; Pedersen 1993, pp. 167–77).

Despite the expansion of public welfare provision, a substantial number of people continued to rely on the means-tested benefits provided by the poor relief system or, as it became known after 1930, public assistance (Harris 2004, p. 203). Although the Ministry of Health did not distinguish between male and female recipients in its published returns, the average number of individuals in receipt of either domiciliary (outdoor) or institutional relief in England and Wales on 1 January and 1 July 1939 was just over 1.2 million, out of a total population of 41 million (Parliamentary Papers 1940, pp. 93–4). However, although the poor law survived after 1918, it did not remain unchanged. In 1918, parliament abolished the clauses which prevented the recipients of poor relief from voting in either local or national elections (7 & 8 Geo. V C. 64, section 9), and in 1927 a Ministry of Health official complained that 'there is now much less reluctance on the part of the community generally to accept assistance from the Guardians who, on their part, have become much more ready to give it' (Harris 1995b, p. 532). This was

Table 2.5 Number of individuals receiving contributory pensions in the United Kingdom under the Widows', Orphans' and Old Age Contributory Pensions Acts of 1925, 1929 and 1936

	65–70 pensions		Widows		Children		Total
	Men	Women	Contributory	Non-contributory	Contributory	Non-contributory	
1926	—	—	49,099	116,085	40,961	230,435	436,580
1927	—	—	107,480	99,648	84,989	197,053	489,170
1928	364,219	180,023	162,749	83,473	124,157	166,153	1,080,774
1929	380,504	201,761	224,644	70,138	166,615	139,826	1,183,488
1930	400,986	243,094	280,171	289,852	206,186	122,425	1,542,714
1931	423,360	254,183	332,345	352,653	238,199	103,782	1,704,522
1932	437,484	262,369	378,793	330,668	263,024	83,267	1,755,605
1933	454,502	272,997	426,477	309,476	283,637	65,284	1,812,373
1934	469,428	285,741	465,055	287,580	291,688	47,676	1,847,168
1935	484,846	298,695	505,363	265,504	295,693	32,996	1,883,097
1936	501,559	296,717	561,168	241,673	293,535	21,041	1,915,693
1937	518,719	310,212	603,376	218,929	291,540	12,375	1,955,151
1938	534,210	323,054	637,948	197,607	286,374	6,760	1,985,953

Source: Parliamentary Papers (1940), pp. 88–9.

another important dimension of the changing relationship between social and political rights during the inter-war period.

Gender and Welfare after 1939

By the end of the 1930s, 'the provision of unemployment benefit, as with other social services, was probably more comprehensive in Britain ... than in any other country which operated a democratic system' (Stevenson and Cook 1994, p. 83). In Marshallian terms, the growth of these services represented a significant expansion of the social rights of British citizens, but it also reflected the reconciliation of social and political rights associated with the Liberal welfare reforms of 1906–11 and the abolition of the pauper disqualification clauses by the Representation of the People Act of 1918. However, these rights were not enjoyed equally by all members of the population. In a number of important respects, women were less likely to enjoy access to social rights than men, and some of the entitlements they did enjoy were directly dependent on their relationship to a male breadwinner.

The years between 1939 and 1945 also played a vital formative role in the development of Britain's welfare state. In June 1941, the Minister-without-Portfolio invited Sir William Beveridge to lead an inquiry into 'the existing national schemes of social insurance and allied services' and the relationship between them (Parliamentary Papers 1942, p. 5). Although the Committee's initial aim was to develop plans for the creation of a unified scheme of national insurance which would incorporate the health and unemployment insurance schemes, together with the existing workmen's compensation scheme, Beveridge insisted that the final proposals could only work if they were linked to a more comprehensive programme of social renewal, incorporating the introduction of family allowances, the establishment of a national health and rehabilitation service, and the maintenance of full employment (Parliamentary Papers 1942, p. 153). He also argued that the achievement of these aims could not be separated from the broader attack on what he called the 'five giants on the road of reconstruction', namely Want, Disease, Ignorance, Squalor and Idleness (Parliamentary Papers 1942, p. 6).

As we have already seen, one of the major limitations of inter-war welfare provision was the gendered nature of the health insurance scheme. The scheme provided insured workers with compensation for loss of earnings due to ill health and free access to a general practitioner; it also offered a maternity benefit for insured women and the wives of insured men, and free accommodation in a tuberculosis sanatorium for insured workers and their dependants. However, the emphasis upon the needs of the insured worker meant that the proportion of adult women who qualified for free general practitioner services was much lower than the equivalent proportion of adult men, and this meant that women were much less likely to seek medical aid when they needed it (Digby and Bosanquet 1988, p. 89; Harris 2004, p. 225). Beveridge went beyond this by arguing that the provision of healthcare was a basic right and should not be dependent on the payment of individual insurance contributions, and this meant that his proposals for the creation of a comprehensive national health and rehabilitation service, and the subsequent establishment of the National Health Service, represented a substantial addition to the healthcare rights of the female population (see Parliamentary Papers 1942, p. 158–9).

However, although contemporary writers described the healthcare proposals as a 'cardinal change' in the development of health service provision (Abbot and Bompas 1943, p. 2), the main purpose of the report was to construct a 'Plan for Social Security', and this plan was much more strongly wedded to the insurance principle. As we can see from Table 2.6, the population was divided into six 'security classes', including 'employees', 'others gainfully occupied', 'housewives', 'others of working age', children and those above working age, but married women were defined as 'housewives' whether they were occupied or not, and this reflected Beveridge's own belief that married women should not be regarded as independent earners, but as individuals who were dependent on their husbands' incomes (Parliamentary Papers 1942, pp. 50–53, 123).

One of the most controversial features of the Beveridge Plan was the 'Married Woman's Option' (Abbott and Bompas 1943, pp. 10–11). Although Beveridge expected women to be employed and to contribute to the scheme before marriage, he also argued that 'most women will not be gainfully occupied' during marriage, and should therefore be given the option of withdrawing from the scheme at that point (Parliamentary Papers 1942, p. 50). Over the next thirty years, approximately three-quarters of married women chose to exercise this option and therefore surrendered their right to independent benefit, and even though the Married Woman's Option was phased out after 1977, its long-term consequences persisted for much longer (Pascall 1986, p. 208).

Although the aim of the Beveridge Report was to establish a basis for 'social security' for the entire population, the social insurance system which emerged after 1945 failed to meet women's needs in at least two main ways. In the first place, the emphasis placed on the relationship between contributions and benefits discriminated against women because they were more likely to be in low-waged, part-time or intermittent employment, and this meant that it became more difficult for them to sustain the contribution records needed to qualify for short-term unemployment benefits. The second major problem concerned the payment of retirement pensions. As we have already seen, many women surrendered their right to an independent pension by accepting the Married Woman's Option, and this continued to limit the pension rights of older women into the present century. However, even after the abolition of the Married Woman's Option, women continued to be at a disadvantage as a result of lower lifetime earnings and the growth of earnings-related pensions, and this problem has been further compounded by the increasing importance of occupational pensions. As Pat Thane (2006, p. 77) has recently observed, occupational pensions and state pensions were the two main 'pillars' of the British pension system after 1945, and 'both have failed older women'.

Table 2.6   The six 'security classes' identified in the Beveridge Report

Class	No. (1,000,000s)	Contribution provisions	Relation to security scheme							Other provisions
			Security provisions							
			Medical treatment	Funeral grant	Retirement pension	Disability benefit	Unemployment benefit	Training benefit	Industrial pension	
I. Employees	18.4	Insured by weekly contribution on employment book	✓	✓	✓	✓	✓	—	✓	Removal and lodging grant; industrial grant
II. Others gainfully occupied	2.5	Insured by contribution on occupation card	✓	✓	✓	✓(b)	—	✓	—	
III. Housewives	9.3(a)	Insured on marriage through the Housewife's Policy	✓	✓	✓	—(c)	—(c)	✓	—	Marriage grant, maternity benefit and grant, widows' benefit, guardian benefit, separation benefit

IV. Others of working age	2.4	Insured by contributions on Security Card	✓	—	—	—	✓	—
V. Below working age	9.6(g)	None	✓	✓	—	—	—	—
VI. Retired above working age	4.3	Insured by contributions made during working age	✓	✓	✓	—	—	✓(e)
Total	46.5							

Notes:

(a) Married women gainfully occupied estimated at 1.4 million are included in the numbers shown for Class III and excluded from the numbers shown in Classes I and II.

(b) After 13 weeks of sickness.

(c) If gainfully occupied and not exempt.

(d) If gainfully occupied even though exempt.

(e) If granted before reaching the age of retirement and if higher than the retirement pension.

(f) Includes removal and lodging grant where needed.

(g) The numbers shown in Class V are on the basis of the present minimum school leaving age, 14. In the report, it is assumed for the purpose of children's allowances that the minimum school leaving age is 15.

Source: Parliamentary Papers (1942), p. 123.

Conclusions

The history of gender and welfare provision in England and Wales over the last two centuries has been closely associated with the concept of dependence and the changing relationship between social and political rights. During the nineteenth century, women were regarded as members of the dependent population, but this also helped to legitimise their entitlement to poor relief. A man who asserted his right to poor relief forfeited his claim to independent status, and this meant that he also surrendered his right to vote. A number of attempts were made to address this issue during the final quarter of the nineteenth century, but these were only partially successful. As a result, the separation of social and political rights was largely maintained until the early years of the twentieth century.

The assumptions which had protected women's welfare rights during the nineteenth century also helped to limit them during the twentieth century. The most important changes introduced by the Liberals between 1906 and 1914 were the establishment of a national system of old age pensions and the introduction of national insurance. The second of these changes provided a mechanism which enabled men to exercise their social rights without surrendering their political rights, but the fact that benefits were directly linked to participation in the labour market meant that these benefits also tended to reinforce the inequalities which existed within it. The persistence of these inequalities also illustrated the limitations of Marshall's view of social citizenship. Although he was right to emphasise the importance of the new welfare measures, he failed to acknowledge the limitations of a view of social citizenship which was based on the career patterns of male workers and defined women by their relationship to a male breadwinner. The significance of this failure was reinforced by the economic, social and cultural changes which affected the development of British society after the Second World War.

References

Acts of Parliament

2 William IV C. 45, *An Act to amend the representation of the people in England and Wales* (1832).

30 & 31 Vict. C. 84, *An Act to consolidate and amend the laws relating to vaccination* (1867).

30 & 31 Vict. C. 102, *An Act further to amend the laws relating to the representation of the people in England and Wales* (1867).

33 & 34 Vict. C. 75, *An Act to provide for public elementary education in England and Wales* (1870).

39 & 40 Vict. C. 61, *An Act to provide for the better organisation of divided parishes and other local areas, and to make sundry amendments in the law relating to the relief of the poor in England* (1876).

48 Vict. C. 3, *An Act to amend the law relating to the representation of the people of the United Kingdom* (1884).

48 & 49 Vict. C. 46, *An Act to prevent medical relief from disqualifying a person from voting* (1885).

5 Edw. VII C. 18, *An Act to establish organisation with a view to the provision of employment or assistance for unemployed workmen in proper cases* (1905).

7 & 8 Geo. V C. 64, *An Act to amend the law with respect to Parliamentary and local government franchises and the registration of Parliamentary and local government electors, and the conduct of elections, and to provide for the redistribution of seats at Parliamentary elections, and for other purposes connected therewith* (1918).

Other References

Abbott, E. and Bompas, K. (1943), *The Woman Citizen and Social Security: A Criticism of the Proposals Made in the Beveridge Report as They Affect Women*, London: Katherine Bompas.

Breiner, P. (2006), 'Is Social Citizenship Really Outdated? T.H. Marshall Revisited', unpublished paper presented at the annual meeting of the Western Political Science Association, Hyatt Regency Albuquerque, Albuquerque, NM, 17 March 2006.

Daly, M. (1998), 'A matter of dependency: Gender in British income maintenance provision', *Sociology*, vol. 28, no. 3, pp. 779–97.

Dicey, A.V. (1962), *Lectures on the Relation between Law and Public Opinion in England during the Nineteenth Century* (1st edn 1905; 2nd edn 1914), London: Macmillan.

Digby, A. and Bosanquet, N. (1988), 'Doctors and patients in an era of national health insurance and private practice, 1913–38', *Economic History Review*, vol. 41, no. 1, pp. 74–94.

Goose, N. (2005), 'Poverty, old age and gender in nineteenth-century England: The case of Hertfordshire', *Continuity and Change*, vol. 20, no. 3, pp. 351–84.

Harris, B. (1995a), 'Responding to adversity: Government–charity relations and the relief of unemployment in interwar Britain', *Contemporary Record*, vol. 9, no. 3, pp. 529–61.

—— (1995b), *The Health of the Schoolchild: A History of The School Medical Service in England and Wales*, Buckingham: Open University Press.

—— (1998), 'Gender, Height and Mortality in Nineteenth- and Twentieth-century Britain: Some Preliminary Reflections', in J. Komlos and J. Baten (eds), *The Biological Standard of Living in Comparative Perspective*, Stuttgart: Franz Steiner Verlag, pp. 413–48.

—— (2000), 'Seebohm Rowntree and the Measurement of Poverty, 1899–1951', in J. Bradshaw and R. Sainsbury (eds), *Getting the Measure of Poverty: The Early Legacy of Seebohm Rowntree*, Aldershot: Ashgate, pp. 60–84.

—— (2004), *The Origins of the British Welfare State: Society, State and Social Welfare in England and Wales, 1800–1945*, Basingstoke: Palgrave Macmillan.

—— (2008), 'Gender, health and welfare in England and Wales since industrialisation', *Research in Economic History*, no. 26, pp. 157–204.

Lees, L.H. (1998), *The Solidarities of Strangers: The English Poor Laws and the People 1700–1948*, Cambridge: Cambridge University Press.

Lewis, J. (1994), 'Gender, the family and women's agency in the building of "welfare states": The British case', *Social History*, vol. 19, no. 1, pp. 37–55.

Lister, R. (2003), *Citizenship: Feminist Perspectives*, 2nd edn, Basingstoke: Palgrave Macmillan.

Macnicol, J. (1998), *The Politics of Retirement in Britain 1878–1948*, Cambridge: Cambridge University Press.

Marshall, T.H. (1950), 'Citizenship and Social Class', in *Citizenship and Social Class and Other Essays*, Cambridge: Cambridge University Press, pp. 1–85.

Parliamentary Debates (1884), *Parliamentary Debates*, 3rd series, vol. 289 (19 June 1884).

—— (1885a), *Parliamentary Debates*, 3rd series, vol. 297 (6 May 1885).

—— (1885b), *Parliamentary Debates*, 3rd series, vol. 298 (12 and 20 May 1885).

—— (1885c), *Parliamentary Debates*, 3rd series, vol. 299 (21 July 1885).

—— (1906), *Parliamentary Debates*, 4th series, vol. 153 (16 March 1906).

Parliamentary History of England (1795), *The Parliamentary History of England*, vol. 32 (9 December 1795).

Parliamentary Papers (1840), PP 1840 (245) xvii, 397, *Sixth Annual Report of the Poor Law Commissioners for England and Wales*.

—— (1859), PP 1859 (2500) ix, 741, *Eleventh Annual Report of the Poor Law Board*, 1858–59.

—— (1878a), PP 1878 (282) ii, 329, *A Bill to remove disqualification by medical relief for infectious or contagious disease.*

—— (1878b), PP 1878–79 (22) iii, 21, *A bill to remove disqualification by medical relief for infectious or contagious disease.*

—— (1884a), PP 1884–85 (206) iv, 77, *A Bill to provide that no person shall be disqualified from voting at Parliamentary elections by the receipt of medical relief for himself or for his family.*

—— (1884b), PP 1884–85 (232) iii, 405, *A Bill to prevent medical relief disqualifying a person from voting.*

—— (1890), PP 1890 C. 6141 xxxiii, 1, *Nineteenth Annual Report of the Local Government Board for 1889–90, with Appendix.*

—— (1892), PP 1892 (317) v, 193, *A Bill to remove disqualification from voting at elections of persons employed on labour by Guardians of the Poor.*

—— (1895a), PP 1895 (18) vi, 11, *A Bill to amend the law relating to the disfranchisement of persons receiving outdoor relief in return for labour.*

—— (1895b), PP 1895 (59) vi, 27, *A Bill to remove under certain circumstances the disqualification of voters in receipt of poor relief.*

—— (1900), PP 1900 (56) ii, 331, *A Bill to relieve members of friendly societies of certain disqualifications from receipt of temporary outdoor relief.*

—— (1901), PP 1901 (51) ii, 385, *A Bill to relieve members of friendly societies of certain disqualifications arising from the receipt of temporary relief.*

—— (1902), PP 1902 (38) i, 955, *A Bill to relieve members of friendly societies of certain disqualifications arising from the receipt of temporary relief.*

—— (1905), PP 1905 (38) v, 543, *A Bill to prevent the disfranchisement of persons receiving poor law relief.*

—— (1906a), PP 1906 (40) v, 561, *A Bill to prevent the disfranchisement of persons receiving poor law relief.*

—— (1906b), PP 1906 (22) iv, 351, *A Bill to remove certain disqualifications at Parliamentary elections.*

—— (1908), PP 1908 (18) iv, 41, *A Bill to remove certain disqualifications at Parliamentary elections.*

—— (1914), PP 1914 Cd. 7444 xxxviii, 1, *Forty-third Annual Report of the Local Government Board for 1913–14.*

—— (1937), PP 1936–37 Cmd. 5556 xxvi, 869, *Twenty-second abstracts of labour statistics of the United Kingdom (1922–36).*

—— (1940), PP 1939–40 Cmd. 6232 xi, 367, *Eighty-third statistical abstract for the United Kingdom.*

—— (1942), PP 1942–43 Cmd. 6404 vi, 119, *Social insurance and allied services: report by Sir William Beveridge.*

Pascall, G. (1986), *Social Policy: A Feminist Analysis*, London: Tavistock.

Pedersen, S. (1990), 'Gender, welfare and citizenship in Britain during the Great War', *American Historical Review*, vol. 95, no. 4, pp. 983–1,006.

—— (1993), *Family, Dependence and the Origins of the Welfare State: Britain and France 1914–45*, Cambridge: Cambridge University Press.

Pierson, C. (1998), *Beyond the Welfare State? The New Political Economy of Welfare*, Oxford: Basil Blackwell and Cambridge: Polity Press.

Pugh, M. (1999), *Britain Since 1789: A Concise History*, Basingstoke: Macmillan.

Slack, P. (1995), *The English Poor Law 1531–1782*, Cambridge: Cambridge University Press.

Stevenson, J. and Cook, C. (1994), *Britain in the Depression: Society and Politics 1929–39*, London: Longman.

Thane, P. (1978a), 'Non-contributory versus Insurance Pensions 1878–1908', in P. Thane (ed.), *The Origins of British Social Policy*, London: Croom Helm, pp. 84–106.

—— (1978b), 'Women and the poor law in Victorian and Edwardian England', *History Workshop*, vol. 6, no. 1, pp. 29–51.

—— (1991), 'Visions of Gender in the Making of the British Welfare State: The Case of Women in the British Labour Party and Social Policy, 1906–45', in G. Bock and P. Thane (eds), *Maternity and Gender Policies: Women and the Rise of the European Welfare States 1880s–1950s*, London: Routledge, pp. 93–118.

—— (2006), 'The "Scandal" of Women's Pensions in Britain: How Did it Come About?', in H. Pemberton, P. Thane and N. Whiteside (eds), *Britain's Pensions Crisis: History and Policy*, Oxford: Oxford University Press and the British Academy, pp. 77–90.

Appendix

Table 2.A.1 Indoor paupers (excluding children, insane paupers and casuals), 1849–1913

| | Males | | | | | | Females | | | | | | All | |
| | Able-bodied | | | Not able-bodied | | | Able-bodied | | | Not able-bodied | | | | |
	Married	Others	Total	Married	Others	Total	Married	Others	Total	Married	Others	Total	Male	Female
1849	1,596	6,322	7,917	1,407	17,628	19,035	1,826	12,285	14,111	1,250	13,277	14,527	26,952	28,638
1850	1,101	5,623	6,724	1,188	17,321	18,509	1,227	10,815	12,041	1,055	12,596	13,651	25,232	25,692
1851	914	4,908	5,822	1,113	17,805	18,917	1,023	10,361	11,384	1,015	12,993	14,007	24,739	25,391
1852	716	4,319	5,034	1,085	18,193	19,277	828	9,834	10,662	1,028	13,048	14,076	24,311	24,738
1853	450	3,377	3,827	1,015	17,946	18,960	608	9,471	10,078	925	13,554	14,479	22,787	24,557
1854	819	4,732	5,551	1,247	19,578	20,824	1,033	11,770	12,803	1,119	15,460	16,579	26,375	29,381
1855	741	4,340	5,081	1,184	20,469	21,652	954	13,123	14,077	1,102	16,159	17,261	26,733	31,338
1856	629	4,169	4,797	1,174	20,870	22,044	861	13,315	14,176	1,087	16,949	18,035	26,841	32,211
1857	546	4,076	4,621	1,118	21,720	22,838	696	12,493	13,189	1,023	16,978	18,001	27,459	31,190
1858	587	4,850	5,437	975	22,041	23,016	587	12,664	13,251	975	16,930	17,905	28,453	31,156
1859	—	—	4,763	—	—	24,797	—	—	11,777	—	—	19,971	29,560	31,748
1860	—	—	4,499	—	—	25,018	—	—	11,354	—	—	19,466	29,516	30,820
1861	—	—	5,932	—	—	26,891	—	—	14,175	—	—	20,928	32,822	35,103
1862	—	—	6,722	—	—	28,706	—	—	15,615	—	—	21,993	35,428	37,608
1863	—	—	7,033	—	—	29,765	—	—	15,224	—	—	22,419	36,798	37,642
1864	—	—	6,009	—	—	29,496	—	—	13,763	—	—	22,205	35,505	35,967

Year											
1865	—	6,215	—	30,272	—	13,478	—	—	22,555	36,487	36,033
1866	—	5,773	—	30,698	—	13,219	—	—	23,249	36,470	36,468
1867	—	6,435	—	32,283	—	14,391	—	—	24,036	38,718	38,427
1868	—	8,141	—	34,535	—	16,013	—	—	25,215	42,676	41,227
1869	—	8,621	—	35,794	—	16,243	—	—	24,719	44,415	40,961
1870	—	9,629	—	37,603	—	15,618	—	—	25,055	47,232	40,673
1871	—	9,496	—	37,869	—	7,134	—	—	25,803	47,365	32,937
1872	—	7,394	—	36,263	—	13,429	—	—	25,386	43,657	38,815
1873	—	6,320	—	36,469	—	12,632	—	—	26,214	42,789	38,846
1874	—	6,082	—	36,703	—	12,104	—	—	26,852	42,785	38,955
1875	—	6,386	—	37,383	—	11,244	—	—	27,246	43,769	38,490
1876	—	5,508	—	38,092	—	10,470	—	—	28,239	43,599	38,709
1877	—	5,886	—	40,698	—	10,932	—	—	30,187	46,584	41,119
1878	—	6,446	—	42,613	—	12,042	—	—	31,366	49,059	43,408
1879	—	7,766	—	46,357	—	12,648	—	—	32,642	54,123	45,290
1880	—	8,939	—	48,690	—	13,893	—	—	33,540	57,629	47,433
1881	—	8,888	—	48,801	—	13,811	—	—	33,988	57,689	47,798
1882	—	8,404	—	48,697	—	13,452	—	—	34,298	57,100	47,750
1883	—	8,271	—	49,415	—	13,031	—	—	35,368	57,686	48,398
1884	—	7,859	—	49,739	—	12,563	—	—	35,928	57,598	48,491
1885	—	8,489	—	50,925	—	12,386	—	—	36,026	59,413	48,412
1886	—	9,699	—	52,682	—	12,796	—	—	36,271	62,381	49,067

Table 2.A.1 Continued

	Males						Females						All	
	Able-bodied			Not able-bodied			Able-bodied			Not able-bodied				
	Married	Others	Total	Married	Others	Total	Married	Others	Total	Married	Others	Total	Male	Female
1887	—	—	10,419	—	—	54,344	—	—	12,784	—	—	36,611	64,763	49,395
1888	—	—	11,328	—	—	55,343	—	—	12,993	—	—	37,086	66,671	50,078
1889	—	—	10,365	—	—	55,042	—	—	12,586	—	—	37,831	65,406	50,416
1890	—	—	—	—	—	—	—	—	—	—	—	—	64,865	49,924
1891	—	—	—	—	—	—	—	—	—	—	—	—	65,063	50,338
1892	—	—	—	—	—	—	—	—	—	—	—	—	65,006	50,919
1893	—	—	—	—	—	—	—	—	—	—	—	—	69,866	52,747
1894	—	—	—	—	—	—	—	—	—	—	—	—	73,718	55,265
1895	—	—	—	—	—	—	—	—	—	—	—	—	76,379	56,183
1896	—	—	—	—	—	—	—	—	—	—	—	—	77,871	56,593
1897	—	—	—	—	—	—	—	—	—	—	—	—	78,500	57,409
1898	—	—	—	—	—	—	—	—	—	—	—	—	79,955	59,184
1899	—	—	—	—	—	—	—	—	—	—	—	—	78,788	59,464
1900	—	—	—	—	—	—	—	—	—	—	—	—	78,558	59,365
1901	—	—	—	—	—	—	—	—	—	—	—	—	79,045	60,764
1902	—	—	—	—	—	—	—	—	—	—	—	—	84,536	63,012
1903	—	—	—	—	—	—	—	—	—	—	—	—	88,191	64,639
1904	—	—	—	—	—	—	—	—	—	—	—	—	93,423	66,884

1905	—	—	—	—	—	—	—	—	—	—	—	99,549	69,066
1906	—	—	—	—	—	—	—	—	—	—	—	102,648	69,424
1907	—	—	—	—	—	—	—	—	—	—	—	105,911	70,820
1908	—	—	—	—	—	—	—	—	—	—	—	104,975	72,315
1909	—	—	—	—	—	—	—	—	—	—	—	114,376	73,918
1910	—	—	—	—	—	—	—	—	—	—	—	114,535	72,815
1911	—	—	—	—	—	—	—	—	—	—	—	112,573	71,031
1912	—	—	—	—	—	—	—	—	—	—	—	109,415	68,953
1913	—	—	—	—	—	—	—	—	—	—	—	103,798	67,717

Notes: These figures are based on the average of the number of paupers receiving outdoor relief on 1 January and 1 July of each calendar year.

Sources: 1849–58: Parliamentary Papers (1859), pp. 196–9; 1859–89: Parliamentary Papers (1890), pp. 366–9; 1890–1913: Parliamentary Papers (1914), p. 87.

Table 2.A.2   Outdoor paupers (excluding children, insane paupers and casuals), 1849–1913

| | Males | | Females | | | | | Totals | |
| | Able-bodied | Not able-bodied | Able-bodied | | | | Not able-bodied | Men | Women |
			Wives of able-bodied men	Widows	Others	Total			
1849	47,467	97,562	37,962	50,930	20,008	108,900	201,642	145,029	310,542
1850	35,689	100,127	28,451	51,910	17,528	97,889	208,892	135,816	306,781
1851	30,534	100,775	24,476	49,388	15,498	89,361	212,130	131,308	301,491
1852	27,525	100,333	21,977	46,355	14,261	82,593	213,088	127,858	295,681
1853	23,171	97,338	18,532	45,227	12,988	76,747	210,556	120,509	287,303
1854	26,837	98,041	21,901	47,457	14,539	83,897	215,238	124,878	299,134
1855	27,923	98,004	22,671	50,363	17,238	90,272	217,128	125,927	307,400
1856	27,175	96,718	22,165	51,502	17,798	91,465	219,536	123,893	311,001
1857	25,532	97,357	20,772	49,871	15,326	85,969	220,996	122,889	306,965
1858	31,492	97,114	25,730	51,495	17,668	94,892	221,530	128,606	316,422
1859	25,146	98,895	—	—	—	87,958	226,380	124,040	314,338
1860	26,114	98,906	—	—	—	86,883	226,889	125,019	313,772
1861	30,667	100,531	—	—	—	92,979	230,235	131,197	323,214
1862	37,530	103,863	—	—	—	103,891	236,729	141,392	340,620
1863	59,889	110,445	—	—	—	137,959	247,462	170,333	385,421

Year								
1864	37,916	108,529	—	—	109,698	245,968	146,445	355,666
1865	33,074	107,637	—	—	102,115	243,808	140,711	345,923
1866	28,174	104,821	—	—	95,298	240,633	132,994	335,931
1867	31,481	106,508	—	—	99,180	245,915	137,988	345,095
1868	37,456	110,049	—	—	108,810	251,704	147,505	360,514
1869	35,852	111,687	—	—	108,354	256,512	147,539	364,866
1870	38,003	114,499	—	—	111,273	262,307	152,502	373,580
1871	36,457	114,847	—	—	108,368	262,800	151,304	371,168
1872	25,392	106,629	—	—	91,739	251,206	132,020	342,945
1873	14,821	97,245	—	—	79,899	237,269	112,066	317,168
1874	16,939	90,271	—	—	72,838	225,099	107,210	297,937
1875	17,313	85,519	—	—	70,146	215,544	102,832	285,690
1876	13,691	78,244	—	—	61,860	201,903	91,935	263,762
1877	13,247	74,691	—	—	59,651	193,774	87,938	253,425
1878	14,562	73,129	—	—	61,418	189,930	87,691	251,348
1879	21,657	74,685	—	—	70,067	189,300	96,342	259,367
1880	19,961	77,051	—	—	69,737	191,643	97,011	261,380
1881	16,142	76,959	—	—	65,813	190,802	93,101	256,614
1882	14,521	77,072	—	—	63,236	190,378	91,592	253,614
1883	14,406	76,327	—	—	62,314	188,865	90,733	251,179
1884	13,279	74,321	—	—	59,966	185,071	87,599	245,036
1885	14,673	74,100	—	—	60,625	184,306	88,773	244,931

Table 2.4.2 continued

	Males		Females						Totals	
	Able-bodied	Not able-bodied	Able-bodied				Not able-bodied		Men	Women
			Wives of able-bodied men	Widows	Others	Total				
1886	16,812	76,202	—	—	—	63,105	187,420		93,014	250,525
1887	16,140	78,122	—	—	—	62,221	190,100		94,262	252,321
1888	16,339	79,732	—	—	—	62,016	192,311		96,070	254,327
1889	14,280	79,695	—	—	—	58,424	193,460		93,975	251,884
1890	—	—	—	—	—	—	—		90,849	246,884
1891	—	—	—	—	—	—	—		87,412	240,795
1892	—	—	—	—	—	—	—		85,604	236,549
1893	—	—	—	—	—	—	—		87,440	240,657
1894	—	—	—	—	—	—	—		90,690	247,094
1895	—	—	—	—	—	—	—		93,625	253,957
1896	—	—	—	—	—	—	—		95,577	258,274
1897	—	—	—	—	—	—	—		96,143	258,946
1898	—	—	—	—	—	—	—		100,839	264,677
1899	—	—	—	—	—	—	—		92,067	254,257
1900	—	—	—	—	—	—	—		89,150	248,795

1901	—	—	—	—	—	86,882	249,373
1902	—	—	—	—	—	88,976	253,196
1903	—	—	—	—	—	90,847	255,854
1904	—	—	—	—	—	94,605	260,394
1905	—	—	—	—	—	103,113	269,599
1906	—	—	—	—	—	101,937	268,976
1907	—	—	—	—	—	101,634	267,435
1908	—	—	—	—	—	102,408	267,417
1909	—	—	—	—	—	101,482	263,676
1910	—	—	—	—	—	94,078	252,969
1911	—	—	—	—	—	72,175	193,758
1912	—	—	—	—	—	62,509	166,554
1913	—	—	—	—	—	58,307	163,091

Notes: These figures are based on the average of the number of paupers resident in workhouses on 1 January and 1 July of each calendar year.

Sources: 1849–58: Parliamentary Papers (1859), pp. 196–9; 1859–89: Parliamentary Papers (1890), pp. 366–9; 1890–1913: Parliamentary Papers (1914), p. 87.

Chapter 3

Scandinavian Gender Equality: Competing Discourses and Paradoxes

Anette Borchorst

In many contexts, the Scandinavian countries (Sweden, Norway and Denmark)[1] have been celebrated for being at the forefront in generating social equality and gender equality, and it has been a recurrent theme in national self-representations that gender equality is a hallmark of the region. In the self-image of these countries, they have 'a passion for equality' (Graubard 1986), and it is true that they have been successful in reducing inequalities in some respects. For instance, they have relatively low Gini coefficients (which measure income inequality) (OECD 2006).

The Scandinavian countries are also ranked among the countries that have the highest level of gender equality, and they have relatively high political representation of women at the national level. This development is related to the fact that the Scandinavian countries are dominated by a universal-breadwinner model, where both men and women are engaged in paid work. When this development took off in the 1970s and 1980s, birth rates declined. This is the case in most Western countries previously characterised by a male-breadwinner model, where married women worked in the family context as housewives. However, it happened relatively early in the Scandinavian countries compared to countries governed by Christian Democratic and Catholic political coalitions.

As demonstrated in Chapter 4, in the Mediterranean countries today, both female labour force participation and birth rates are low. The ageing of populations constitutes a serious challenge here and in many other European countries, and low fertility is considered a threat to the sustainability of the welfare states in the long run. Therefore, the EU Commission as well as the OECD recommend governments to stimulate female employment and high fertility at the same time. This has been done in the Scandinavian countries (OECD 2009; European Commission 2009). It seems obvious to conclude that the combination of high female labour force participation and high fertility in the Scandinavian countries may be explained by the welfare policies on childcare and parental leave that were adopted in the 1980s and 1990s. Chapters 9 and 10 also demonstrate how the lack of policies like parental leave and low-cost daycare facilities for pre-school children contribute

---

1   The five Nordic countries (the three Scandinavian countries plus Finland and Iceland) share many characteristics, but in this chapter I will focus on those of Scandinavia, since they are the most similar.

to the low number of women (especially with children) in gainful employment in Mediterranean countries.

The Scandinavian welfare states have been labelled 'woman-friendly' (Hernes 1987). The term implies that they have been responsive to women's claims, have adopted a range of policies that have increased women's options, and that women have gained a voice in the public and political spheres. The broad political mobilisation of women from the late 1960s through the 1970s and 1980s put pressure on the political system, and the feminist movement influenced the public and political agendas, where a range of new issues related to human reproduction appeared.

However, competing discourses reveal that gender equality is a contested issue. Scandinavian gender equality is far from an unambiguous success, and the dominant discourse about a gradual and linear development towards more gender-balanced societies is clearly not accurate, despite the dominant idea about being 'on the road' to gender equality (Skjeie and Teigen 2005). New paradoxes have emerged in relation to the universal-breadwinner model as the dominant vision of gender equality. Increasing multiculturalism has made the previously fairly homogeneous countries much more diverse, and the Scandinavian countries have been less successful in reducing ethnic minority/majority inequality than in reducing class and gender inequality. The grand vision of gender equality has difficulties acknowledging differences between groups of women and between groups of men.

This chapter focuses on the Scandinavian experiences in generating gender equality, and it critically addresses woman-friendliness as discourse and practice. I will set out by briefly introducing the historical trajectory of the welfare states and the significance of gender equality, after which I will present two competing discourses within feminist research about the achievements in Scandinavia in terms of gender equality, one far more positive and optimistic about the state than the other. In the following section, I will contrast recent discourses about the potential of woman-friendly policies to tackle the challenges welfare states face in the light of ageing populations and globalised economies. One discourse is at the European level, in the form of policy recommendations for the implementation of the Lisbon Strategy from 2000. Another discourse unfolded in relation to the Danish Welfare Commission in 2004. After this, I will look at differences between the three Scandinavian countries and the visions of gender equality that have been predominant as policy rationales. Finally, I will address the role of multiculturalism in the Scandinavian welfare models, and I will conclude with some reflections on the Nordic experiences as models for other countries.

The Historical Trajectory

Comparative welfare state literature has highlighted the historical trajectory of the Scandinavian welfare states. Roughly speaking, social equality was introduced as a political value of the societies during the latter part of the nineteenth century and the beginning of the twentieth century. The welfare states were expanded due to pressure from the peasant movement, the labour movement and the women's movement (Christiansen et al. 2006). The social democratic parties led the way towards the adoption of redistribution policies aimed at alleviating class differences. The *right-wing* parties have also supported universalist as well as tax-based and welfare-based benefits, and the welfare policies have by and large been based on broad political alliances during the expansive years. The social partners have been an integral part of the compromise, and corporatism in the form of institutionalising the influence of the social partners on a broad range of policies has in some periods been a significant phenomenon of the welfare architecture. Yet level and form differ in the three countries.

In the early years of the welfare states, women were excluded from citizenship in terms of civil (freedom of speech and so on) and political (suffrage and so on) rights, and they received lower social benefits than men. Feminist organisations pushed for reforms for women, and a number of milestones were reached in the early twentieth century (Bergqvist et al. 1999, p. 296), among other things because the political systems were responsive to forces in civil society such as women's organisations. This was facilitated by co-operation between experts in law, feminist organisations and politicians (Melby et al. 2007) who engaged in policy learning.

Scandinavia: Woman-friendly or a Renewed Gender System?

According to a very influential discourse, Scandinavian welfare states have a woman-friendly potential. The concept was launched by Norwegian political scientist Helga Hernes in 1987, and features two important aspects. On the one hand, it reflects the idea that the Scandinavian welfare states have been responsive to changing political forces in civil society and have given room for women's agency. The feminist organisations have been influential in putting central issues, like women's rights and reproductive rights, on the public and political agendas, within political parties and as autonomous organisations and movements. On the other hand, 'woman-friendliness' refers to the impact of political decisions on women's daily lives:

> A woman-friendly state would not force harder choices on women than on men, or permit unjust treatment on the basis of sex. In a woman-friendly state women will continue to have children, yet there will also be other roads to self-realization open to them. In such a state women will not have to choose futures that demand greater sacrifices from them than are expected of men. It would be, in short, a state where injustice on the basis of gender would be largely eliminated without an increase in other forms of inequality, such as among groups of women. (Hernes 1987, p. 15)

The changing boundary between public and private was a central issue in Hernes's account, and feminist scholarship has for many years argued that a public–private dichotomy, especially with regard to the division between family and state, has cemented a patriarchal order. Hernes argued in her book that the development towards 'reproduction going public' was a key element in the woman-friendly potential that increases women's options compared to men's. This definition also highlights the role of options in relation to women's motherhood and responsibility for reproduction and care.

In the years after it was published, her book served as an eye-opener for feminist state theorists. It marked a break with the previous rather pessimistic view about the state among feminist scholars that had stressed women's marginalisation and their dependency on the patriarchal state. These interpretations were often generated from analysis of welfare states rooted in a liberalist paradigm (see, for instance, Pateman 1987). The change towards a focus on the empowerment and inclusion of women was stimulated by the increasing presence of women in politics, especially in Norway and Sweden.

Hernes's arguments for Scandinavian exceptionalism resonated with the development in welfare state research at large, which took a comparative turn during the late 1980s and early 1990s. This development implied increasing academic attention to differences between welfare states and the role of politics in institutionalising specific welfare and gender models (Esping-Andersen 1990).

'Woman friendliness' was a catchy term, but the analytical strength and empirical validity of the concept have been questioned. Hernes's conceptual framework was normatively biased towards the political culture, institutions and gender model of the Scandinavian countries. It was premised on a vision of a universal-breadwinner model, which considers breadwinning as the primary route to gender equality (Borchorst and Siim 2008).

It is interesting that almost at the same time as Hernes wrote her book, Swedish historian Yvonne Hirdman (1990) reached conclusions about the development in the Swedish welfare state that contrasted starkly with Hernes's analysis. In the final report from the Swedish power study, Hirdman argued that the gender system had remained intact due to its two operating logics: gender segregation and hierarchy based upon a male norm. Scandinavian feminist scholars often depict Hirdman and Hernes as the pessimist Cassandra versus the optimist Pollyanna, but Hirdman has questioned this interpretation (Hirdman 1996). She explains their different conclusions about the Scandinavian development as resulting from their different focuses: Hirdman concentrates on the labour market, Hernes on the welfare state.

Hernes held indeed a rather optimistic view on the ability of the state to improve gender equality, but she was pessimistic about the potential for achieving gender equality in the market. Another explanation of the opposing conclusions is that Hernes highlights the role of women's agency, whereas Hirdman downplays the significance of actors and underlines the role of structures of the gender system.

Hirdman's rather pessimistic interpretation of gender equality in Swedish society was coloured by the lack of a comparative perspective, since Sweden was in many respects in the forefront of gender equality internationally, but she was much more successful than Hernes in capturing the continuous gender hierarchy. Interestingly enough, this rather dark picture of Sweden has contributed to keeping the issue of gender equality high on the political agenda.

A central element in Hernes's interpretation of Scandinavian developments is the synergy between women's agency and political presence, political decisions on welfare benefits and services, and women's policy machinery. She emphasises the combination of 'feminisation from below' through mobilisation of women in political and cultural activities, and the response 'from above' in terms of institutionalisation. She characterised this as 'state feminism', which is different from the typical way of defining this concept as referring exclusively to women's policy machineries (Outshoorn and Kantola 2007, pp. 2–3).

Expert Discourses: Woman-friendly Policies as the Solution or the Problem?

The concept of woman-friendliness has been quite influential, and still plays a role today. However, it is subject to competing discourses, and is framed both as a solution to future challenges in Western welfare states and as part of the problem. In the following, I will illustrate this via two discourses. One was triggered by the presidency of the European Council, which asked welfare state experts to provide policy recommendations for the central Lisbon strategy from 2000. The contrasting discourse was launched by the Danish Welfare Commission.[2]

The first discourse was prompted by attempts to make the Lisbon strategy operational. The strategy aimed to meet the common challenges posed by increased globalisation and the ageing of populations, and the goal was to make the EU the most competitive and knowledge-based economy in the world. The document contained benchmarks for various indicators, for instance 60 per cent women's employment by 2010 (Lisbon European Council 2000). The Belgian EU presidency found that combating inequality was a central issue, and asked four welfare state experts to provide recommendations to make the Lisbon strategy operational and to be 'explicit on the underlying issues of social justice' (Esping-Andersen et al. 2002, Foreword, p. ix). The experts, who mainly had a background in sociology and were inspired by the influential power resource school in welfare state research, concluded that achievement of social equality and gender equality was central to compliance with the Lisbon objectives. They argued that women-friendly and family-friendly policies like affordable childcare, paid maternity and parental leave and so on should be defined as social investment, since they 'yield a substantial collective return to society at large' (Esping-Andersen et al. 2002, p. 94). It is striking that neither inequality between ethnic minority and majority

---

2   Sweden also set up a welfare commission in the year 2000, and it had a very different approach to welfare and gender than the Danish. Norway has not had a welfare commissions in recent times.

groups nor immigration were considered as solutions to labour demand problems. It is also noteworthy that a special chapter was devoted to gender inequality, since the issue had so far largely been ignored by mainstream welfare state research. Gøsta Esping-Andersen emphasised the significance of generating gender equality through public policies:

> It is uncontroversial to promote better opportunities for women, not only because they respond to women's demands but also because their employment may yield increasing social returns. In many countries women constitute a massive untapped labour reserve that can help narrow future age dependency rates and reduce associated financial pressures. Moreover, as women's educational attainment exceeds men's, clearly there exists an often large, untapped productive reservoir. We also know that female employment is one of the most effective means of combating social exclusion and poverty. All this implies that 'women-friendly' policy is, simultaneously, family- and society-friendly. If it yields a private return to individual women, it also yields substantial collective return to society at large. It should, accordingly, be defined as social investment. (Esping-Andersen et al. 2002, p. 94)

This quote illustrates that woman-friendliness has become part of the public and political discourse at the European level. It was defined as affordable childcare, parental leave and provisions for work absence when children are ill, and the policies were labelled as win–win solutions with the capacity to foster social inclusion and gender equality, and improve economic competitiveness at the same time.

The win–win interpretation of woman-friendly policies stands in stark contrast to the second discourse that frames welfare policies as a problem per se. It was forwarded by the Danish Welfare Commission in a debate about Danish welfare reforms in 2004. The Commission, which consisted mainly of neo-classical economists, was set up in 2003 by a right-wing government. Its task was quite similar to the one assigned to the EU experts: to analyse future challenges to the Danish welfare system and provide policy recommendations for the Danish government. It was open to explanations linking the expansion of the Danish welfare state to the large-scale entry of women into the labour force, but for the main and most important part of the analysis, it adopted a narrow utilitarian approach to welfare in interpreting the development of the Danish welfare state.

The Commission calculated net contributions (taxes) and net deductions (take-up rates of services and benefits) of the Danish population over a life span, and it concluded that a Danish citizen, on average, is a net recipient of 800,000 DDK (Velfærdskommissionen 2004). The figures were broken down by gender, and it was concluded that a newborn girl, over her lifetime, can expect to receive 2.4 million DDK from the welfare state, whereas a newborn boy will contribute 800,000 DDK. The explanation was that women take much more parental leave than men, and they live longer.

In the final recommendations, the Commission did not suggest cutbacks in welfare service and childcare services. It did, however, frame women's pregnancy, births and responsibility for children as a cost to society, and the argument inspired the newspapers to label women as policy-takers and money-spenders, and it triggered headlines in the newspapers like 'Women cost big bucks', 'Men pay the bill'.

It is interesting that the two groups of experts shared the same overall objectives of improving economic competitiveness and tackling the challenges of the ageing society, but they ended up with contrasting views about woman-friendly policies. The Danish Welfare Commission saw the welfare architecture as problematic for the economy, whereas it was highlighted as a good model by the EU experts.

Neither the EU experts nor the Danish Welfare Commission successfully influenced the policy agendas. The European Council became dominated by governments of right-wing observance and was influenced by a neo-liberal discourse, which does not consider social equality as a central parameter for economic competitiveness. The Danish Welfare Commission did not suggest cutbacks in woman-friendly policies and did not gain much influence on the political agenda of the right-wing government. Hence, at the level of political practices, the differences may not be as profound as the discourses indicate.

Scandinavian Gender Equality Paradoxes

The Scandinavian countries have given women a voice in the public sphere. First of all, women obtained political rights relatively early, but it was not until the 1970s that they reached a critical mass in the national parliaments. During the past three decades, the five Scandinavian countries have been in the world's top five in terms of female political participation. Today, they are no longer placed together in the lead,[3] as other countries have adopted a fast-track approach to gender quotas (Dahlerup 2006).

Another important factor is that the political system has been relatively responsive to forces in civil society like women's organisations that have been influential in generating reforms for women throughout the twentieth century.

In terms of employment, it is noteworthy that Sweden and Denmark reached the EU Lisbon targets for women's employment in the late 1970s, thirty years before the EU's deadline, and today the Scandinavian countries are in the top ten among OECD countries in terms of female employment (OECD 2009). However, it is also clear that neither this nor the fact that today more women than men complete higher education have generated gender equality. The labour markets have become even more gender-segregated after the large-scale entry of women, and the gender pay gap has stabilised during the last two decades (European

---

3   See <http://www.ipu.org/wmn-e/world.htm> (accessed 8 May 2011).

Commission 2009). Furthermore, the share of female managers is low, especially in Denmark (World Economic Forum 2009).

It is also debatable whether women's options that Hernes emphasised as central to woman-friendliness have been improved, because the pressure for integration in paid employment is very strong. Furthermore, women often lose control over future conditions of choice when they become pregnant, give birth and care for small children. The right to care for the newborn has been extended through parental leave, but for older children, the right to receive care is much stronger than the right to provide care, since most children are cared for in childcare facilities (Knijn and Kremer 1997). At the same time, women are subject to a child penalty, and they lose pay increases, career opportunities and pension for every child they have (Nielsen et al. 2003).

Woman-friendliness and Multiculturalism

In recent years, a new debate about the woman-friendliness of Scandinavian welfare states has appeared in relation to the development towards multicultural societies. When Hernes published her book, the countries were still rather homogeneous in terms of ethnicity, but since the 1980s and 1990s, they have become much more diverse, and it has been questioned whether the grand story about Scandinavian gender equality glosses over differences among women (de los Reyes et al. 2003; Siim 2007; Borchorst and Siim 2008).

Both Hernes and Hirdman ignored the fact that gender inequalities intersect with other types of differentiation, such as class and ethnicity, whereby the dynamics and the character of exclusion and marginalisation differ. The concepts of woman-friendliness and the gender system are both based on the premise that women have common and collective interests. As demonstrated in the first quote, Hernes did, however, emphasise the problem with differences among women. Also, immigration had not yet become a political problem and a key issue in the public debates in Scandinavia. Today, the question is whether all groups of women have the same interests in specific care policies and care arrangements. This also highlights the issue of *options* that was central to Hernes's concept of woman-friendliness.

Hernes's conclusion about 'reproduction' going public is also debatable. The public–private split is subject to ongoing negotiations, and it has been rearticulated in some countries, for instance in Denmark, where a 'daddy quota' that earmarks part of the parental leave for the father has been framed as coercion and unwanted interference with the autonomy of the family, whereas age restrictions for marrying foreigners have not been framed in the same way (Borchorst 2006; Siim 2008).

Furthermore, women from ethnic minorities have a limited political presence, and relatively few immigrant or minority organisations for women have obtained a voice in the political debate. Ethnic minorities are subject to much stereotyping; minority women are constructed as passive victims, and the headscarf is used to draw distinctions between 'us' and 'them' (for Danish media, see Andreassen

2005). The Danish debate appears to be much more polarised than the Swedish and Norwegian. A former Danish prime minister and several ministers of gender equality have claimed that women from ethnic minorities have not benefited from the gender equality that majority women enjoy, for cultural reasons (Siim and Skjeie 2008; Borchorst and Siim 2008; Borchorst and Teigen, 2009).

One or Three Models?

In this chapter, the Scandinavian countries have so far been treated as one coherent model. They appear relatively similar in large-scale comparisons, and they have all witnessed a combination and a synergy of forces from below and from above, which is also true of the two remaining Nordic countries. However, closer analysis reveals considerable differences in the gender-political models and discourses of the three countries (Bergqvist et al. 1999; Borchorst et al. 2002).

Sweden has the most institutionalised model and Denmark the most bottom-up-oriented model of women's political influence and the level and strength of state influence on gender equality policies. The Norwegian gender-political model falls between the two others.

In Sweden, the feminist influence has been and is strongest within the political parties. It is remarkable that the majority of the Swedish political parties today call themselves 'feminist'. Gender is highly politicised, and there is a strong discourse about women's structural oppression, which may be attributed to, among other things, the influence of Yvonne Hirdman's analysis of the gender system (Hirdman 1990).

Denmark's bottom-up-oriented gender model now has a weak input from the bottom, since the feminist movement is relatively weak. The extra-parliamentary feminist movement was very strong in the 1970s and 1980s, but feminist issues never gained ground in the political parties. Today, gender issues are placed low on the political agenda, and the political significance of gender is limited. There is a strong belief that gender equality has already been achieved, except for minority women.

In Norway, there is relatively strong institutionalisation of gender equality compared to Denmark, and medium political significance for gender. The Christian party has played a much more central political role than similar parties in the two other countries. The stronger role of religion in Norway has nurtured a more ambivalent gender equality policy. During the 1970s and 1980s, Norwegian politics was characterised by a rhetoric of gender differences (Skjeie 1992), and Norwegian women were integrated in politics before they entered the labour market on a large scale. The processes in Sweden and Denmark were simultaneous.

Family and gender policies in the three countries are guided by different policy logics and visions of gender equality (Borchorst 2008). Apart from the universal-breadwinner model that has been promoted through expansion of public childcare facilities, parental leave and so on, a second vision seeks to revaluate women's care work, for instance by adopting cash-for-care schemes. Finally, a third vision seeks to integrate men in care (Fraser 1997, ch. 2).

Norway has the most ambivalent model, since its policies are based on all three visions. The country has adopted cash-for-care schemes and expanded childcare facilities. Furthermore, Norway was the first country in the world to adopt a 'daddy quota', which may be regarded as a very small step towards the third vision that seeks to strengthen men's caring role.

In Sweden, the universal-breadwinner model has been the dominant policy rationale, but Sweden has adopted a 'daddy quota' *and* subsequently prolonged it. In Denmark, the predominant vision has been the universal-breadwinner role. For a few years Denmark had a 'daddy quota', but it was abandoned in 2001 (Borchorst 2006).[4] Yet the Scandinavian experience demonstrates that integrating women into employment does not generate gender equality in itself, unless men participate on an equal level in care work (see Chapter 11 in this volume). The differences in Scandinavian men's take-up rate of parental leave clearly reflect that 'daddy quotas' are successful in integrating men in care.[5]

Differences between the three countries seem even greater when it comes to policies for integrating minorities. Systematic research in this area is still lacking, but it seems safe to conclude that there is no Scandinavian model in this area, and discourses on diversity and multiculturalism are even more varied. The countries also differ in the relative share of foreign citizens and asylum seekers.

Conclusion and Perspectives

From the 1960s until the 1980s, the Scandinavian countries were at the forefront in terms of women's political representation and employment rates, and it is also quite obvious that Hernes's notion of woman-friendliness has become quite influential in the public debate, also at a European and an international level (see, for example, Chapter 9 in this volume). During some periods, the countries have presumably functioned as laboratories that generated experiences which have served as a vision for political actors and civil society organisations in other countries. Today, it is clear that the Scandinavian countries diverge in several respects, both in terms of gender equality and welfare state models, and even more so regarding the discourses on gender equality among ethnic minorities. Furthermore, they are not in the front line in all areas. In some areas, such as family-based violence and trafficking, Denmark and Norway are not very proactive. Further, in Sweden, dissatisfaction is high among couples regarding how they share paid work and

---

4   Iceland today has the longest 'daddy quota', which is three months. Icelandic fathers have a take-up rate of 34 per cent (Social Protection in the Nordic Countries 2008/2009   table   3.7   http://nososco-eng.nom-nos.dk/filer/publikationer/Social%20 Protection%202010.pdf, accessed 2. August 2011).

5   Ibid.

housework (see Chapter 11 in this volume). The Scandinavian experience may still contribute to reflections about what works and what does not, but it is important to bear in mind that context, timing and political opportunity structures matter, and that makes it difficult to copy policies from one country to another.

First of all, ideas travel, and the Scandinavian experience demonstrates that policy learning may work across countries. Some legal reforms have been adopted following close co-operation between experts, organisations and political parties, and during the last century the Scandinavian countries have engaged in what resembles the open method of co-ordination in the EU (implemented in employment, pensions and gender equality). It sets up common benchmarks for the countries, which may choose different means to reach them. In the Scandinavian countries, this method has been in practice for many years, but in a less formalised way, driven by actors devoted to gender equality and supported by the Council of Scandinavian Ministers.

The region has also been influenced by international organisations. The UN recommendations to establish policy machineries for women, the effort to implement the CEDAW convention and to further gender mainstreaming have been central. The close co-operation on gender equality within the EU that today includes many different areas is also of great importance.[6]

Finally, the Scandinavian experience demonstrates that the universal-breadwinner vision has obvious shortcomings. It is often driven by a narrow utilitarian policy logic that restricts women's options and makes gainful employment imperative. It is also clear that with the emerging multiculturalism, which is a relatively new phenomenon in Scandinavia, diversity has become a challenge to the grand vision of gender equality in Scandinavia.

References

Andreassen, R. (2005), *The Mass Media's Construction of Gender, Race, Sexuality and Nationality. An Analysis of the Danish News Media's Communication about Visible Minorities 1971–2004*, PhD dissertation, Department of History, University of Toronto.

Bergqvist, C. et al. (eds) (1999), *Equal Democracies? Gender and Politics in the Nordic Countries*, Oslo: Scandinavian University Press, Council of Nordic Ministers.

Borchorst, A. (2006), 'The Public–private Split Rearticulated: Abolishment of the Danish Daddy Leave', in A.L. Ellingsæter and A. Leira (eds), *Politicising Parenthood in Scandinavia: Gender Relations in Welfare States*, Bristol: Policy Press, pp. 101–20.

—— (2008), 'Woman-friendly Policy Paradoxes? Childcare Policies and Gender Equality Visions in Scandinavia', in K. Melby, A.-B. Ravn and C. Carlsson

---

6   Norway is not a member, but participates in a restricted way.

Wetterberg (eds), *The Limits of Political Ambition? Gender Equality and Welfare Politics in Scandinavia*, Bristol: Policy Press, pp. 27–42.

—— and Siim, B. (2008), 'Woman-friendly policies and state feminism: Theorizing Nordic gender equality', *Feminist Theory*, vol. 9, no. 2, pp. 207–24.

Borchorst, A. and Teigen, M. (2009), *Who is at Issue – What is at Stake? Intersectionality in Danish and Norwegian Gender Equality Policies*, ECPR Joint Session of Workshops, Lisbon, Portugal, 14–19 September 2008.

Borchorst, A., Christensen, A.-D. and Siim, B. (2002), 'Diskurser om køn, magt og politik i Skandinavien' ('Discourses on Gender, Power and Politics'), in A. Borchorst (ed.), *Kønsmagt under Forandring*, Copenhagen: Hans Reitzels Forlag, pp. 246–66.

Christiansen, N.F., Petersen, K., Edling, N. and Haave, P. (eds) (2006), *The Nordic Model of Welfare: A Historical Reappraisal*, Copenhagen: Museum Tusculanum Press.

Dahlerup, D. (ed.) (2006), *Women, Quotas and Politics*, London and New York: Routledge.

de los Reyes, P., Molina, I. and Mulinari, D. (2003), *Maktens olika förklädnadar. Kønn, klasse og etnicitet i det post-koloniale Sverige*, Stockholm: Atlas.

Esping-Andersen, G. (1990). *The Three Worlds of Welfare Capitalism*, Oxford: Polity Press.

—— et al. (2002), *Why We Need a New Welfare State*, Oxford: Oxford University Press.

European Commission (2009), *Report on Equality Between Women and Men 2009*, <http://ec.europa.eu/social/main.jsp?catId=421&langId=en&pubId=86&type=2&furtherPubs=yes> (accessed 8 May 2011).

Fraser, N. (1997), *Justice Interruptions. Critical Reflections on the 'Postsocialist' Condition*, New York and London: Routledge.

Graubard, S.R. (ed.) (1986), *Norden: The Passion for Equality*, Oslo: Universitetsforlaget.

Hernes, H.M. (1987), *Welfare State and Women Power: Essays in State Feminism*, Oslo: Norwegian University Press.

Hirdman, Y. (1990), 'Genussystemet', in *Demokrati och Makt i Sverige*, Maktutredningens huvudrapport, SOU 1990:44, pp. 73–114.

—— (1996), *Key Concepts in Feminist Theory. Analyzing Gender and Welfare*, Aalborg: Aalborg University, FREIA paper 34.

Knijn, T. and Kremer, K. (1997), 'Gender and the caring dimension of welfare states: Towards inclusive citizenship', *Social Politics*, vol. 4, no. 3, pp. 328–61.

Lisbon European Council (2000), *Presidency Conclusions*, 23–24 March.

Melby, K. et al. (eds) (2007), *Inte ett ord om kärlek: Äktenskap och politik i Norden ca. 1850–1930*, Stockholm: Makadam förlag.

Nielsen, H.S., Simonsen, M. and Verner, M. (2003), *Does the Gap in Family-friendly Policies Drive the Family Gap?*, Working Paper no. 2000–01, Aarhus: School of Economics and Management, Aarhus University.

OECD (2006), *OECD Factbook*, Paris: OECD.

—— (2009), *OECD Factbook*, Paris: OECD.

Outshoorn, J. and Kantola, J. (eds) (2007), *Changing State Feminism*, Basingstoke: Palgrave Macmillan.

Pateman, C. (1987), 'The Patriarchal Welfare State', in A. Gutman (ed.), *Democracy and the Welfare State*, Princeton, NJ: Princeton University Press.

Siim, B. (2007), 'The challenge of recognizing diversity from the perspective of gender equality: Dilemmas in Danish citizenship', *CRISPP – Critical Review of International Social and Political Philosophy*, vol. 10, no. 4, pp. 491–511.

—— (2008), 'Dilemmas of Citizenship: Tensions between Gender Equality and Respect for Diversity in the Danish Welfare State', in K. Melby, A.-B. Ravn and C. Carlsson Wetterberg (eds), *Gender Equality as a Perspective on Welfare: The Limits of Political Ambition*, Bristol: Policy Press, pp. 149–65.

—— and Skjeie, H. (2008), 'Tracks, intersections and dead ends: State feminism and multicultural retreats in Denmark and Norway', *Ethnicities*, vol. 8, no. 3, pp. 322–44.

Skjeie, H. (1992), *Den Politiske Betydningen av Kjønn: En Studie av Norsk Topp-politik*, Oslo: Institut for Samfunnsforskning.

—— and Teigen, M. (2005), 'Political constructions of gender equality: Travelling towards a gender balanced society?', *NORA, Nordic Journal of Feminist and Gender Research*, vol. 13, no. 3, pp. 187–97.

Velfærdskommissionen (2004), *Fremtidens Velfærd Kommer Ikke af Sig Selv*, Copenhagen: Velfærdskommissionen.

World Economic Forum (2009), *The Global Gender Gap Report*, Geneva: WEF, <http://www.weforum.org/pdf/gendergap/report2009.pdf> (accessed 8 May 2011).

Chapter 4

Too Much Family and Too Much Gender Inequality: Women's and Men's Total Work in Mediterranean Countries

Lina Gálvez Muñoz, Paula Rodríguez Modroño
and Mónica Domínguez-Serrano

The Mediterranean countries are characterised in terms of gender as having the lowest female activity rates and the lowest fertility rates. This is indicative of not only a highly unequal society, but a non-sustainable socio-economic system, since the fertility level is far below the replacement rate – the birth rate which is needed to enable the population to reproduce itself and maintain its numerical strength. As highlighted by Livi-Bacci (2001) for the Italian case, we are facing a situation of *too few children, too much family*. However, what is not always emphasised is that these countries are also the ones with a more unequal distribution of unpaid care work. Time use data allow us to show how unpaid care work that takes place outside the marketplace represents an essential and distinctive part of the Mediterranean economy, and how this work is unevenly distributed among women and men. This unequal distribution of care work inside the family is contributing to maintain fertility rates at lower levels than in other Western European countries, as these Mediterranean nations have not yet completely developed public childcare facilities to reduce the family burden that is placed almost entirely on women, and to the unsustainability of a society in which women in general, and employed mothers in particular, bear an extremely high workload. We use the term 'unpaid care work', following Elson (2000), to cover all the unpaid services provided within a household for its members, because care is not only caring for children, the elderly or the disabled; it is also caring for able-bodied adults, including adult males.

Is this because of the prevalence of a male traditionalist culture, or could we find some institutional settings that allow for family models of varying degrees of gender equality? Women and men make important choices about how to allocate their time and their relationship with the provision and share of well-being. But their choices are significantly constrained by the different restrictions and social determining factors which women and men experience, and the limits dictated by the institutional environment in which they live. Each society will combine the provision of welfare among the state, the market, the family and the community in a different and dynamic way, having a differentiated impact on well-being distribution by gender. Public policies play a differentiated and essential role, shaping the behaviour of other agents and the institutional environment. As Addis (1999) points out, welfare states play an important role in the modernisation of gender roles, by either encouraging or discouraging women's involvement in the labour market and influencing the patterns of such participation, and also by shaping gender relations.

Since some countries converge and others differ on the institutional arrangements that contribute to the sum total of societal welfare, they have been grouped in the literature in what have been called 'welfare regimes', 'welfare systems' or the most comprehensive grouping of mixed economies of welfare, 'care diamonds', since not only are the state and the market included as providers of well-being, but also the family and civil society.[1] In the latter, the accent is on the diversity of sites in which welfare is produced and the decisions taken by society to privilege some forms of provision over others (Razavi 2007, p. 20).[2] What states do and the conditions on which benefits are made available carry other implicit objectives and consequences which support different types of family and gender relations. Time use data allow us to look for the differentiated gender impact of the mixes of welfare provision among the different providers of well-being such as the state, the family, the market and civil society; different sharing patterns will have different outcomes in terms of gender relations and equality.

One of the strengths of the welfare regime literature has been its cross-national comparative dimension, based on regime analysis: clusters of countries around dominant institutional patterns. However, when including time use data, the clusters do not have the same composition as when they were first established by Esping-Andersen.[3] This is because they were created to characterise the relationship between state and economy across advanced capitalist countries. In fact, despite the centrality of care to human welfare, it was absent in the first wave of comparative social policy research (Razavi 2007, p. 18). The proposed three-way classification of welfare capitalism into liberal, corporatist/conservative and social democratic was used as a starting point, to which the Mediterranean regime was later added when the importance of the family as an institution in the provision of welfare was acknowledged.

Institutional development and public policies in Mediterranean countries (as well as in some Eastern European countries, where the transition to a

---

1   For a recent study which highlights the importance of the role played by civil society in welfare provision, see Harris and Bridgen (2007), pp. 1–18.

2   As Razavi (2007, p. 20) says: 'the role of the state in the welfare architecture is of a qualitatively different kind, compared to, say, families or markets, because the state is not just a provider of welfare, but also a significant decision maker about the responsibilities to be assumed by the other three sets of institutions'.

3   For a cluster analysis of time use by gender in the European context, see 'Work and time use by gender in European welfare systems' in a special issue of *Feminist Economics* on 'Time Use and Unpaid Work' (Galvez et al. 2011).

capitalist society resulted in a withdrawal of the state, increases in inequality and a deterioration of labour market conditions for certain population groups), have evolved in a less female-friendly environment than in other welfare regime types such as the Nordic ones, where there are a more even distribution of total work by gender and higher fertility rates, although, as shown by Anette Borchorst in Chapter 3 of this volume, the Nordic countries are far from homogeneous or achieving a gender-equal model. Policies will influence the feasibility of the crucial issue of combining work and family through different arrangements involving time, money or services. But policies also fundamentally shape labour market institutions and regulations, as well as general levels of employment, leading to spatial and temporal variations in the return to education and the degree of uncertainty.

Previous work, including time use data, on welfare regime comparisons shows no regime effects on unpaid work and leisure time. The only significant difference regarding time use was found on hours of paid work, which were shorter in the so-called social democratic regime than in the liberal one. The authors associated these results with the need to provide time for the consumption of high value-added leisure and services and the necessity to engage in care work, since there was not a significant amount of cheap labour available (Gershuny and Sullivan 2003). However, the sample of countries was limited and their allocation to different welfare systems predetermined. In fact, in the European context, prior to the Time Use Survey (TUS) promoted by Eurostat and carried out in 2002–2003, whose main results were made available in 2004, comparative studies presented limitations related to the different methodologies that forced a reduction in the sample of countries or cases, or conditioned the results.[4] The existence nowadays of consistent surveys for different countries not only allows us to make international comparisons, but also to extend our investigations into the causes of the uneven time use between women and men, and how we could link such differences to the particular institutional settings present in those countries or groups of countries, as we do in this chapter with the Mediterranean group.[5] The Mediterranean group is limited in this sample to Italy and Spain, which are the countries that completed the TUS 2002–3003 and for which we have homogeneous data. However, as it is possible to see in other chapters of this volume, these two countries share

---

4   This happened in the studies based on the European Community Household Panel (ECHP), the Multinational Time Use Study (MTUS) and the European Harmonized Time Use Survey, an important piece of work by the ESRC Research Centre on Micro-social Change, <http://www.iser.essex.ac.uk/research/misoc/research-theme/time-use> (accessed 8 May 2011). See Joesch and Spiess (2006), Burda et al. (2006) and Burda et al. (2007).

5   A recent OECD publication pays attention to differences in leisure time by gender in OECD countries, but without giving a clear understanding of what is leisure, or, come to that, what is work: OECD (2009), *Society at a Glance 2009: OECD Social Indicators*, <http://www.oecd.org/els/social/indicators/SAG> (accessed 8 May 2011). See especially ch. 2 on measuring leisure: <http://www.sourceoecd.org/pdf/societyataglance2009/812009011e-02.pdf> (accessed 8 May 2011).

some common patterns with other Southern European countries regarding gender inequalities and welfare state developments, such as Portugal and Greece.

The aim of this chapter is, on the one hand, to use the homogeneous time use data to fill the gap, noted by previous feminist literature, created by the failure of public policy regimes literature to address issues of gender beyond labour market behaviour. On the other hand, this chapter sets out to show the inter-relationship between paid and unpaid work, focusing on the Mediterranean countries, which are the ones showing a more unequal share of total work by gender, in order to further the development of the institutional framework helping to advance gender equality. Including time use in welfare regime analysis allows us to see the complete picture, showing how unpaid care work is at the core of gender inequality in all countries. There are welfare systems which present a higher provision of state services and benefits for the majority of the population, together with a more stable labour market and public policies oriented towards work–life balance issues, which are the ones that account for the most egalitarian distribution of unpaid care work and of total work time between the genders. These countries are also the ones showing higher fertility rates nowadays. However, some recent literature highlights the importance of labour market conditions for explaining fertility rate differences instead of 'female-friendly' states or policies (Esping-Andersen 2007). The explanations about what is understood by 'female-friendly policies' differ among feminist and non-feminist scholars.[6] This allows us to build up some public policies regarding labour market and work–life balance policies that will help to solve the care crisis and the lower fertility rates without decreasing women's well-being and autonomy.[7]

This introduction is followed by four sections. In the next section we will deal with feminist economics advances on the concept of work and unpaid work, and on gendering welfare regimes. In the following section, we will analyse the similarities and differences found in all the countries studied. In the next section, we will concentrate on the special characteristics of the Mediterranean countries included in our sample (Spain and Italy), and we will offer our conclusions in the final section.

---

6   For a discussion on the label 'female-friendly' regarding a welfare state, see Chapter 3 in this volume by Anette Borchorst, who explains how competing discourses in Nordic countries reveal that gender equity is a contested issue far from the homogeneous idea derived from the concept of female-friendliness. In fact, she contrasts the recent discourses about the potential of woman-friendly policies to tackle the challenges welfare states face in the light of population ageing and globalised economies.

7   There are many studies showing that the common basic preference for the number of children is on average 2.2–2.4 (for example, Bien 2000; Van de Kaa 2001) over the standard total fertility rate in developed economies.

Gendering the Definition of Work in Time Use Surveys

Until very recently, standard definitions of work only corresponded to a Western male experience. As a result of this narrow definition, feminist economists have concentrated on defining and enlarging the concept and measurement of work (Benería 2003). As a matter of fact, we could define work as the creation of goods and services that meet human needs for the benefit of oneself or others, in the present and regarding future generations (Picchio 2003). We produce things in order to care for ourselves and for our families, but we sometimes forget that the process of caring is also a process of production. Building upon this idea, we agree with Folbre (2008, pp. 99–101) that the activities that should be included in a work definition should follow Reid's (1934) third-person criterion: work can be defined as an activity that one could in principle pay a person outside the family (a third person) to perform.[8] As Elson (2005, p. 2) says, the fact that much unpaid care work is done for love does not mean that we always love doing it. So work, or total work, is composed of paid and unpaid work. As a matter of fact, leisure is defined as time spent free of obligation and necessity. For example, the quantity of leisure has been defined as 'all activities that we cannot pay somebody else to do for us and we do not really have to do at all if we do not wish to' (Burda et al. 2006, p. 1).[9]

Elson (1999) establishes the term 'unpaid care work' to include housework, care of persons and 'community' work which are sustaining life to reproduce the labour force. Folbre (2008, p. 96) argues:

> time, like money, can be denominated in standardized units and tallied in spreadsheets. But an hour of time is not nearly as homogeneous as a unit of money, and many family activities are conceptually difficult to measure … measuring the amount of time devoted to the care of others is far more difficult,

---

8   As Folbre (2008) argues, on the one hand neoclassical economic theory defines work in terms of motivation. Work is a means to an end, an activity undertaken for the purpose of generating income. Classical political economy, on the other hand, defines work in terms of its results, rather than motives. Neither of these definitions is entirely satisfactory. Motivation is difficult to observe. Human needs are difficult to define. However, the third-party criterion is not without inconsistencies. Some activities are not defined as work even though, in principle, a third party could be hired to perform them. Sexual services are commonly bought and sold, but consensual sex is usually undertaken with the presumption of mutual pleasure. Studying is often subjectively experienced as work rather than leisure. It could reasonably be considered work even if it does not satisfy the third-person criterion. Another classificatory problem is posed by sleep and personal care activities. Unlike leisure, sleep and personal care are necessary activities of personal maintenance.

9   Although some very recent time use studies have categorised *all* sleep as leisure (see Aguiar and Hurst, 2007; Engler and Staubli 2008), and bearing in mind that some sleep is voluntary, we do not consider it so in our analysis, where sleeping is included in self-care activities.

because care is an emotionally laden, complex interaction that is not always
reported as a specific activity.

Unpaid care work includes all activities needed by households, including tasks
outdoors, which are not exchanged in the market.[10] As a matter of fact, it is
important not to divorce unpaid care work from other types of unpaid work such
as cooking, cleaning or shopping which are done for the entire family and account
for, following time use studies, the biggest amount of unpaid work time and the
biggest inequalities by gender. Since due to data constraints we are not including
voluntary work, the term we will use in this chapter is *unpaid care work*.

Although we acknowledge that any definition that distinguishes leisure from
work is a matter of judgement, we consider that total work is formed by both
market and unpaid care work, including care work that can be hired in the market,
in our measurement of total work time. Nevertheless, other authors such as Aguiar
and Hurst (2007) have not included care time in their measure of total work time
and leisure in the US from 1965 to 2003. By not including care, they have found
a dramatic increase in leisure time from six to nine hours per week for men and
from four to eight hours per week for women. This increase in female leisure
time was possible even with increased market working time due to a decrease
in time allocated to work associated with the home of ten hours per week. Their
explanation for not including care time in household production is the difficulty
of distinguishing between care which is considered as work and that which is
regarded as free time spent with the family. The same could be true for certain
individuals when talking about cooking or gardening, however, these cases, too,
were not considered by these authors here. One person could enjoy caring for
another, just as other people could enjoy the jobs they do for pay.

In addition, there is another reason for including care when considering total
work.[11] In the TUS, care time is underestimated. In fact, an important proportion of
time devoted to care is already implicitly included in leisure activities. Otherwise,
how can we explain the important number of hours that women – and not men –
allocate to walking in parks or being in amusement parks, while men spend much

---

10   Technically, unpaid care work is the equivalent to 'non-SNA work': care of
persons for no explicit monetary reward. The largest amount of unpaid care is carried
out within the household, but it is not confined to the household since the individuals
also perform unpaid care for other families and for the community. This is the definition
recently adopted by the UNRISD Project 'The Political and Social Economy of Care in a
Development Context' (Razavi 2007). However, in this chapter we concentrate on unpaid
care work, excluding voluntary work since time use gender ratios on voluntary work do not
differ very much by country and by groups of countries. Unpaid care work is at the heart of
gender inequality in all countries, showing very slow changes with time, though there are
significant welfare system differences or different labour market settings and conditions.

11   We also group study together with working time because it is included as such
in the database. However, differences among genders are not important, and as a matter of
fact, they do not affect total time work differences among men and women.

more time doing sports.[12] Aguiar and Hurst (2007) found that female working time narrowed when childcare was included in total work especially in the period 1993–2003. Such a change in their long-term analysis shows a preference towards a quality education in childrearing while technology and changing consumption patterns have made possible a decrease in home work time. However, it could also show an increased female consciousness in some countries of childcare as a task – even if a pleasant one – rather than a natural path for being born female. Differences in self-awareness by women in each country could be derived from different results in international surveys.

In any case, childcare work is underestimated in this TUS survey, as many women consider it such a natural activity that they do not take that time into account.[13] Although using the TUS allows for a deeper analysis of the inequalities between women and men, and therefore an improvement in the implementation of public policies designed to eradicate this inequality, it also demonstrates important limitations related to the maintenance of a pattern of activity and time which is still mercantile and androcentric. This in turn reveals the unsustainability of our socio-economic system, which will not be rectified unless we achieve gender equity. The TUS identifies work with employment when including it under the category 'work' only when it is paid work, whereas unpaid care work is labelled 'home and family', without considering that both types of work are related and are included in gender-non-neutral processes.

Comparative Time Use Analysis in Europe[14]

Time use distribution by gender shows important similarities all over Europe. Female specialisation in non-market work is common to all countries. However, in some countries, such as the Nordic ones, total work is more egalitarian by gender than in other groups of countries, such as the Mediterranean ones, which show a very unequal distribution. Despite the fact that 'woman-friendliness' is a contested issue regarding the challenges welfare states are facing with ageing populations and economic globalisation, a comparative analysis regarding both paid and unpaid care work shows the existence of countries which are more 'woman-friendly' than others in terms of well-being and autonomy. Different institutional

---

12   Gálvez et al. (2008) show, using micro data from the Spanish survey, that time use differences by gender in care work increase when a woman and a man live together – married or not – but they do not increase so dramatically when having the first child. This therefore shows the impact of care for the independent – for the household – and not just for the dependent members of the family on patterns of time consumption.

13   On this topic, see the analysis of TUS 2002–2003 for Catalunya by Carrasco et al. (2005), and the comparison with Durán (2006).

14   This section relies on a previous publication by the authors, Domínguez et al. (2011).

settings and public policies have different impacts on gender equality. This is because there is an interdependence between the diverse work processes and the state's organisation which determines an unequal distribution of time and work between women and men, and consequently, an unequal social status.[15] We will first deal with the similarities and then differences among countries and groups of countries in our sample.

Time use data for the countries for which we have homogeneous data – Belgium, Italy, Slovenia, Germany, Latvia, Finland, Estonia, Lithuania, Sweden, Spain, Hungary, the United Kingdom, France, Poland and Norway – show that gendered inequalities still exist in European countries. Gender is a determining factor in the allocation of time between paid and unpaid care work as well as free time. The first common characteristic in time allocation by gender in EU countries is that, if we add paid work time and unpaid work time in housekeeping and care, women work for longer each day than men do. Only in Sweden do men and women spend the same amount of time in total work. In Norway and the United Kingdom, women work for only a few more minutes every day than men. Those countries in which we find the largest difference, where women work at least one hour more each day than men, are the Eastern European and Mediterranean ones: Lithuania, Slovenia, Latvia, Estonia, Hungary, Italy and Spain. In Spain, for example, women work 1 hour and 5 minutes more than men, which, when multiplied by 365 days per year, means an annual difference of 395.42 hours of overload, and therefore, considerably reduced opportunities for women to develop other capabilities, especially over their life span, following the capabilities approach used by Addabbo et al. in Chapter 5 of this volume.

This higher female workload leads to the second common characteristic in the European countries studied: European women have less free time.[16] In Lithuania, Italy and Slovenia, this difference in free time by gender amounts to one hour per day, and in Spain 48 minutes (see Table 4.1). Less free time for women reduces the opportunities for women to develop their personal and social lives. It should be emphasised that we are taking the mean time spent in each activity in an average day, including working days, weekends and holidays, which explains, for example, that the working time is far below that of an ordinary working day. Also, we are including in this table all those aged 20–74 years, whether employed or not.

Third, men continue to be over-represented in the market economy, and women in the non-market economy. In these 15 European countries, women in general work longer than men in unpaid care tasks, and less in the market. In all European countries, as fewer women than men work in the market full-time or at all, the female average hours spent in housework and care exceed those allocated in their paid jobs. The opposite phenomenon happens with men. In all EU countries, the

---

15   On this interdependence, see Picchio (2001).

16   Burda et al. (2006) and Burda et al. (2007) find no important differences in total workload by men and women in their sample of countries, except for some exceptions such as Italy, Spain and France.

Table 4.1   Time use activities of women and men aged 20–74 years expressed in hours and minutes per day (hours:minutes)

WOMEN	Be	De	UK	Fr	Ee	Lv	Lt	Hu	Pl	Si	Fi	Se	No	It	Es
Work total	6:39	6:16	6:48	7:01	7:35	7:37	8:10	7:30	7:14	7:57	6:45	6:54	6:40	7:26	7:21
Paid work and study	2:07	2:05	2:33	2:31	2:33	3:41	3:41	2:32	2:29	2:59	2:49	3:12	2:53	2:06	2:26
Unpaid care work	4:32	4:11	4:15	4:30	5:02	3:56	4:29	4:58	4:45	4:58	3:56	3:42	3:47	5:20	4:55
Travel	1:19	1:18	1:25	0:54	1:06	1:20	1:04	0:51	1:06	1:02	1:07	1:23	1:11	1:14	1:05
Sleep	8:29	8:19	8:27	8:55	8:35	8:44	8:35	8:42	8:35	8:24	8:32	8:11	8:10	8:19	8:32
Meals and personal care	2:43	2:43	2:16	3:02	2:08	2:10	2:22	2:19	2:29	2:08	2:06	2:28	2:08	2:53	2:33
Free time	4:50	5:24	5:04	4:08	4:36	4:09	3:49	4:38	4:36	4:29	5:30	5:04	5:51	4:08	4:29
MEN	Be	De	UK	Fr	Ee	Lv	Lt	Hu	Pl	Si	Fi	Se	No	It	Es
Work total	6:08	5:56	6:36	6:25	6:28	6:59	7:04	6:26	6:37	6:47	6:17	6:54	6:38	6:01	6:16
Paid work and study	3:30	3:35	4:18	4:03	3:40	5:09	4:55	3:46	4:15	4:07	4:01	4:25	4:16	4:26	4:39
Unpaid care work	2:38	2:21	2:18	2:22	2:48	1:50	2:09	2:40	2:22	2:40	2:16	2:29	2:22	1:35	1:37
Travel	1:35	1:27	1:30	1:03	1:17	1:28	1:13	1:03	1:13	1:09	1:12	1:30	1:20	1:35	1:16
Sleep	8:15	8:12	8:18	8:45	8:32	8:35	8:28	8:31	8:21	8:17	8:22	8:01	7:57	8:17	8:36
Meals and personal care	2:40	2:33	2:04	3:01	2:15	2:10	2:25	2:31	2:23	2:13	2:01	2:11	2:02	2:59	2:35
Free time	5:22	5:52	5:32	4:46	5:28	4:48	4:50	5:29	5:25	5:34	6:08	5:24	6:03	5:08	5:17

Note: Belgium (Be), Italy (It), Slovenia (Sl), Germany (De), Latvia (Lv), Finland (Fi), Estonia (Ee), Lithuania (Lt), Sweden (Se), Spain (Es), Hungary (Hu), United Kingdom (UK), France (Fr), Poland (Pl), Norway (No).

Source: Eurostat National Time Use Surveys.

average number of remunerated working hours for men is far greater than their hours of unpaid care work. The difference is usually two hours more for men in the labour market than in care work (see Figure 4.1), almost the same time that women must allocate in excess to unpaid work than to their paid jobs in the market. Therefore, we can see that, in general terms, patriarchal work specialisation still survives in Europe – something that must be taken into consideration as a central issue in macroeconomic models and policies.

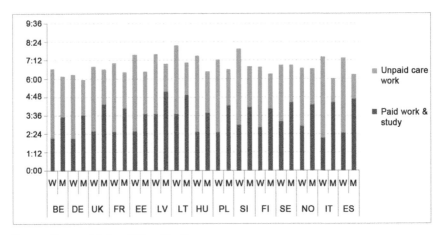

Source: Eurostat National Time Use Surveys.

Figure 4.1   Working time of women and men aged 20–74 years expressed in hours and minutes per day (hours:minutes) (left bar women; right bar men)

These results of the TUS show that nowadays, the highest gender inequality is not in paid working time, as there has been increased incorporation of women into the labour market, but in the differences in time spent by each gender in unpaid care work. This is explained by the fact that equality policies and women's movements have focused on improving women's access to the labour market rather than achieving a more egalitarian division of care work, which has been a more recent battle. Nowadays, women have improved their presence in the labour market, but they have not been able to reduce their work at home very much, thus bearing the double burden of paid and unpaid care work. When they have been able to reduce it, this has been by buying it in the labour market (see also Chapter 6 in this volume) rather than improving substantially their partner's sharing of unpaid family and care work. The main duty for women continues to be the maintenance of their households and the care of dependent – and independent – people.

After the hours of sleep, unpaid care work constitutes the main activity of women of, in this order, Italy, Estonia, Hungary, Slovenia, Spain, Poland, France and Lithuania, spending a daily average of five hours in unpaid care work. On the contrary, Sweden, Norway, Finland and Latvia are the countries where women allocate fewer hours to care work, with an average of 3 hours and 50 minutes. Although men have fewer incentives – with the recent exception of some modern social values which are redefining masculinity and the institutional setting which favours more egalitarian families – to involve themselves in unpaid care work, they do not seem to offer resistance to having another salary in the family, mainly due to changes in consumption patterns and the transformations taking place in labour markets since the crisis of the 1970s. These changes have entailed a greater instability in employment and better job opportunities for women related to the service economy, and mainly, with women's better qualifications that have been reflected in an increase in their wages and have changed their opportunity cost. Governments have not offered any resistance either, as they benefit from the increase in social security taxes without a significant increase in the average cost of social transferences over total public expenses. In fact, the Lisbon agenda for 2010 included a compromise to increase women's activity rate, still particularly low in countries such as Italy or Spain.

In fact, past and present evidence proves that the unequal distribution of non-market care work takes place in the form of more work for women than for men, even in those households in which women are those that contribute a higher income to the family budget (Brines 1994; Gálvez 1997; Akerlof and Kranton 2000). Longitudinal analyses using time use surveys prove that in spite of the increase in women's participation in the labour market, male working time in the household changed very little in the last decades of the twentieth century (Aguiar and Hurst 2007). In any case, empirical evidence demonstrates that women do more and men less care work than we might expect from the Beckerian model of total specialisation in order to obtain the greatest relative efficiency, and that bargaining models (Chiappori 1988; Chiappori 1992), and therefore social norms in the division of work appear to be better explanatory variables than those following the economic theory explanation.[17]

In addition to these characteristics shared by most of the European countries, there are some different patterns in time allocation by gender among the various

---

17   The basic underlying assumption of the neoclassical analysis of the family is that it is a unit whose adult members make informed and rational decisions that result in maximising the utility or well-being of the family. Simple neoclassical models based on the seminal work of Gary Becker and Jacob Mincer from the 1960s onwards suggest that there are considerable efficiency gains to the traditional division of labour in which the husband specialises in market work and the wife specialises in home work. However, historical and contemporary research shows that in most of the cases, when women specialise in market work, men do not specialise in care work. In a recent survey published by Gálvez and Matus (2010) regarding the impact of the new law for gender equality in Spain on work–life balance measures on Andalusian businesses, employed women married or cohabiting with unemployed or inactive men were the ones reporting more problems balancing their professional and personal life. This means specialisation could work in one sense but not in the other, because of the maintenance of gender stereotypes.

groups of European countries considered in our analysis which are highly related to institutional development and labour market characteristics. Some countries show similarities in their behaviour as well as in their institutional development. For example, the countries in which time allocations to care work are more evenly shared between women and men overcame the phase of low fertility rates and have now higher total fertility rates (see Table 4.2), whereas in the Mediterranean countries, in which women continue to bear a heavy domestic overload as men dedicate much less time to care work than women, a decline in the number of children has been the option chosen by many couples, or solely by women, with the subsequent future problems of ageing and maintenance of the present welfare states. Italy and Spain have experienced a small increase in their total fertility rates (TFR) in recent years, and this increase has been mainly due to immigrants' high fertility rates and some pro-natalist policies. However, the TFR was only 1.46 in Spain in 2008 and 1.37 in Italy in 2007. Of course, this has consequences for women's well-being, as they are forced to choose in many cases between their professional careers or their maternity – a trade-off which is not experienced by their male counterparts.

The most evident differences among groups of countries are between the Nordic countries and the rest. The Nordic countries – Finland, Norway and Sweden – are those with the smallest gender differentiation in the distribution of time, whereas the Mediterranean nations, Spain and Italy, plus Estonia, still maintain a very uneven distribution of activities between men and women. In the Nordic countries, female economic activity rates are higher than in other groups of countries, although there is a high presence of part-time employment (see Table 4.3). The growth of the state provision of services has developed together with female labour opportunities in the public sector. However, this has implied an important gender labour segregation by economic sector and dependency from the state. Comparative fertility studies point out to stable labour market opportunities as the main key for explaining differences by country (Ahn and Mira 1999; Esping-Andersen 2007). In fact, especially in Mediterranean countries, women are more likely to have children if they are either housewives or in stable and well-paid employment (Adsera 2004; González and Jurado 2007).

Table 4.3 also shows how part-time employment is one of the ways in which women try to balance their professional and personal lives. In fact, the percentage of women who work in part-time jobs increases when women live in couples, and increases even more when they have dependent-aged children (OECD 2007). The problem with this kind of work is that usually wages are lower, with the consequent loss of economic autonomy, which can have serious implications in situations such as divorce and over the life span in terms of pensions. These jobs offer fewer possibilities for promotion, and the accumulation of human capital and experience is lower than in full-time jobs. Therefore, in each group of countries we are facing different models of gender discrimination related to employment patterns and institutional incentives. In fact, the Lisbon target of increasing female activity rates cannot be achieved by using part-time contracts as the strategy. Part-time work fails

Table 4.2   Fertility and mean age at first child, 2005

	Be	De	UK	Fr	Ee	Lv	Lt	Hu	Pl	Si	Fi	Se	No	It	Es
Mean age of women at birth of first child	27.6	29.1	29.8	28.5	25.2	24.9	24.9	26.7	25.8	27.7	27.9	28.6	27.7	29.6	29.3
Total fertility rates	1.7	1.34	1.78	1.94	1.50	1.31	1.27	1.31	1.24	1.26	1.80	1.77	1.84	1.32	1.35

Source: Eurostat and UNECE

Table 4.3   Activity and employment rates for people aged 25–74 years

2006	Activity rates		Employment rates		Unemployment rates		Part-time employment rates		Involuntary part-time employment
	Women	Men	Women	Men	Women	Men	Women	Men	Women
Be	55.9	71.3	51.5	66.8	7.9	6.2	41.9	6.9	11.9
De	61.0	74.3	55.0	67.0	9.7	9.6	48.2	8.6	19.1
UK	62.6	77.2	60.4	74.2	3.6	4.0	42.3	7.8	5.9
Fr	62.4	73.2	57.3	68.4	8.2	6.6	29.8	5.0	28.4
Ee	68.4	78.9	65.2	74.5	4.7	5.6	10.4	3.8	22.6
Lv	64.4	77.4	61.1	72.0	5.2	6.9	7.9	4.4	31.9
Lt	64.4	74.8	61.1	70.8	5.1	5.4	12.1	7.8	32.7
Hu	52.7	69.1	49.1	64.9	6.9	6.1	5.6	2.5	24.0
Pl	55.5	72.3	48.4	64.4	12.8	10.9	11.8	5.9	27.3
Si	62.8	73.9	58.9	70.9	6.2	4.1	8.8	4.9	8.0
Fi	67.3	73.1	62.8	68.8	6.6	5.8	15.2	7.1	33.5
Se	71.1	78.6	67.5	74.6	5.1	5.0	38.4	10.1	21.5
No	70.3	79.2	68.6	77.1	2.5	2.7	41.4	10.2	19.2
It	46.2	71.0	42.8	67.9	7.4	4.3	26.2	4.2	N/A
Es	54.6	77.3	49.0	73.2	10.2	5.3	22.1	3.3	32.4

Source: Eurostat and LFS.

to challenge women's traditional specialisation in housework and childcare, both of which are very time-consuming activities. Gender equality policy on limiting labour hours of men and women and reducing the gender wage gap is crucial if gender equality is to be achieved in participation in the caring roles.

Our data also show that things do not change much when just looking at the employed population by gender. Labour market situations in European countries are quite different, and in fact, countries also differ if only the employed population is analysed. The analysis of time use differences in the employed population shows how the Beckerian gender specialisation argument does not work – see footnote 17. Our focus on labour market participation is based on our understanding of this participation as crucial for gender equality, and well illustrates the intersection of women's multiple status as clients and consumers of welfare services, as employees and as political citizens, and signals both opportunity and dependence associated with welfare state developments (O'Connor 1993, p. 507). What is more important is that female participation in labour markets is a key aspect for achieving autonomy, although this can only be pursued by universalism in the welfare state system, since women's increasing participation in the participation in the labour market is not always accompanied by a more even distribution of care work, with men experiencing a larger total workload.[18]

Gender differences in the distribution of unpaid care work do not vary substantially when women are employed in the labour market. If we only take into account those women and men who are employed, in an average day women continue to have a total workload which is higher than men, with women working up to around one hour more in some countries like Italy, Hungary, Slovenia and Spain (see Table 4.4). Only UK and Swedish employed women work in total 2–3 minutes per day less than employed men. Once again, in the Mediterranean and Eastern European countries, women's total working time is higher than the European average. The Spanish female working population works an average of 8 hours and 26 minutes daily (including holidays and weekends) – 16 minutes more than the average European woman, and 55 minutes more than Spanish male workers.

One of the main problems women face is that the division of labour within households is relatively unchanged, despite the increasing female activity rates, and the transfer of care services to the public sector or to the market, either wholly or partially, depends on the welfare regime and purchasing power. Work in the labour market is still configured on the assumption of an ideal worker who has no care work, as it has historically happened with male workers. However, the difference between employed women and men is somewhat smaller than the difference between all women and men aged 20–74 years. This suggests that gender inequalities are somewhat reduced, but in a very insufficient way, when women enter the labour market and their bargaining and purchasing power increase. But what makes this lower level of female care work feasible is not an increase in male care work, but that women reduce theirs by replacing it with other people's work, remunerated. In fact, when a person works in the market, it reduces the time available for domestic tasks, and this happens for both genders, but at a different level for women and men. The average time that employed women do not spend in care work compared to women who do not work in the market is 50 minutes in Europe, 1 hour and 26 minutes in Spain, and 1 hour and 29 minutes in Italy, whereas in the case of men it is 21 minutes less in Europe, 17 minutes less in Spain and 25 minutes in Italy. That is to say, the amount of care work performed by men is so low that they can do very little to reduce the time dedicated to these

---

18   According to Iversen and Rosenbluth (2006, p. 1): 'Mainstream political economy has tended to treat the family as a unit when examining the distributional consequences of labour market institutions and of public policy. In a world with high divorce rates, we argue that this simplification is more likely to obscure than to instruct. We find that labour market opportunities for women, which vary systematically with the position of countries in the international division of labour and with the structure of the welfare state, affect women's bargaining power within the family and as a result, can explain much of the cross country variation in the gender division of labour as well as the gender gap in political preferences.'

Table 4.4   Daily average time in these activities of female and male workers expressed in hours and minutes (hours:minutes)

WOMEN	Be	De	UK	Fr	Ee	Lv	Lt	Hu	Pl	Si	Fi	Se	No	It	Es
Work total	7:45	7:03	7:34	8:12	8:17	8:54	9:19	8:37	8:44	8:47	7:41	7:37	7:12	8:30	8:26
Paid work and study	3:53	3:52	4:06	4:32	4:13	5:46	5:55	4:43	4:46	4:23	4:20	4:05	3:46	4:39	4:57
Unpaid care work	3:52	3:11	3:28	3:40	4:04	3:08	3:24	3:54	3:58	4:24	3:21	3:32	3:26	3:51	3:29
Travel	1:30	1:27	1:33	1:05	1:15	1:26	1:07	1:02	1:10	1:09	1:16	1:28	1:17	1:28	1:22
Sleep	8:16	8:11	8:25	8:38	8:23	8:21	8:13	8:18	8:08	8:12	8:22	8:05	8:07	8:00	8:11
Meals and personal care	2:36	2:31	2:07	2:57	2:06	2:06	2:16	2:21	2:14	2:02	2:02	2:23	2:02	2:44	2:28
Free time	3:53	4:48	4:21	3:08	3:59	3:13	3:05	3:42	3:43	3:50	4:39	4:27	5:22	3:18	3:33

MEN	Be	De	UK	Fr	Ee	Lv	Lt	Hu	Pl	Si	Fi	Se	No	It	Es
Work total	7:18	6:57	7:36	7:37	7:20	8:07	8:10	7:34	8:03	7:44	7:31	7:40	7:08	7:23	7:31
Paid work and study	5:03	5:05	5:42	5:44	5:00	6:41	6:31	5:25	6:10	5:20	5:32	5:17	4:56	6:13	6:11
Unpaid care work	2:15	1:52	1:54	1:53	2:20	1:26	1:39	2:09	1:53	2:24	1:59	2:23	2:12	1:10	1:20
Travel	1:43	1:31	1:36	1:10	1:20	1:31	1:17	1:10	1:15	1:14	1:17	1:32	1:23	1:40	1:23
Sleep	8:01	8:00	8:11	8:24	8:22	8:16	8:08	8:08	7:59	8:06	8:12	7:52	7:53	7:58	8:15
Meals and personal care	2:35	2:21	1:55	2:58	2:11	2:08	2:23	2:30	2:14	2:07	1:55	2:05	1:58	2:52	2:31
Free time	4:23	5:11	4:42	3:51	4:47	3:58	4:02	4:38	4:29	4:49	5:05	4:51	5:38	4:07	4:20

Source: Eurostat National Time Use Surveys.

tasks when they work in the market. However, women must reduce their care working time to be able to enter the labour market, even though this reduction does not compensate for the increase in working time in the market.

Employed people's total work continues to be unevenly distributed by gender. Men spend an average of 75 per cent of their time in paid work, whereas women spend only 55 per cent of their total working time, with an average of two hours more than men invested in care tasks in all EU countries. In Table 4.5, we can appreciate better this gender difference in time distribution between paid work and unpaid work. Therefore, if we understand work as an activity that incorporates all the necessary tasks for the support of human life, we cannot speak of under-utilisation of female labour, but of over-exploitation. In fact, as Elson (1999) points out, labour markets are gendered institutions operating at the intersection of the productive and reproductive economies. Participation in the labour market does not automatically empower women. Elson affirms that discrimination against women may persist because, in the absence of institutional changes, it is profitable. Practices, perceptions, norms and networks are aspects of dynamic processes which contain elements of both continuity and transformation.

It seems clear that the best solution would be a more equitable distribution of care work, since the incorporation of women into the labour market by itself only partially improves the unequal gender distribution of working time. In general, European female employees spend less time than male workers in all activities except for care work, to which they dedicate on average twice the male time. Italian and Spanish women are those who must devote more time to housekeeping and the family in comparison, by three times the amount done by men. The reason for this unequal distribution is that traditional social and cultural attitudes have not yet been overcome, and the Mediterranean well-being system based on family support is not only diminishing women's access into the labour market, but is also perpetuating the gender occupational segregation, and it is limiting women's opportunities to develop their professional careers, reducing fertility rates and diminishing their quality of life and health, as we will analyse in the next section.

Mediterranean Countries as Examples of an Unsustainable Social and Economic System

If the Nordic countries are the ones showing a more egalitarian time use by gender, we find the opposite when looking at the Mediterranean countries, which together with some Eastern European countries show the most unequal picture. Other sources beyond the European TUS support these results. According to the European Barometer of 1996, Spanish women were those that suffered the most uneven distribution regarding the amount of care work. Only 12 per cent experienced an egalitarian distribution, whereas the European average was 25 per cent. As Álvarez and Miles (2006, p. 7) point out, Spaniards are conscious of that inequality, since 35 per cent of women (the highest percentage, along with

Table 4.5   Gender differential in time use structure of employed women and men

	Be	De	UK	Fr	Ee	Lv	Lt	Hu	Pl	Si	Fi	Se	No	It	Es
Work total	1.06	1.01	1	1.08	1.13	1.1	1.14	1.14	1.08	1.14	1.02	0.99	1.01	1.15	1.12
Paid work and study	0.77	0.76	0.72	0.79	0.84	0.86	0.91	0.87	0.77	0.82	0.78	0.77	0.76	0.75	0.8
Unpaid care work	1.72	1.71	1.82	1.95	1.74	2.19	2.06	1.81	2.11	1.83	1.69	1.48	1.56	3.3	2.61
Travel	0.87	0.96	0.97	0.93	0.94	0.95	0.87	0.89	0.93	0.93	0.99	0.96	0.93	0.88	0.99
Sleep	1.03	1.02	1.03	1.03	1	1.01	1.01	1.02	1.02	1.01	1.02	1.03	1.03	1	0.99
Meals and personal care	1.01	1.07	1.1	0.99	0.96	0.98	0.95	0.94	1	0.96	1.06	1.14	1.03	0.95	0.98
Free time	0.89	0.93	0.93	0.81	0.83	0.81	0.76	0.8	0.83	0.8	0.91	0.92	0.95	0.8	0.82

Note: Differential = women's time divided by men's time.

Source: Eurostat National Time Use Surveys.

Ireland) and 28 per cent of men agreed that the distribution of care work is the most important area of work which needs to be focused on in order to provide equal opportunities for women.

It seems that the great differences in the distribution of unpaid care work between women and men in the Mediterranean countries still represent the main barrier to access of Spanish and Italian women to the labour market on equal terms with men, limiting women's capacity to get a job and be promoted.[19] In fact, Spain and Italy also share other common characteristics which are strongly correlated with this unequal time use by gender. The first is the lowest female activity rates in the labour markets. The microeconomic theory of the family predicts a negative relationship between fertility and women's employment at the individual level. However – and this is the other strong common characteristic among Spain and Italy – both countries also have the lowest fertility rates in the world. In fact, there seem to be difficulties in balancing market and non-market work, as the average age of mothers at birth of their first child is the highest of all countries. This is also related to an increase in the price of housing and a preference for housing property, as well as lack of housing rent that leads sons to achieving independence from their family home later than elsewhere.[20] Children cost money and time, and the burden of labour market adjustment to the arrival of children falls overwhelmingly on mothers.

These low fertility rates combine with the importance of the family in the provision of welfare. Indeed, the family continues working as the main supplier of care in this socio-economic system.[21] In the two Mediterranean countries in our sample, Spain and Italy, the state still attaches to the family unit the maximum responsibility in the production of welfare, so this restricts the process of defamilialisation of individuals (Moreno 2007). In fact, the common characteristics that we find in the Mediterranean countries could be explained by the prevalence of a male traditionalist culture, or – perhaps – by the existence of institutional settings that allow for more or less gender-egalitarian family models (see also Chapters 6, 9 and 10 in this volume). Maybe it is in the way men and women combine between them paid work and unpaid work, including care work that the TUS allows us to see, where the role of institutions is likely to manifest itself most concretely (Baizán 2007, p. 94).

---

19   For other Southern European countries, see other chapters in this book, especially Chapter 9 by Sara Falcão Casaca and Sónia Damião.

20   This is not independent of increasing precariousness in the labour market, especially for young people, and the existence of dual labour markets. Nor is it independent of the lack of social services for the reconciliation of work and family and personal life.

21   Laat and Sanz (2006) have found – using the multi-country ISSP94 household survey – that within countries, more children are born in households which have a more unequal distribution of time, but women's participation in the labour market is smaller. However, consistent with the presence of social externalities, countries with less egalitarian views have lower average fertility.

The Mediterranean countries are the ones in which the direct, and especially the indirect, costs of childcare and elderly care are greater. McDonald (2002) notes that the key explanations behind low fertility lie in the combination of changed female roles and preferences on the one hand, and the resilience of traditional family and gender roles on the other. The process of individualisation of citizenship rights has occurred slowly in these countries, as is evidenced by the belated and limited development of non-transferable paternity rights or the possibility of joint tax returns – something that, according to de Villota (2009), represents strong fiscal discrimination and discourages the participation of the second family earner – usually women – in the labour market. In these countries, the legacy of totalitarian regimes is still felt in the way in which risks are distributed between the state, family and market through family responsibility for care, social policy and the composition and behaviour of their labour markets. In addition, it must be taken into account that family matters have been considered to be within the private sphere by reducing the implementation of public policies in the context of the family. This lack of family policies results in the persistence of the traditional family which takes on the burden of care, and it is associated with low female activity rates (Trifiletti 1999). In the Mediterranean countries, the 'economic gift' is the greatest, as the family acts as a substitute for the state.[22] Table 4.6 gives an example of how the different EU social protection schemes offer greater or fewer opportunities to individuals – mainly women – to reconcile market work and caring work.

Despite the fact that we should not concentrate on childcare alone when talking about care, we agree with Esping-Andersen (2007, p. 24) that gender symmetry is much easier to achieve in an institutional setting such as the Danish one, which is not zero-sum: the marginal additional caring burden is quite limited considering that children are usually in full-day external care. In Spain or Italy, on the other hand, couples can easily face zero-sum conditions, and this means that gender symmetry will require a very large sacrifice on the part of the male – so large that it will almost inevitably cut into the working day. When we add to this the very long working hours in the Spanish case, it is easy to see why the margin for raising the father's contribution to home production or childcare is narrow. In fact, the constraints on parenthood and work–life balance differ dramatically from one country to another, reflecting the relevant time use gender symmetries.

---

22   The 'economic present' or 'economic gift' is the mechanism by which non-paid women's services allow men to develop their professional careers and limit those of women. It is the opposite situation to the Cinderella tale: the prince does not bring wealth to her, but a decrease in her potential income. Motivated men perform better when married, but ambitious women are better off without a spouse or a committed relationship. Wives who do not work in the labour market not only assume all housework, but also commit themselves to promoting their spouses' careers, for example by agreeing to move to follow work, helping them in their social lives or arranging their diaries (Hufton 1997, pp. 89–90).

Table 4.6   Number of full-time employed persons aged 20–49 years taking time off over the last 12 months for family sickness or emergencies

2005	No		Yes, 'special leave' days remunerated		Yes, 'special leave' days not at all remunerated		Yes, other arrangements always used	
	Women	Men	Women	Men	Women	Men	Women	Men
Be	252.5	616.3	50.6	72.9	21.2	23.7	30.8	50.1
De	4.813.6	9.546.4	133.6	296.6	106.4	212.8	169.3	294.5
UK	3.583.0	6.605.5	737.5	988.9	239.2	453.1	348.1	681.6
Fr	4.392.9	7.316.7	456.5	445.5	77.6	112.1	998.9	1.406.7
Ee	157.1	189.9	13.4	2.1	2.5	2.5	16.2	14.4
Lv	238.2	309.4	28.1	15.1	12.6	19.0	31.6	12.2
Lt	420.9	503.3	10.2	NA	7.2	NA	64.7	39.2
It	3.408.1	6.130.4	565.4	910.7	91.8	186.2	347.0	580.2
Es	3.454.3	7.039.6	568.9	659.9	90.7	125.2	805.0	1.560.9
Hu	899.6	1.225.3	151.8	106.2	44.5	67.1	150.9	161.3
Pl	3.783.2	5.063.3	240.5	161.0	47.4	74.6	216.7	190.1
Si	261.8	335.6	40.9	21.8	—	—	12.7	11.8
Fi	472.8	619.6	96.8	86.3	8.6	12.6	46.7	62.4
Se	533.5	886.1	146.5	253.4	13.7	25.7	83.6	168.8
No	153.9	243.8	66.4	94.3	5.0	12.4	71.2	100.8
It	3.408.1	6.130.4	565.4	910.7	91.8	186.2	347.0	580.2
Es	3.454.3	7.039.6	568.9	659.9	90.7	125.2	805.0	1.560.9

Source: Eurostat Labour Force Survey, special module on reconciliation between work and family life (2005).

Italy and Spain display strong cash transfer and corporatist core worker-oriented welfare states, where public transfers are directed mainly at the elderly, and where universal child and housing allowances are almost non-existent.[23]

---

23   In Spain, from 2007 to 2010, there has been a direct cash transfer of 2,400 euros for having a baby without considering income differences of the family, although fertility literature considers that direct income transfers, such as family allowances, have virtually no effect on fertility (Gauthier and Hatziu 1991), and even less on changing traditional sexual division of labour patterns within the family (Tobío 2008).

Parents could be supported in their childrearing labours by the provision of time (maternity, paternity and parental leave, plus care leave, career breaks and flexible working time patterns), money (family allowance, housing allowance, tax allowance, plus social security and social assistance) or services (nursery places for small children, school and after-school services). In Italy and Spain, the use of extended family support and the externalisation of housework and care work in the market are pursued when possible.[24] The externalisation of care work is clear in the cases of Italy and Spain when comparing the share of care work by gender among the total population over age 20 and the population in occupations. In Spain, the incorporation of women into the labour market and the balancing of working life with family and personal life without the co-responsibility of their male counterparts have been possible due to the low wages of an increased population of female immigrants (Gálvez and Marcenaro 2008).

Women and men face direct and indirect individual costs for having babies – especially women, who are the ones facing high indirect costs during their life cycle.[25] Daycare should reduce mothers' earnings depreciation, and paid maternity, paternity and parental leave will compensate for lost wages, and potentially also diminish interruptions (Del Bocca 2002). Where daycare is mainly supplied through markets, its cost becomes a regressive tax on mothers' labour supply, and in this case, the classical fertility–education correlation should change, since high-income (usually highly educated) households may substitute with purchased care. The marginal cost of daycare changes dramatically where it is predominantly publicly provided and subsidised, as in the Nordic countries (Esping-Andersen 2007).

In the Mediterranean countries, no explicit family policy exists, and public expenditure on families with children is very low. In addition, the offer of childcare services for children under three is relatively low compared to other European countries (see Table 4.7), although parental leave in Italy is comparatively

---

24   In the particular case of Spain, a study on family networks in Southern Spain (Fernández and Tobío 2006) has shown that the belief that the nuclear family disappeared with industrialisation and urbanisation is not true since family networks continue to be essential for sustaining the economic and social system. In Spain, in general terms, women dedicate much more effort than men to child and elderly care, mainly in domestic tasks performed inside the household. Male carers present a participation rate slightly above that of women only in the case of support in order to go out or to arrange business. In addition, there is a higher percentage of male carers than women who dedicate less than 7 hours per week to the aid of relatives, whereas women have the highest percentages, more than 40 hours per week. In this sense, in Italy, and especially in Spain, this situation is possible due to the low economic activity rates of women who are now grandmothers because of the low levels of female activity rates in the post-war decades. However, this situation will change in the coming decades as the new grandmothers may still be working women.

25   We also need to consider the increasing care burden of old people, which is also mainly shouldered by women within the family. In Spain, the 2007 dependency law established the possibility of providing paid assistance to old infirm people by another member of the family through a monetary allowance.

Table 4.7   **Main childcare-related reasons given by employed women aged 20–49 years for not working or not working more (% of total respondents)**

Employed women	Be	De	UK	Fr	Ee	Lv	Lt	Hu	Pl	Si	Fi	Se	No	It	Es
Lack of childcare services at special times	0.2	0	0	0	0	0	0	0	0	0	0	0	0	0.1	0.5
Lack of childcare services during the day or at special times	0	0	0	0.2	0	0	0	0	0	0	0	0	0	0	0.1
Childcare services are too expensive	0.3	0	0.5	0.2	0	0	0	0	0	0	0	0	0	0.3	0.5
Other reason not linked with the lack of suitable childcare services	0.7	0.5	1.0	5.5	0	0	0	0.5	0.2	0	0	2.2	1.1	1.9	1.8

Source: Eurostat. Labour Force Survey, special module on reconciliation between work and family life (2005).

generous with respect to Spain (Naldini and Jurado 2006). Paternity leave is a relative novelty in Spain, having only been implemented in 2007, and is still short, only 15 days, and we do not yet know its real impact. Children have a high opportunity cost for mothers and high direct costs for the family. A welfare system favouring mothers would be one which decreases direct consumption costs, but if gender equality is to be promoted too, the need will be to reduce the opportunity costs of motherhood and to raise the relative bargaining status of the wife. It is essential to look at labour market policies. Policies will influence the feasibility of achieving the crucial needs of combining work and family through different arrangements involving time, money or services. Policies also, however, fundamentally shape labour market institutions and regulations, as well as the general levels of employment, leading to spatial and temporal variations in the returns to education and the degree of uncertainty (Esping-Andersen 2007).

In Spain and Italy, labour markets are characterised by closed employment relations whose consequences are large numbers of insecure jobs – fixed-term and part-time contracts – for young people and women. In both countries, the young find getting a secure job very difficult (Mills and Blossfeld 2005). This, combined with the difficulties they experience accessing decent housing, also results in their starting their families later – a further potential stress in addition to the ongoing employment difficulties. Spain is the EU leader in terms of the incidence of precarious fixed-term contracts, as well as suffering very high levels of youth unemployment. In fact, stability in the labour market and well-paid jobs are essential key issues for improving women's bargaining power in the family and their chances of buying in housework and care work.

However, the solution cannot be to increase female part-time jobs, as in Nordic countries, because this does not challenge the traditional sexual division of labour. In fact, difficulties re-entering the labour market after the interruption due to childbirth differ widely across countries, according to their levels of unemployment and labour market regulations. In addition, time costs are by no means limited to periods out of employment or (paid) maternity leave, but include periods of part-time work subsequent to childbirth. Part-time working often involves less pay per hour of work and limited opportunities for promotion. Furthermore, this type of job tends to contribute to the segregation of women in the labour market (they are often jobs which are held by women), and probably also to maintaining the sexual division of labour inside households (Baizán 2007).

Conclusions

Mediterranean countries are characterised in terms of gender as being those that have lower female activity rates and the lowest fertility rates among European countries. The TUS data allow us to add a new aspect to the study of gender inequalities and social reproduction of the population by highlighting the fact that they are also the countries that show a more unequal distribution of unpaid care work – together with some Eastern European countries. Italian and Spanish women must employ more time in housekeeping and the family in comparison to men, by a factor of three. This unequal distribution of care work is damaging women's capabilities and labour market opportunities, and imposing on them an unsustainable burden that is harming further progress in equality.

Despite the fact that recent decades have seen an increase in female activity rates – though not yet to the level seen in Scandinavian countries – this increase has not been accompanied by the implementation of appropriate systems of family support, which, combined with precariousness in labour markets, especially for young people, and increasing housing costs, is restraining these countries' fertility rates to lower levels compared to Central and Northern Europe. In the coming years, it will be possible to see the effects of important institutional transformations regarding gender equality in the case of Spain, which have been approved since

2007 and have just begun to be developed. However, the global economic crisis led to the withdrawal in January 2011 by the Spanish government of maternity benefits that were initiated just three years earlier.

The international comparison shows that there are institutional settings in which gender symmetry is much easier to achieve: as in the case of the Nordic countries compared to the Mediterranean countries. Those institutional settings point specifically to: first, a greater public responsibility for the provision of care, especially through services and regulations on time flexibility; second, better overall conditions in the labour market which allow men, but also women, to access the labour market and to achieve careers and financial autonomy through labour market participation, and third, the development of public policies that will help directly or indirectly in the reconciliation of work and family policies and opportunities. What states do and the conditions on which benefits are made available carry other implicit objectives and consequences which support different types of family and gender relations. Time use data allow us to look for the differentiated gender impact of the mixes of welfare provision among the state, the family, the market and civil society.

References

Addis, E. (1999), 'Gender in the reform of the Italian welfare state', *South European Society and Politics*, vol. 4, no. 2, pp. 122–49.

Adsera, A. (2004), 'Changing fertility rates in developed countries: The impact of labor market institutions', *Journal of Population Economics*, vol. 17, no. 1, pp. 17–43.

Aguiar, M. and Hurst, E. (2007), 'Measuring trends in leisure: The allocation of time over five decades', *Quarterly Journal of Economics*, vol. 122, no. 3, pp. 969–1,006.

Ahn, N. and Mira, P. (1999), *Job Bust, Baby Bust: The Spanish Case,* FEDEA Working Papers 99-06.

Akerlof, G.A. and Kranton, R.E. (2000), 'Economics and identity', *The Quarterly Journal of Economics*, vol. 115, no. 3, pp. 715–53.

Álvarez, B. and Miles, D. (2006), 'Husbands' housework time: Does wives' paid employment make a difference?', *Investigaciones Económicas*, vol. 30, no. 1, pp. 5–31.

Baizán, P. (2007), 'The Impact of Labour Market Status on Second and Higher-order Births', in G. Esping-Andersen (ed.), *Family Formation and Family Dilemmas in Contemporary Europe*, Madrid: Fundación BBVA, pp. 93–128.

Benería, L. (2003), *Gender, Development and Globalization: Economy as if All People Mattered,* New York: Routledge.

Bien, W. (2000), 'Changing Values among the Future Parents of Europe', paper presented at the European Observatory on Family Matters, Seville, 15–16 September 2000.

Brines, J. (1994), 'Economic dependency, gender and the division of labour at home', *The American Journal of Sociology*, vol. 100, pp. 652–88.

Burda, M.C., Hamermesh, D.S. and Weil, P. (2006), *The Distribution of Total Work in the EU and US*, Institute for the Study of Labour (IZA) Working Paper 2,270, August.

Burda M.C., Hamermesh, D.S. and Weil, P. (2007), *Total Work, Gender and Social Norms*, Institute for the Study of Labour (IZA) Working Paper 2,705, March.

Carrasco, C., Domínguez, M. and Mayordomo, M. (2005), *El treball de les dones a Catalunya*, Barcelona: Consell de Treball, Econòmic i Social de Catalunya.

Chiappori, P.-A. (1988), 'Rational household labour supply', *Econometrica*, vol. 56, pp. 63–89.

—— (1992), 'Collective labour supply and welfare', *Journal of Political Economy*, vol. 100, pp. 437–67.

de Villota, P. (2009), 'A Proposal for a Discrimination Index for a Non-neutral Fiscal Policy', in B. Harris, L. Gálvez and H. Machado (eds), *Gender and Well-being in Europe: Historical and Contemporary Perspectives*, Aldershot: Ashgate, pp. 141–56.

Del Bocca, D. (2002), 'The effect of child care and part-time opportunities on participation and fertility decisions in Italy', *Journal of Population Economics*, vol. 15, no. 3, pp. 549–73.

Durán, M.A. (2006), *El valor del tiempo*, Madrid: Espasa.

Elson, D. (1999), 'Labour markets as gendered institutions: equality in efficiency and empowerment issues', *World Development*, vol. 27, no. 3, pp. 611–27.

—— (2005), 'Unpaid Work, the Millennium Development Goals, and Capital Accumulation', paper presented at UNDP-Levy Institute conference 'Unpaid Work and Economy: Gender, Poverty, and the Millennium Development Goals', The Levy Economics Institute of Bard College, 3–5 October 2005.

Elson. D. (2000), *Towards a gendered political economy*, Basingstoke: Macmillan Press.

Engler, M. and Staubli, S. (2008), *The Distribution of Leisure Time Across Countries and Over Time*, University of St. Gallen, Department of Economics, Discussion Paper no. 2008–14, <http://ssrn.com/abstract=1233842> (accessed 8 May 2011).

Esping-Andersen, G. (1990), *The Three Worlds of Welfare Capitalism*, Princeton, NJ: Princeton University Press.

—— (2007), 'Introduction: The Contemporary Fertility Puzzle', in G. Esping-Andersen (ed.), *Family Formation and Family Dilemmas in Contemporary Europe*, Madrid: Fundación BBVA, pp. 13–32.

European Commission (1998), 'Equal opportunities for women and men in Europe?' (results of an opinion survey), *Eurobarometer*, vol. 44, no. 3.

—— (2004), *Guidelines on European Harmonised Use Time Surveys*, Luxembourg: OPOCE.

Eurostat (2004), *How Europeans Spend their Time: Everyday Life of Women and Men*, Luxembourg: OPOCE.

Eurostat (2005), *Statistics in Focus*, 4/2006, Luxembourg: OPOCE.

Fernández, J.A. and Tobío, C. (2006), *Andalucía: Dependencia y solidaridad en las redes familiares*, Seville: IEA.

Folbre, N. (2008), *Valuing Children: Rethinking the Economics of the Family*, Cambridge, MA: Harvard University Press.

—— and Nelson, J. (2000), 'For love or for money – or both?', *Journal of Economic Perspectives*, vol. 14, pp. 123–40.

Gálvez, L. (1997), 'Breadwinning patterns and family exogenous factors: Workers at the Tobacco Factory of Seville during the industrialization process (1887–1945)', *The International Review of Social History*, vol. 5 (December), pp. 87–128.

—— and Marcenaro, O. (2008), *Conciliación: Un reto para los hogares andaluces*, Actua 26, Seville: Centro de Estudios Andaluces.

—— and Matus, M. (2010), *El impacto de la Ley de Igualdad en las medidas de conciliación de las empresas andaluzas*, Seville: CCOO.

Gálvez, L., Rodríguez-Modroño, P. and Domínguez-Serrano, M. (2008), "A Comparative Analysis on "Total Work" by Gender in EU Countries", paper presented at Symposium 4th Gender and Well Being: The Role of Institutions from Past to Present, Madrid, 25-27/06/2008.

Gálvez, L., Rodríguez-Modroño, P. and Domínguez-Serrano, M. (2011), "Work and time use by gender in European welfare systems". Feminist Economics 17 (4), 2nd special issue on Unpaid Work, Time Use, Poverty, and Public Policy. Routledge pub. (October).

Gauthier, A.-H. and Hatziu, J. (1991), 'Family benefits and fertility', *Population Studies*, vol. 38, pp. 295–306.

Gershuny, J. and Sullivan, O. (2003), 'Time use, gender, and public policy regimes social politics', *International Studies in Gender, State and Society*, vol. 10, no. 2, pp. 205–28.

González, M.J. and Jurado, T. (2007), 'Is there a minimum set of conditions for having a baby? The experience of the 1955–1982 Female cohort in West Germany, France, Italy and Spain', in G. Esping-Andersen (ed.), *Family Formation and Family Dilemmas in Contemporary Europe*, Madrid: Fundación BBVA, pp. 33–92.

Harris, B. and Bridgen, P. (2007), 'Introduction: The "Mixed Economy of Welfare" and the Historiography of Welfare Provision', in B. Harris and P. Bridgen (eds), *Charity and Mutual Aid in Europe and North America since 1800*, New York: Routledge, pp. 1–18.

Hufton, O. (1997), 'La investigación europea sobre tiempo y género', *Revista Internacional de Sociología*, vol. 18, pp. 83–98.

Iversen, T. and Rosenbluth, F. (2006), 'the political economy of gender: Explaining cross-national variation in the gender division of labour and the gender voting gap', *American Journal of Political Science*, vol. 50, no. 1, pp. 1–19.

Joesch, J.M. and Spiess, C.K. (2006), 'European mothers' time spent looking after children: Differences and similarities across nine countries', *International Journal of Time Use Research*, vol. 3, no. 1, pp. 1–27.

Laat, J. and Sanz, A.S. (2006), *Working Women, Men's Home Time and Lowest–low Fertility*, ISER Working Paper 2006–23, Colchester: ISER.

Livi-Bacci, M. (2001), 'Too few children and too much family', *Daedelus*, vol. 130, no. 3, pp. 139–56.

McDonald, P. (2002), 'Low Fertility: Unifying the Theory and Demography', paper presented at the Population Association of America Meetings, Atlanta, GA, 9–11 May 2002.

Mills, M. and Blossfeld, H.-P. (2005), 'Globalization, Uncertainty and the Early Life Course: A Theoretical Framework', in H.-P. Blossfeld, E. Klijzing, M. Mills and K. Kurz (eds), *Globalization, Uncertainty and Youth in Society*, London: Routledge, pp. 1–24.

Moreno, A. (2007), *Familia y empleo de la mujer en los regímenes de bienestar del sur de Europa*, Madrid: CIS.

Naldini, M. and Jurado, T. (2006), 'The South European Family Model', in P. Nikiforos Diamandouros, R. Gunther and H.-J. Puhle (eds), *Democracy and Cultural Change in the New Southern Europe*, Strasbourg: Council of Europe Publishing.

O'Connor, J. (1993), 'Gender, Class and Citizenship in the comparative analysis of welfare state regimes: Theoretical and methodological issues', *British Journal of Sociology*, vol. 44, no. 3, pp. 501–18.

OECD (2007), *Babies and Bosses, Reconciling Work and Family Life: A Synthesis of Findings for OECD Countries*, Paris: OECD.

Picchio, A. (2001), 'Un enfoque macroeconómico "ampliado" de las condiciones de vida', in C. Borderías and C. Carrasco (eds), *Tiempos, trabajos y género*, Barcelona: Universitat de Barcelona.

—— (2003), *Unpaid Work and the Economy: A Gender Analysis of the Standard of Living*, London: Routledge.

Razavi, S. (2007), *The Political and Social Economy of Care in a Development Context: Conceptual Issues, Research Questions and Policy Options*, Gender and Development Programme Paper no. 3, June, Geneva: United Nations Research Institute for Social Development.

Reid, M. (1934), *Economics of Household Production*, New York: John Wiley & Sons.

Tobío, C. (2008), 'Redes familiares, género y política social en España y Francia', *Política y sociedad*, vol. 45, no. 2, pp. 87–104.

Trifiletti, R. (1999), 'Southern European welfare regimes and the worsening position of women', *Journal of European Social Policy*, vol. 9, no. 1, pp. 49–64.

Van de Kaa, D.J (2001), 'Postmodern Fertility Preferences: From Changing Value Orientation to New Behavior', in R.A. Bulatao and J.B. Casterline (eds), *Global Fertility Transition*, Supplement to PDR 27, New York: Population Council, pp. 290–332.

Chapter 5

A Social-reproduction and Well-being Approach to Gender Budgets: Experiments at Local Government Level in Italy

Tindara Addabbo, Giovanna Badalassi, Francesca Corrado
and Antonella Picchio

This chapter illustrates a new approach to gender budgets based on Amartya Sen and Martha Nussbaum's[1] capability approach, as experimented with in Italy since 2002 at local government level. Following the method first discussed in Addabbo et al. (2010), this chapter places public budgets in an *extended reproductive well-being approach* to the economic system (Picchio 2003; Bakker 2007). We consider this approach the most appropriate for dealing with gender inequalities because it includes unpaid work as a major component of the total work of women and men, it places the process of social reproduction of the population among the structural processes of the economic system as a condition of its sustainability, and it assesses gender inequalities from the standpoint of a multi-dimensional concept of well-being as defined by a list of the individual capabilities and effective functionings[2] of women and men.[3]

We think that well-being gender budgets (WBGBs) can also be applied to other countries and at different levels of government. They could, in fact, become a key to a greater co-ordination of policies and a basis for social participation in public debate on both the concept and the actual experience of women's and men's well-being in a given territory.

---

1   See Sen (1983; 1985; 1991; 1993), Nussbaum and Sen (1993).
2   Functionings refer to observable achievements like being in good health or being educated.
3   This approach has been applied at various levels of local government in Italy. In particular, we might note the cases of the Emilia-Romagna Region in 2003, which included the gender budgets of the Modena Provincial District and Modena City Council (Regione Emilia Romagna 2003), the Modena Provincial District in 2004 (Dalfiume 2006), the Bologna Provincial District in 2007 and 2008 (Addabbo et al. 2007a; Addabbo et al. 2009), the Forlì City Council (Corrado and Saltini 2009), the Piedmont Region in 2007 (Badalassi 2007), the Modena City Council in 2004, 2006 and 2008 (Addabbo and Saltini 2009) and the Lazio Region in 2008 (Addabbo et al. 2007b). The approach has also been used in the training of public administrators on gender budgets, organised by the Lazio Region and by Forlì City Council.

In the first section, we present the macro framework and the conversion process of means and services into individual and collective well-being; the following sections describe the tools used to apply WBGBs, showing cases of their application by some local governments in Italy. The second section introduces the list of capabilities and the criteria followed to define it, while in the third section we discuss how to build a context analysis by using WBGBs presenting a system of indicators. In the next section we show how WBGBs can be applied to analyse the distribution of public expenditure, and finally, we draw our conclusions.

A Well-being Approach to Gender Budgets

A government budget is a comprehensive account of public expenditures and revenues. As such, it is a highly political document that assesses a specific distribution of resources, work (both paid and unpaid), responsibilities and power relationships between institutions and residents in the territory. It also reflects inherent political and social tensions, often disguising them through linguistic obscurity. Gender budgets provide new ground for gender mainstreaming because they make it possible to enter the general policy framework and the overall distribution of monetary resources.

The new mainstreaming challenge first of all requires the analytical framework to be engendered: that is, to provide a feminist perspective on the value system, micro and macro analyses, policies and measures which are able to take women's experiences and gender inequalities into proper account at the systemic level. To do so, we need to move on all three levels that define the economic system: the macro structure, the relationship between ends and means, and the concept of human living conditions.

When public budgets are viewed from a gender perspective, it becomes clear that ignoring the differences between women and men, and their unequal living conditions, is a cause of inequity and inefficiency. Gender budgets based on the well-being approach define the multi-dimensional nature of these inequalities, and reveal a methodological confusion between ends and means. The first problem to face is an analytical one: in the macroeconomic framework on which budgets are constructed, the complexity and diversity of the individual and social processes by which public resources are converted into actual well-being are methodologically disregarded; means are mistaken for ends, and the whole perspective is blind to women's experience and responsibility in sustaining the actual process of the social reproduction of living conditions.

In order to accommodate a feminist shift of perspective on the budget framework, we must clarify certain concepts and analytical tools. With regard to living conditions, Sen uses a particular definition of well-being which avoids reducing it to a mere package of goods and services, defined as 'standard of living' (Sen 1987b). Following the lines of the classical humanist tradition, he refers to the normative experience of a 'good life', characterised by a range of capabilities whereby women and men, both individually and in relation to others, may enhance the value of their lives (Sen 1993). According to this view, the criteria of value refer both to a moral context, in a given time and place, and to the exercise of autonomy and individual liberty. The criteria of value are neither constant over time nor exclusively local, because the cultural, moral, political and religious frameworks in which people think about their own lives are being ineluctably globalised given the current trends towards nomadism and cultural fluidity.

The worst fault of the dominant economic and political perspective comes from thinking of women as a social group rather than as protagonists in human society who, like men, are segmented by social conditions, profession and so on. Even more serious, from both the symbolic and practical point of view, is the fact that women are seen as a social service infrastructure whose natural role is to make life sustainable in the home, while their role in sustaining social capital and an economic system based on severe inequalities is hidden from theory.

The different processes whereby resources are converted into sustainable individual and collective well-being should be kept in mind when formulating and implementing public policy; it should not be assumed that providing equal means will suffice to obtain equal results in terms of the quality of life of different people (Sen 1993).[4] Disparities are caused not only by unequal distribution, but also by the fact that well-being is so complex and variegated that it cannot be assumed that everybody accesses and uses resources in the same way. While policies should not get caught up in endless details, policy makers must always bear in mind that real people have bodies, are in necessary and responsible relationships with other people, and have different individual and social characteristics. This is important from a policy point of view because such differences can markedly affect the use of goods, commodities and services, and – above all – results. Figure 5.1 is an attempt to represent the complexity of the process that converts goods and services into the well-being of those who live in a given area.[5] This figure shows the process of converting goods, commodities and services into actual well-being. It also indicates feedback from final individual well-being to the general context, taken as historically given in the picture, but changeable in time and place through agency, social participation and political action. Individual and group capabilities are deployed in the transformations of the social context, and freedom and agency contribute to the introduction of new social practices.

Visualising the conversion process highlights the role of unpaid domestic and care work in transforming goods to provide a better standard of living (cooking food, washing clothes, and so on), and the role of caring in forming and maintaining individual capabilities, for example being healthy, educated,

---

4   A dynamic relationship exists between individual well-being and collective well-being, since belonging to different groups is important for specific dimensions of life and for their importance in the qualification of the social context. On this issue, see Stewart (2005).

5   The diagram is an elaboration of an earlier one proposed by Robeyns (2003).

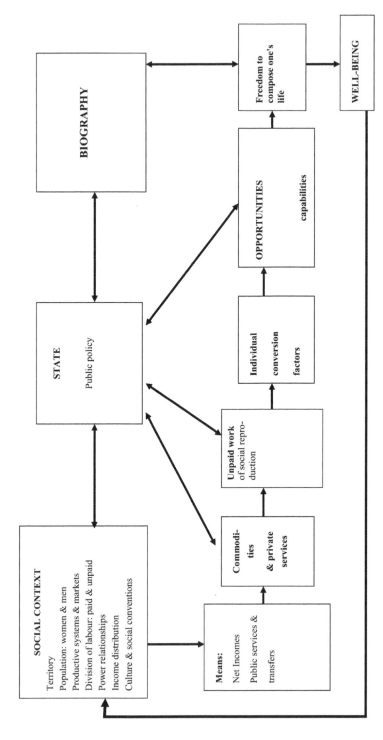

Figure 5.1 Conversion circular process of means into a well-being state

responsible, sociable and so on (Picchio 2003). Figure 5.1 also shows freedom as an essential component of the quality of life. This dimension is crucial for women because it includes their struggles to be recognised as autonomous subjects, and not instrumentally as social infrastructure.

Because the very process of living is so complex and people have such strong aspirations for a sustainable life worth living, the attainment of well-being ultimately remains a creative individual practice of composing their own lives. The context, however, defines the space of opportunity and equity that makes it possible to pose the question 'Equality of what?' between men and women. Hence it becomes a public responsibility to remove the obstacles that block equal access to opportunities and to sustain the quality of individual lives. Public choices, if not constrained by utilitarian welfare optimisation and its constraints (as argued by Sen in *Ethics in Economics*), as shown in Figure 5.1, can play a major role in pragmatically regulating the whole process of the conversion of means into a capability expansion and in sustaining what individuals and groups can effectively do and be.

Moreover, careful attention to the activities and mutual relationships of men and women in the private sphere sheds light on the process that enables both of them on a daily basis to take part in the public sphere: accessing resources and acting politically. The relationship between private (domestic) spaces and public ones is an interdependent, dynamic and circular one, fundamental to the sustainability of the economic and social system. It is also at the heart of the issue of gender relationships, given that the ultimate responsibility for the process of adapting the quality of life to the modes of production and distribution of resources (both private and public) is allocated to women, and this means the quality of life of adult men as well as of children and the elderly. The traditional role of women whereby they have ultimate responsibility for the quality of life is becoming less and less sustainable with the present dramatic shift of resources from wages to profit and financial return, which has hard-hitting effects on real wages and security of employment, and puts deferred wage components (pensions) and social wages (services and public transfers) at risk.

Recognising the existence of subjects with different experiences of life depending upon which sex they are follows a principle of realism that underscores our analytical perspective, extending it to dimensions that are usually hidden or set aside. If one takes account of women's experience in the daily processes that enable people to live, work and act in society throughout their lives, the analysis becomes much more complex yet also more concrete and relevant to people's lives and to the sustainability of the economic and social system. This broadening of the perspective can also enhance the effectiveness of policies which otherwise suffer from a lack of accountability with regard to a dramatic reality that constantly takes policy makers by surprise.

WBGBs allow for a level of gender mainstreaming that offers new possibilities, not only for re-reading all policies in terms of gender, but also for showing the analytical connections that shape the budgetary framework.[6] The traditional perspective, on the basis of current economic theory, defines the nature of consumption, investment and capital, and determines which issues lie at the centre of the productive system and which lie at its margins as social questions. In the traditional theoretical picture, the exclusive field of observation is the market – that is to say, only paid work and the exchange of commodities and services, not responsibilities, unpaid domestic or care work, or the real lives of people. In this reductive economistic picture, even motivations for public action hardly fit in, because it is an analytical system methodologically hostile to the state, especially when it is concerned with protecting the quality of life, and the lives themselves, of those who depend on wages. Lastly, the overall picture is totally blind to the enormous mass of unpaid work that women do in the process of social reproduction of the population. This is not included among the great processes that structure the economic system according to neoclassical economic theory – as if workers did not exist in flesh and blood, did not have relationships and care responsibilities, and their ability to do things did not need to be formed and continually sustained.[7]

WBGBs allow for a reassessment of the political and administrative budgeting processes. In this regard, together with all gender budgets, they are part of a growing tendency towards greater transparency at various institutional and social levels, as well as a greater accountability for policy results.[8] What WBGBs do is to specify good living as the ground for policy valuation.

Women have, in fact, a particular interest in making visible the chain of responsibilities with regard to the well-being of the population and bringing it to public attention, because normally it is tacitly assumed that women are ultimately responsible for the sustainability and quality of the living conditions of all.

Having presented the approach in this section, and clarified why it is important to use gender budgets to shift the focus directly onto women's and men's well-being, in the following sections we will analyse the models and the tools used for doing this.

Well-being Gender Budgets: The List of Relevant Capabilities

In the WBGB, local government functions, powers and political aims are used to draw up a list of significant dimensions to express the administration's responsibility for the quality of life of the population. There are several ways of

---

6   For connections between budgets and analytical frameworks, see Galimberti (1970).

7   Elson (2004); Elson and Cagatay (2000); Picchio (1992; 2003); Sen (2000).

8   On recent developments of performance budgets, also proposed by the OECD, and for a critical assessment of the possibility of effectively engendering them, see Klatzer (2008).

compiling the list.[9] They may lead to different results, and the process of defining a list of capabilities can be more or less participatory, open to different strata of civil society and/or to administrators, and it may take place inside and/or outside the administration itself. The process can help to spread awareness in society of the role of gender auditing, and to stimulate public reflection about what a 'good life' means for people of different sexes belonging to different classes and ethnic groups. The list forms a good basis for defining indicators of empirically observable functionings, gathering useful information for a context analysis and evaluating the impact of policies over time on the various dimensions of well-being for different subjects and groups.

In the different experiences of WBGB, the working group GenderCAPP, to which the authors belong, has experimented with different ways of formulating the list based on the functions and politico-administrative structures of each local government and on its programmes and budgetary documents. These tools make it possible to see the different responsibilities assumed by different sectors of a given local government with regard to specific capabilities. Here, as examples, we present the capabilities listed in the WBGB of the Province of Rome. This list is drawn, as in the original case of the Province of Modena, from the list of departments that constitute the provincial administration, and takes into account their specific institutional functions such as training, school buildings safety or roads (Addabbo et al. 2010). The list was then discussed and agreed with political representatives and administrators on the basis of their main objectives and programmes.

Having Access to Knowledge (Education, Training and Information)

One of the objectives is providing access to lifelong training and education. The province is responsible for some aspects of education and most training, including that of adults, and within the powers assigned to it by law and by delegation from the administrative region, for measures designed to favour access to the labour market (including training policies). The remit of this capability also includes information and communication services.

Living a Healthy Life

All the functions linked with the environment, road safety, and some social services directly sustain this capability, which is also indirectly influenced by all the policies dealing with sports, school buildings and so on. With regard to this

---

9   One may start from a 'universal' list like that defined by Nussbaum (2003), or follow the approach described by Robeyns (2003) of defining and justifying capabilities in relation to the context, or – as suggested in Addabbo et al. (2010) – define a list based on the functions of the public administration being audited, taking account of the aims stated in the statute and other documents (such as the Mandate Budget) which set its objectives.

capability, however, the direct role of the province is limited because, in Italy, health policies are largely the responsibility of the region.

Working and Carrying Out Business Activities

This covers paid work and self-employment. The province has a department dealing with labour and employment centres that directly influences this capability. In this regard, a gender perspective can show that this capability is strictly inter-related with the development of other capabilities, such as the one usually overlooked by economic analysis: caring for others. The provincial council can intervene in the development of the capability to work and do business by the direct exercise of its powers over active and passive labour policies, by supporting women's enterprises, by acting indirectly in the spheres of education and training, and by forging links with other agencies which are more directly responsible for care services. Ensuring the maintenance of effective transport systems and roads can also prove to be necessary to sustaining this dimension.

Having Access to Public Resources (Services and Allowances)

Access to public resources by using services or receiving subsidies is the focus of this objective, in the development of which the provincial government participates directly through services and subsidies provided for families or individuals and by defining criteria of access to public resources and/or of the provision of public goods and services.

*Living and Working in Safe and Suitable Places and in an
Eco-compatible Environment*

The objective here is to ensure the adequacy and security of all the private and public spaces in which human life goes on: workplaces, houses, schools, transport systems. Thus, this capability may be affected by provincial functions involving planning and urban development, public buildings, safety regulations, the environment, roads and transport.

Travel

This refers to the individual's ability to move within the province. The provincial administration affects this capability through its transport policy, roads and territorial planning. This capability interacts with other important ones (like the capability to work, to be educated and trained, to care for oneself and others) by allowing and facilitating movements in daily life, with due care for their safety and suitability. In the interlinking of different capabilities, the differing behaviour of women and men may be seen, along with their movements and motivations.

Caring for Others

This capability includes care work done both for one's relatives, whether within or outside the nuclear family, as well as for others as unpaid voluntary work. If the municipal government has direct responsibility for children's services and care work in the community, the province can influence and sustain caring both through sub-provincial agencies and through functions linked to the labour market, for example by improving the work–life balance and adopting practices that facilitate care for workers' relatives who need it. The administration can help to sustain caring by designing policies which facilitate the gender distribution of unpaid family work, and by giving direct support to care. Similarly, supporting the voluntary sector and working with associations already present on the territory may influence caring.

Caring for Oneself

This capability includes both the chance to have time for oneself, and the ability to use that time for recreational, cultural and sports activities. Policies dealing with sport, free time, tourism and culture can help enable people to enjoy their lives. Indirectly, they can give people more free time to spend on these activities through territorial planning, constructing roads and regulating road traffic to shorten both the time and length of journeys, and facilitating access to structures (sports halls, theatres, museums). There is a clear nexus between this capability and others, such as living a healthy life (consider the positive impact that sport can have on health). Needless to say, cultural activities directly affect knowledge and imagination, and potentially work and business activities.

Participating in Public Life and Living in an Equitable Society

This capability can be affected by policies that influence participation in social life, political representation and access to power, and the promotion of equal opportunities for women.

The proposed list does not give an order of priorities, nor is it immutable in relation to civil society. However, it is drawn from the reading of policies and motivations contained in various preparatory and budget documents and from discussion with administrators. Our research group sees its role as providing the administration with a mirror, a tool for self-reflection on its responsibilities for the well-being of the population and its sections, both as a whole and with regard to specific dimensions. In this way, we bring to the fore the real aim of public intervention: the well-being of the resident population. This goal often gets lost in economic analyses, those on which public accounts are based, which assume spontaneous processes of optimising resources at individual and social level (Sen 1987a). Once the public aims and functions are restored, the accounts also become clearer, as the new framework favours transparency, accountability and public debate on the notion of a 'good life', correcting the inversion between means and ends and recognising the complexity of human lives. A well-being analysis of the budget can also clarify political power relationships.[10] This 'self-reflective analysis' can also be carried out by including a participatory process opening a public discussion on the very meaning of well-being and its dimensions, in which civil society (made up of organisations as well as individuals) can reflect collectively on its experiences of life and the values attributed to them.

In order to extend the approach to other government levels in order to verify the impact of their public policies on the well-being of men and women, a more comprehensive list of area-specific capabilities would be required. In this case, by reading the capabilities transversely, across the network of different local governments present on the territory with different responsibilities, institutional mechanisms and often different policies, one may work out to what degree the result derives in each case from a failure to face up to a political commitment or from inadequate or inefficient action. From this examination, it might emerge that the list of capabilities ought to be more exhaustive and closer to the well-being of the inhabitants, or that the allocation of resources does not lead to adequate results in terms of the actual functionings of different individuals or even entire sections of the resident population.

Well-being Gender Budgets: Context Analysis

Having defined the different capabilities that may be affected by the local-government budget subjected to auditing, we now turn our attention to the context, both with reference to the indicators of capabilities and/or functionings and with respect to the available factors that – according to Sen and Nussbaum's approach (Nussbaum and Sen 1993; Sen 1983; Sen 1985; Sen 1991; Sen 1993; Sen 2005) – may allow for the conversion of capabilities into observable functioning. This context analysis is useful when providing suggestions for public policies regarding well-being and the redressing of gender inequalities. At this point, as well as showing possible indicators of functionings and indices of deprivation with regard to the capability as well as indicators on the effective 'doings and beings' of women and men, we may also indicate some conversion factors relative to the Province of Rome – social context factors, part of which fall under the administration's responsibility, which may influence individual processes of the conversion of means and services into actual well-being.

The indicators of functionings are then disaggregated by gender, and one proceeds to analyse the gender gap in order to highlight the observable inequalities and assess the development in the analysed context of conversion factors. Context analysis will require not only statistical analysis of existing survey and

---

10   By the term 'political', we mean here primarily the politics of living conditions and the processes of social reproduction, not only party politics.

administrative micro data, but also qualitative analysis based on interviews and focus groups with special attention to the inequalities observed by gender and on the conversion factors that the local government can promote.

With regard, for example, to the capability of working and carrying out business activities in the Province of Rome, the analysis of specific employment rates by sex and territory has revealed a problem when converting a potential (which we cannot observe directly) into actual behaviour and states of being. The lower rate of female employment may be caused by obstacles which are more frequently encountered by women than they are by men. Thus, the low employment rates could be used as a gender indicator of deprivation in the capability of working and conducting business activities, when the difficulty of getting a job results in a primary indicator of 'deprivation' in the gender difference in unemployment rates. On average, the rate of unemployment in the Province of Rome is in line with the national one, but that of women is higher. The fact that women find it much harder to find employment is revealed not only by the elaboration of data from sample-based sources (ISTAT Labour Force Survey data), but also by elaborations of data from administrative sources (applicants and those who find jobs through provincial employment centres). The indicators utilised as the effective use of the capability of working and carrying out business activities do not, however, relate only to access to employment (a dimension which we consider particularly important for the provincial administration, given the powers assigned to it), but also to the quality of employment: rank, hours, work schedules, contractual modalities, earnings and other employment conditions. The variables observable at provincial level show a gender bias against women, both in access to top positions and also in standard work contracts (full-time permanent employment). The greater importance for women of non-standard contracts is a signal also to the designers of economic policy who set themselves targets for equality and face the urgency of adopting policies to guarantee the stabilisation of labour, for instance by offering non-standard workers more access to training. This would increase the likelihood that when women accept non-standard jobs, when entering or returning to paid employment, they will not find themselves ensnared in the same old mechanism. The analysis of individual time use has also shown the importance of taking account of unpaid housework and care work; in fact, in the Province of Rome, on average women spend about 15 hours a week on the care of children or other relatives, and about 13 on housework (Provincia di Roma 2005, ch. 2, section II). The number of hours of women's housework and care work does not seem to vary significantly with their professional status, which shows the importance of women's double role in Rome, as elsewhere. The burdensomeness of paid work is shown partly by the high number of women who consider the total number of working hours excessive (Provincia di Roma 2005, pp. 164–7), and by the lower rates of participation by women in on-the-job training courses outside normal working hours. We take these as indicators of the greater time burden for women of unpaid domestic and care work, a fact that should be considered by those designing labour policies and implementing them.

Context analysis can highlight information on differences and inequalities by gender with respect to the development of capabilities; hence it provides the administration with a picture of reality on which to intervene, and gives administrators and civil society a view of the critical nature of certain dimensions of women's and men's well-being on which to reflect in political and public participatory forums. Through context analysis, one may also account for the real processes of conversion of means into functionings with special reference to the role played by public government. Public employment centres providing assistance to the unemployed in the process of searching for employment in this regard can help the conversion of the capability of working and conducting business activities into functionings. Thus, it is an essential step for interpreting budget documents and for evaluating policies in terms of the well-being of those who live in the area.

Well-being Gender Budgets: The Allocation of Public Expenditure

In reading budget documents from the point of view of the WBGB, one may use matrix methods linking monetary expenditure to the political objectives of the specific policies in order to evaluate their different impacts on different people, relating the local administration to the women and men directly or indirectly affected by the public choices. In particular, as mentioned above, this method defines a 'matrix of capabilities' by crossing the vertical columns of capabilities considered important for the territorial context with the horizontal lines representing the organisational structure of the local government itself.

The list of capabilities and organisational structures will differ between local governments, so a different specific matrix is required in each case. The matrices are constructed to take account of the structural characteristics of each administration, involving, as explained earlier, not only the juridical framework, but also the specific programmatic and political objectives as well as the policies and characteristics of each administrative area. The matrix is completed with the accounting of current expenditure, organised by capabilities (see Figure 5.2). This demonstrates how matrices can also be used in accounting as a tool for shifting the analytical field from the administrative structure directly to the well-being of the resident population, thus correcting the present distortion in the relationship between means (allocated resources) and ends (well-being) – in fact, reversing its direction. One problem encountered in using the matrix concerns the attribution of single capabilities to the different functions of the administration. One way to cope with this problem (followed in Figure 5.2) is to attribute capabilities to the areas, or sectors, or departments to which they primarily belong. For example, policies affecting labour correspond primarily to the capability to work; policies for transport to the capability to move about the territory; policies for training to the capability to acquire knowledge; health policies to the capability to live a healthy life. This direct attribution makes it possible to allocate expenditure according to specific 'doings and beings' so that the administration can reflect on the effect of

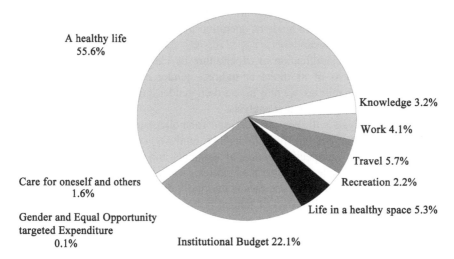

Figure 5.2   Distribution of expenditures by capability – Piedmont Region, 2006

expenditures on specific dimensions of people's well-being, and evaluate their consistency not only in terms of its administrative functions, but also in terms of its political, programmatic and statutory objectives.

By applying this criterion, current expenditures in the final budget of the Piedmont Region were distributed among capabilities as shown in Figure 5.2, where the regional centres of responsibility are translated into corresponding capabilities.

However, with regard both to the interaction between the different capabilities and to the different responsibilities of each area, we noted above that often the action of several administrative sectors or policies can have a bearing on the same capability. For example:

- Labour policies can directly affect the capability to work and do business, but in so far as they allow accumulation of human capital on the job, they also influence the capability for knowledge and education.
- Training policies also favour the capability to work and to access resources, in so far as they have a positive effect on trainees' probability of finding employment.
- Health policies can affect not only the capability to live a healthy life, but also the capability to care for others.
- Transport policies, in so far as they facilitate mobility between places of work and life, can influence not only the capability to move about, but also the capability to care, to work, to live a healthy life and to enjoy recreation.

An analytical accounting approach that refers to the specific objectives of the local government's various projects could also allow for a more detailed distribution of expenditure by the same sector to several capabilities, thus leading to the possibility of an integrated mode of operation in administrative processes and in the system of governance.[11]

Therefore, the classification of expenditure by capability and/or capabilities involves an analysis of its direct or indirect gender impact. Having allocated expenditure to capabilities, we may assess their gender impact by using the system of indicators used in the context analysis.

Context analysis will then also be used for policy suggestions targeting the critical aspects that emerge from the context analysis, and assessing the impact of public policies on specific aspects of women's and men's well-being.[12] The emphasis on real people, on gender inequalities, on the development of capabilities and on the conversion process of means into individual functionings allows us to assess at a local level the effect of budget policies on resources and well-being, also taking account of the need for co-ordination among different public and private institutions operating in the same territory. For instance, in the case of early discharge of hospital patients, which may be a burden on families, especially women, in terms of the work of caring for convalescents, the transfer of costs is invisible unless the analysis of individual time budgets and the different gender distribution of care work in the household are taken into account. In our view, moreover, only an integration of regional health policies with municipal policies concerned with domiciliary care can guarantee the opening up of the political space for intervention, which would otherwise be lost when passing from the public to the private sphere. Furthermore, the capability approach makes the costs visible in terms of the well-being for both the caregiver and the care receiver, and the gender approach clarifies who the subjects most exposed to the risk of deprivation are in several important dimensions of well-being.

Conclusions

WBGBs constitute an original proposal that shifts the assessment of policies from the usual analysis of means to an analysis of the quality of life of women and men, taking into proper account their sex, different gender life experiences and social conditions. It is an innovative perspective that has been received with interest at local government level because it frames public accounts on the basis of a direct

---

11   This analysis is provided in Addabbo and Saltini (2009) with reference to Modena City Council's public budgets.

12   For example, we have analysed the criteria for access to children's services at the local level which, according to the WBGB approach, may be considered important factors in the conversion of the mothers' (and fathers') capability to work into actual employment. This highlights the need to facilitate access to services for one-parent families, and to avoid penalising the children of non-standard workers through difficulties of access to childcare services.

relationship between the public administration and residents in the territory they administer. Sen's capability approach, although not immediately easy to grasp, becomes more comprehensible when its experiential nature becomes clearer. The concept of multi-dimensional well-being is in fact recognisable in everyone's experience of the complexity of living as sexed individuals embedded in a social context and positioned in a network of human relationships, socially necessary for their human sustainability.

By presenting some of the results of these Italian local governments' experiments in well-being gender budgets, we aim to open a discussion on the pros and cons of our way of approaching the assessment of the gender impact of public policies because we think that WBGBs could become a key to greater co-ordination of policies and a basis for social participation in a public debate on the very notion and effective experience of women's and men's well-being, which always takes place in a specific territory. Our proposals need to be discussed in a wider forum, together with the possibility of their application to other countries and at different government levels.

The novelty of WBGBs does not lie in choosing well-being as the basis for policies, for in theory that is already the public aim *par excellence*. What is new is the use of a framework of economic analysis that recognises new connections and highlights the actual results of policies precisely in terms of the state of well-being: in other words, revising the usual hierarchy between economic and social data.

What must be confronted is the picture of the normal functioning of the system, including the social reproduction of those sections of workers which are strong. Hidden fundamental aspects, hitherto heaped onto the backs of women and shut away in domestic negotiations and psychological depressions, must be revealed. To this picture we must add the further problems involved in the reproduction of weak sections of the population that are not self-sufficient.

To summarise the proposed gender budget approach from a well-being perspective, we may indicate its methodological characteristics as follows:

- It assumes that human subjects who live and act in society are male and female, and hence physically and historically two subjects in relation to each other. As subjects, they are also marked by many social inequalities of class and rank and by differences of age, ethnic origin, religion and so on.
- It conceptualises well-being as a complex of dimensions, defined capabilities, and a sub-complex of functionings determined by the free and effective exercise of individual capabilities by real people, located in a social, moral, territorial and historical context.
- It evaluates public policies from two points of view: (1) inequalities of gender, and (2) well-being as a complex of potentialities for a good life.
- It uses women's experience of life as a relational and social process to define the effective complexity of well-being.
- It takes account of the processes that give access to resources and enable people to compose the dimensions of their own lives according to their

criteria of value.

- The list of capabilities we adopt refers specifically to the politico-administrative structure, taking account of the functions and objectives contained in the statutory mandate and in the budget documents of the local governments concerned.
- The list is proposed by those who drafted the WBGB and discussed with representatives of the administration; however, it can and should also be discussed and agreed in wider circles with the participation of civil society, thus gaining in clarity and political significance.
- It attempts to account for the real costs involved in the policies, ensuring that expenditures are adequate to the declared well-being objectives.

A context analysis enables gender budgets on the basis of well-being to be created, as it helps to highlight the different dimensions of gender inequalities and their effects on an individual's sense of well-being. Bringing together the relationship between the well-being of women and men with the division of labour, the distribution of incomes and redistribution of public resources in a specific territory is not a simple operation. It is not merely a question of focusing on the dimensions of well-being and gender inequalities, but also of articulating possible connections and causal relationships to assess the impact of economic policy on human lives.

Beyond recognising the methodological and analytical difficulties due to the innovative and experimental nature of the approach adopted, from the experience acquired through the gendered reading of both the context and the budget documents of some Italian local governments, a number of important points emerge which, in this concluding section, are interesting to highlight.

One initial element concerns the shift of budget analysis towards an area that makes it possible to evaluate the coherence between the well-being policy objectives, as stated at the political programmatic stage, and the political choices actually made, together with the adequacy of the resources allocated to the implementation of the goals set.

The second important element, which at present has yet to be sufficiently explored, is that of being able to identify a direct relationship between the expenses that impact directly on the well-being dimensions of women and men residing in a given territory, and the main items of aggregate spending of local governments: staff expenses and the costs linked to servicing debt.

As far as staff expenses are concerned, the notion of well-being as the underlying goal of the public institution and the assessment of results in terms of the actual quality of life of real people, seen in terms of their different conditions and access to resources, introduces a new notion of efficiency in resource management as well as the chance to reflect on the potential capacities and actual functionings of the public institution itself (planning, carrying out research, building networks, communicating, allocating resources, and so on).[13]

Furthermore, particularly in times of financial crisis, it becomes more important than ever to give immediate visibility (even at the accountability stage) to the problematic relationship to be found between the resources destined for the market and the financial resources used for managing debts, and those resources to be used for the services necessary to provide a good quality of life to those living in the territory. The lack of direct visibility of and accountability for the structure of the distribution of resources, the progress of policy results and the effective use of resources risks maintaining a situation in which the ultimate responsibility for the quality of life and the process of social reproduction is passed down to women, shutting off the ensuing tensions into a politically invisible domestic space.

In this approach, which shifts both the analytical focus and the accountability framework, gender impact is considered not only with reference to levels deemed as female areas (reproductive health, equal opportunities, childcare services and so on), but is also used to show the non-neutrality of all expenditure, starting from the apparently neutral financial costs (Bakker and Gill 2003; Elson 2004).

One of the aims of WBGBs is to guarantee greater transparency of the accounts, connecting expenditure and possibly revenues directly to the living experience of the women and men, adopting an approach that directly links the aims of well-being with the allocation of public resources. An essential element of this transparency is that which makes it possible to identify and highlight the programmes, the areas and the sectors that have an impact on well-being and in which a gender gap in well-being emerges.

It follows that the gender gap may be read in terms of discrimination and deprivation on the level of potential capabilities and individual functionings, thus making it possible to capture the quality of life of women and to better answer the question, 'Equal in what?'

The WBGB thus lends itself to a preventive and/or a final balance analysis of the overall management of public activities, focusing on individuals, men and women, who live in relation to each other, in a specific social context with regard to productive structures, markets, the distribution of income, social norms

---

13   In the case of the Province of Bologna and that of Rome, a number of matrices were drawn up showing the capacities of the provincial authorities in which what the administration is able to do was placed directly in relation to the dimensions relevant to well-being. In this perspective, the actual policy results regarding the lives of different people must come together to provide a generally well-balanced and sustainable way of living. The re-composition of the overall state of well-being is not obtained *a posteriori* as the sum of separate and unconnected results provided by various structures, but must be thought out and planned *a priori*, with a clear idea that, for example, those people who travel on public transport must be able to reconcile paid work and their care responsibilities in space and time, as well as being able to access other public and private services (healthcare institutions, transport links, schools, theatres, gyms and so on).

and conventions, as shown in Figure 5.1. In this way, starting from real and circumstantiated situations examined in a broad contextual analysis, bringing together the production of means and the social reproduction of the population within the same macroeconomic framework, it becomes possible to pragmatically think, design and implement public choices in a continuous reflective process on the adequacy of the results and the efficiency of the means employed to obtain them. Public choices may therefore be measured against an explicit value system and the clarity of the goals that are to be achieved, with a direct assumption of responsibilities with regard to the quality of lives of different people, and not negatively affected by false notions of market self-regulation and the separation of the logics of means and the ethics of goals (Sen 1987a).

Lastly, the WBGB is designed to be a participatory budget, in the sense of an instrument of dialogue with civil society, which may then foster the construction of new democratic relationships between the local authority and its citizens, with a view to political and social equality. The list of capacities lends itself to an open discussion between representatives of the administration, local associations and individuals, ensuring a level of participation, for instance, on behalf of women in a participatory process that at present often excludes them not only because of their own time constraints, but also because of a lack of motivation caused by a perception that these concerns are far from their own real lives. A form of social participation, directly focused on the effective experience of a good life, may prove to be a key factor for the sharing of ideas and good practices of individual and collective living. It can also provide a public space for discussing expenditure priorities and taxation criteria that could have a real impact on people's lives and making the state political representatives and administrators accountable for their responsibility in the processes of social, territorial and urban planning.

Until now in Italy, the only instance of a participatory WBGB took place in a school as part of the project entitled 'De-strutturazione del bilancio scolastico nell'approccio ben-essere: Che genere di bilancio?' ('De-structuring the school budget as part of the well-being approach: What kind of budget?').[14] This project involved the students of two fifth-year classes of the Istituto Cattaneo in Modena, and provided them with the opportunity to take part in a direct democracy experience, based on analysis of the school budget documentation. In this way, the students were given the chance to assess the teaching plans, to reflect on the mainstays of their own well-being and analyse the responsibilities assumed by the school on their behalf as well as the institutional capacities which were actually activated in order to respond to these needs effectively. This created a discussion space that led to the identification of critical elements of their life experience and the school environment, as well as the recognition that alongside the most highly valorised potential capacities, there were also other aspects of individual potential that were not sufficiently supported.

---

14   It must be noted that in Italian, the word *genere* means both 'gender' and 'kind'.

References

Addabbo, T. and Saltini, S. (2009), *Gender Auditing del Bilancio del Comune di Modena Secondo l'Approccio dello Sviluppo Umano*, research report, Modena and Reggio Emilia: Comune di Modena and GenderCAPP.

Addabbo, T. Lanzi, D. and Picchio, A. (2004), 'On sustainable human development: Gender auditing in a capability approach', *Materiali di Discussione del Dipartimento di Economia Politica*, no. 467 (September).

Addabbo, T., Lanzi, D. and Picchio, A. (2010) 'Gender Budgets: A Capability Approach', Journal of Human Development and Capabilities, vol. 11, no. 4, pp. 479–501.

Addabbo, T., Badalassi, G., Corrado, F., Ferrari, E. and Picchio, A. (2007a), *Amministrazione Provinciale di Bologna: Rendicontazione in chiave di benessere di donne e uomini*, research report, Modena and Reggio Emilia: GenderCAPP.

Addabbo, T., Corrado, F., Galaverni, M., La Rocca, D., Misiti, M., Picchio, A. and Squillante, D. (2007b), *Bilancio di genere della Regione Lazio in un approccio sviluppo umano*, research report, Modena and Reggio Emilia: GenderCAPP, Regione Lazio.

Addabbo, T., Badalassi, G., Corrado, F. and Saltini, S. (2009), *Rendicontazione in chiave di benessere di donne e uomini*, GenderCAPP, final research report, Bologna: Provincia di Bologna.

Badalassi, G. (ed.) (2007), *Bilancio di genere della regione Piemonte 2006*, Turin: IRES Piemonte, Regione Piemonte, IGF, no. 3,000.

Bakker, I. (2007), 'Social reproduction and the constitution of a gendered political economy', *New Political Economy*, vol. 12, no. 4, pp. 541–56.

—— and Gill, S. (eds) (2003), *Power, Production and Social Reproduction*, Chippenham: Palgrave Macmillan.

Corrado, F. and Saltini, S. (2009), *Amministrazione Comunale di Forlì: Rendicontazione in chiave di benessere di donne e uomini – Progetto di fattibilità*, research report, Comune di Forlì, Modena and Reggio Emilia: GenderCAPP.

Dalfiume, M. (ed.) (2006), *Oltre le Pari Opportunità, Verso lo Sviluppo Umano: Il Bilancio di Genere Nella Provincia di Modena*, Milan: Angeli.

Elson, D. (2004), 'Gender Equality, Public Finance and Globalization', in J.K. Boyce et al. (eds), *Human Development in the Era of Globalization: Essays in Honor of Keith B. Griffin*, Cheltenham: Edward Elgar.

—— and Cagatay, N. (2000), 'The social content of macroeconomic policies', *World Development*, vol. 28, no. 7.

Galimberti, F. (1970), *Politica fiscale e struttura dei bilanci pubblici*, Padua: Cedam.

—— and Cagatay, N. (2000), 'The social content of macroeconomic policies', 35 World Development, vol. 28, no. 7, pp. 1347-1364.

Klatzer, E. (2008), 'The Integration of Gender Budgeting in Performance-based Budgeting' Watch Group, Gender and Public Finance, paper presented at the conference 'Public Budgeting Responsible for Gender Equality. Presupuestación Pública Responsable con la Igualdad de Género', Bilbao, 9–10 June 2008.

Nussbaum, M. (2003), 'Capabilities as fundamental entitlements: Sen and social justice', *Feminist Economics*, vol. 9, nos 2–3, pp.33–59.

—— and Sen, A.K. (eds) (1993), *The Quality of Life*, Oxford: Clarendon Press.

Picchio, A. (1992), *Social Reproduction: The Political Economy of the Labour Market*, Cambridge: Cambridge University Press.

Picchio, A. (ed.) (2003), *Unpaid Work and the Economy*, London: Routledge (2nd edn 2006).

Provincia di Roma (2005), *La qualità della vita delle donne nella provincia di Roma*, Rome: Provincia di Roma, Ufficio per la promozione della qualità della vita nella Provincia di Roma, Assessorato alle Politiche del lavoro e della qualità della vita e Eures Ricerche Economiche e Sociali.

—— (2008), *Studio propedeutico per il Bilancio di genere della Provincia di Roma*, Rome: Provincia di Roma.

Regione Emilia Romagna (2003), *Studio di fattibilità per la costruzione del bilancio delle amministrazioni pubbliche secondo un'ottica di genere*, final research report, Bologna: SCS Consulting, January.

Robeyns, I. (2003), 'Sen's capability approach and gender inequality: Selecting 17 relevant capabilities', *Feminist Economics*, vol. 9, nos 2–3, pp. 61–92.

Sen, A.K. (1983), *Resources, Values and Development*, Oxford: Blackwell.

—— (1985), *Commodities and Capabilities*, Amsterdam: North Holland.

—— (1987a), *On Ethics and Economics*, Oxford: Blackwell.

—— (1987b), *The Standard of Living*, Cambridge: Cambridge University Press.

—— (1991), 'Welfare, preference and freedom', *Journal of Econometrics*, vol. 50, no. 1, pp. 115–29.

—— (1993), 'Capability and Well-being', in M. Nussbaum and A. Sen (eds), *The Quality of Life*, Oxford: Clarendon Press.

—— (2005), 'Human rights and capabilities', *Journal of Human Development*, vol. 6, no. 2, pp. 151–66.

Sen, G. (2000), 'Gender mainstreaming in finance ministries', *World Development*, vol. 28, no. 7, pp. 1379–1390.

Stewart, F. (2005), 'Groups and capabilities', *Journal of Human Development*, vol. 6, no. 2, pp. 185–204.

PART II
Gender, Well-being and the Provision of Care: The Family and the Household

PART II

Chapter 6

Home Care and Cash Transfers: The Search for a Sustainable Elderly Care Model

Annamaria Simonazzi

Projections of sharp increases in the demand for long-term care (LTC) have prompted the search for new organisational solutions aimed at cost efficiency to ensure both availability of resources and long-term financial sustainability. Two common trends, uniting otherwise still very different care systems, have been observed in Europe: a shift to home care away from institutional care, and a shift from in-kind to cash transfers. The ultimate aim of this policy shift is to strengthen families' caring capacities and transfer more weight onto informal care. In fact, home or community care (whether formal or informal) is considered to be far cheaper than institutional care, and is also usually preferred by the elderly. With families at the limit of their caregiving capacity, monetary benefits and other non-monetary support schemes are increasingly provided to care-users and their families as support for their caring activities. When combined with monetary transfers, this policy shift seems to meet both cost-efficiency and customer satisfaction requirements (Lundsgaard 2005).

Cost considerations pushing towards encouraging and supporting a greater role of the family may run counter to other economic and social trends and goals pushing in the opposite direction. Demographic developments, changing family structures and the drive among women for emancipation and higher participation in the labour market will give rise to an increase in the demand for formal long-term care services. Governments may be caught between two apparently conflicting goals: a higher female activity rate and a greater reliance on home care. The impact of these policy changes on the division between formal and informal care, on the one hand, and caregiving and female employment on the other may vary widely across different countries with different care regimes and labour market models.

The various systems also differ in the conditions regulating monetary benefits, such as those who are entitled to them and how they must be spent. The range varies from freely disposable monetary transfers that can be treated by families as income support (as is the case of the dependence allowance in Italy and Austria) to tightly controlled benefits conditional upon the employment of regular paid carers (as in the case of France, Belgium or the Netherlands) (Ungerson and Yeandle 2007). The differences in their effects can be equally large (Simonazzi 2009). By reducing the cost of market care, tied monetary transfers encourage the creation of a formal market (which, in turn, may or may not entail good working conditions).

Conversely, untied cash payments provide a support for family income that may or may not be used to hire formal or informal carers. The effect can be either an increase in the 'informal', but subsidised, family care, with possible negative effects on female labour market participation, or an increase in the demand for paid care (subsidised market demand). When the latter is the case, unconditional monetary transfers may encourage the development of a particular form of home-based, often irregular, low-paid care, generally accessed privately through the market (such as the employment of female immigrant carers in the Mediterranean countries, in Austria, and increasingly in Germany).

The aim of this chapter is to analyse the impact of different models of subsidised home care and cash-for-care schemes on women's incentive to care and on the features of the care labour market. In particular, it will analyse how cash payments in different employment and care models affect the trade-off between caregiving and female employment, and on working conditions in the care labour market. The next section examines the factors regulating the choice between formal and informal care; the third and fourth sections analyse how labour market institutions and the features of care regimes affect the opportunity cost of caring and the cost of paid care. The final section focuses on how monetary transfers affect the division between formal and informal care, and its effects on the quality of care jobs; this is followed by the conclusions.

The Cost of Care

The decision to provide care is influenced by several motivational factors, such as love, duty and guilt. Regardless of the motivation, provision of care clearly conflicts with alternative allocations of the carer's time, namely leisure and paid work. While all care systems rely heavily on informal carers (mostly female family members) for the provision of home care, on the assumption that it is the cheapest solution, carers' time is often not even included in cost calculations.

If we leave 'non-economic' motivations aside, the choice between providing care directly or buying care in the market is regulated by the carer's opportunity cost relative to the price of care. The trade-off between caregiving and paid work can be illustrated by a simple budget constraint:

$$P_c L_{pc} + X = w(T - L_l - L_{uc})$$

with $T = L_l + L_{uc} + L_w$

$$wL_w = P_c L_{pc} + X$$

$$C = L_{pc} + L_{uc}$$

where P_c = the price of formal/market care; w = the wage rate that the carer can command in the labour market, that is, the opportunity cost of care; L_{pc} and L_{uc} = the amount of paid and unpaid (family/informal) care respectively (hours of care); T = the total time available; L_l = leisure; L_w = time spent on paid work; X = the value of the main carer's contribution to the family income;[1] C = total time of care.

Generally speaking, if the family carer's opportunity cost is greater than the price of formal care, he or she will buy formal care; otherwise, the carer will provide care him- or herself. Any factor that reduces the cost of care, relative to the carer's opportunity cost, will favour the demand for market care (regular or irregular).

In practice, the carer may face income constraints, which increase with the intensity of care. If the required amount of care (in value) exceeds the income that could otherwise be earned in the labour market, the carer must either reduce consumption (X), shifting a part of the resources to buy care, or reduce leisure to increase the total time of work (L_w) (assuming that he or she is not rationed on the labour market) or to provide care him- or herself. An alternative arrangement is offered by solutions that can reduce the price per hour of care, such as those adopted by the Mediterranean countries with a 'migrant in the family' or live-in migrant carer.[2] Technology can provide yet another alternative for cost reduction by drastically reducing the labour content of care, as is the case in high-labour cost countries.[3] Monetary subsidies can relax the budget constraint, making it possible to consume a greater amount of paid care or to supplement the family income.

Formal and informal care are usually complementary activities. In no care regime does formal care, whether public or private, completely obviate the need for family care (Bonsang 2008): while in the Scandinavian countries informal, family care complements public care, in other care regimes the family must search for ways to combine public and private resources to complement its own caring. Fixed and inflexible working schedules may restrict carers' choices in their allocation of time, preventing them from deciding how much care work to offer. If reduction in working hours is unavailable, outright exit from paid work may be

---

1   We are assuming that there are no other sources of income, such as elderly persons' pensions or other family members' income, or savings to draw upon. Alternatively, we may redefine X as the difference between the family's normal consumption – X* – and the family's sources of income other than the main carer's – that is, her contribution to the family's necessary consumption.

2   When, as in Italy, home paid care is organised on a live-in, round-the-clock basis, the pay is often set on a monthly basis; when account is taken of all the hours during which the minder is on call, this amounts to an extremely low wage per hour. Bettio and Solinas (2009) have found that the cost-effectiveness of home care in Italy, compared to Ireland and Denmark, is based on low wages and/or long hours for the paid carers, and low opportunity costs of family care.

3   Bettio and Solinas (2009) have found that Italy and Denmark have approximately the same percentages of total cost for home paid care, but Italy provides 43.6 hours of care versus 12.3 for Denmark.

the only option. Similarly, carers may also be rationed by the availability of formal care services (Spiess and Schneider 2003).

We conclude that the opportunity cost of family carers and the cost of paid care will vary with the conditions governing the labour market (such as employment opportunities, the market wage, flexible working time arrangements and other measures aimed at reconciling caregiving and wage-earning) and the features of the care regimes (such as the different weight of formal and informal carers and of public care provision, flexible and affordable market care, the availability of cheap migrant labour, and monetary and non-monetary schemes aimed at supporting informal caregiving). Highly diverse conditions in labour markets and care regimes will result in large differences between countries in the division between family and market care, as well as in the quality and conditions of care jobs.

The Opportunity Cost of Caring and the Labour Market

Although the negative correlation between caregiving and employment is fairly well documented, the causality running from caregiving to employment is more problematic (Fevang et al. 2008). In the Eurobarometer survey on health and long-term care (European Commission 2007), only a small proportion of respondents declared that they had given up paid work in order to take care of an elderly parent: 2 per cent had quit their jobs completely, and 3 per cent had switched from full-time to part-time work. This proportion is low in all the countries surveyed, including those care regimes where care is still mostly a 'family business'. These results may be a consequence of the combined effect of low activity rate and carers' old age, but they may also reflect the increasing private marketisation of care due to the difficulties in reconciling the various demands on the family carer (see Bettio et al. 2006). In fact, although the traditional male-breadwinner model has been substantially eroded throughout Europe, making room for various earner models, cross-country differences in female participation rates are still relevant. Employment patterns and welfare and care regimes still affect the female activity rate (see Table 6.1), the division between formal and informal care, and the urgency of the reconciliation issue. This is all the more true because the commitment to care tends to come at a fairly advanced stage in a carer's life, reaching its peak when women are well into their fifties. However, demographic change, smaller families and increased female participation in the formal labour market have all put a strain on the capacity of the family to provide care. Women's increasing engagement in paid employment poses a serious challenge to the reconciliation between caring and paid work. How serious the challenge is depends largely on the features of the national employment and care models.

The first empirical research on the impact of caregiving on labour market participation decisions, based on US data,[4] provided mixed evidence. The trade-off

---

4   See Jenson and Jacobzone (2000) and Crespo (2008) for overviews.

Table 6.1   Female employment rates 1960–2007, people aged 15–64 years

		1960	1980	2000	2007	Men 2007	Lisbon Distance*
Nordic		40.5	64.3	70.3	71.9	77.3	11.9
	Denmark	42.7	66.2	71.6	73.2	81.0	13.2
	Finland	54.9	65.0	64.2	68.5	72.1	8.5
	Norway	26.1	58.4	74.0	74.0	79.7	14.0
	Sweden	38.1	67.6	70.9	71.8	76.5	11.8
Anglo-Saxon		43.1	54.5	64.7	65.5	77.3	5.5
	UK	43.1	54.5	64.7	65.5	77.3	5.5
Mediterranean		30.8	40.1	40.9	49.7	73.9	-10.3
	Greece		30.7	41.7	47.9	74.9	-12.1
	Italy	28.1	28.4	39.6	46.6	70.7	-13.4
	Spain	21.0	28.4	41.3	54.7	76.2	-5.3
Rest of Europe			41.0	57.0	62.3	74.9	2.3
	Austria		52.4	59.6	64.4	78.4	4.4
	Belgium	29.6	35.0	51.5	55.3	68.7	-4.7
	France	42.9	50.0	55.2	60.0	69.3	0.0
	Germany	35.0	34.8	58.1	64.0	74.7	4.0
	Ireland		32.3	53.9	60.6	77.4	0.6
	Netherlands		35.7	63.5	69.6	82.2	9.6
	Portugal		47.1	60.5	61.9	73.8	1.9
EU average 15				54.1	59.7	74.2	-0.3

Note: * Lisbon distance is the difference between the female employment rate in 2007 and the Lisbon target of 60%.

Source: 1960 and 1980: Pissarides et al. (2005) on OECD data; 2000 and 2007: EU (2008b); Norway: OECD.StatExtracts (2009).

between labour supply and caregiving decisions was often small, or not statistically significant. Evidence from EU countries is equally mixed. Differences in the unit of analysis – the trade-off is measured either in terms of reduction in hours spent on paid work (Carmichael and Charles 1998), or as a shift from employment to non-participation or from full-time to part-time work – make meaningful comparisons difficult. In fact, differences in the functioning of labour markets and in working time arrangements may restrict the range of choice in the allocation of time, and account for the differences in results. However, a general finding is that the intensity and duration of care are key factors affecting the trade-off. No significant differences are found across Nordic and Southern EU countries in the trade-off between intensive caregiving and labour market participation of adult working women (Crespo 2008; Spiess and Schneider 2003): intensive caregiving affects labour market participation negatively in both groups of countries, though possibly with a different timing (see also Fevang et al. 2008 for Norway).[5] Low income or education and availability of social services are other important factors. Re-entering employment after a caring episode may prove almost impossible, owing to the erosion of skills and human capital. This explains both informal carers' preference for reducing the number of hours worked rather than leaving the labour market altogether (after adjusting for the carer's age and the intensity of the care required) and the key role played by institutional factors, such as availability of flexible working arrangements, job protection, training, and support structures, in reconciling care and paid work (Jenson and Jacobzone 2000; Carmichael et al. 2008).

We can conclude that intensive caregiving negatively affects women's employment in all employment and care regimes, although the opportunity cost of caregiving varies across countries with female activity rates and working arrangements. In the Southern European familistic countries, given the low activity rate of women in the older age bracket (54–65), the trade-off between care and paid work does not yet appear quantitatively conspicuous (see Figure 6.1). Reconciling work and care may become more difficult in the future, when the increase in the female activity rate, by now very high in the younger cohorts, will start to have an effect along the life cycle. Various estimates suggest that these cohort effects are substantial (Pissarides et al. 2005: 60; Simonazzi et al. 2009),[6] and may combine with those produced by pension reforms aimed at postponing the retirement age in substantially increasing the number of working carers. This implies that the opportunity cost of care will increase substantially for those countries (like the Mediterranean and the 'Bismarckian' regimes) which still rely most heavily on the

------

5   Spiess and Schneider (2003) found that starting caregiving significantly reduces work hours for women in Northern European countries (except Ireland), but has no effect in Southern European countries. By contrast, the increase in the intensity of care reduces women's labour supply in Southern Europe and Ireland, but has no such effect in Nordic countries. The authors suggest that this result can be explained by the different role played by the extended family and by public care services in the two groups of countries: the family can better tackle the emergency when the care need abruptly arises, but cannot cope with its increasing intensity, where the more comprehensive Nordic care regime performs better. It should be noted that the results derive from the ECHP surveys of 1994 and 1996: since then, a huge increase in the use of an immigrant labour market to supply care in the Mediterranean countries may have somewhat reduced the trade-off in the intensive stage of care (Bettio et al. 2006).

6   According to Pissarides et al. (2005, p. 60), for the Mediterranean countries as a whole, the cohort effects can result in an increase in the female employment rate of some 6–7 percentage points. In the case of Italy, by 2010, the employment rate was estimated to be 49 per cent, up from a level of 41.3 per cent in 2001 and 46.4 per cent in 2007.

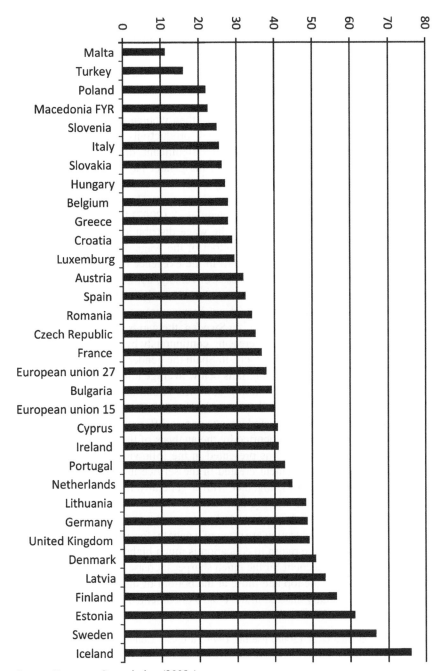

Source: European Commission (2008a)

Figure 6.1   Employment rates of female population aged 54–65, 2007

family to provide care – all the more so if the increase in the level of education of younger cohorts of women raises the level of their potential earnings.

Wage Gaps, Sticky Floors and the Cost of Care

It is widely documented that men earn more than women even after controlling for measurable characteristics related to their productivity (Dolton et al. 2008). Comparative studies show that there are significant differences across EU countries in the extent and the structure of the gender pay gap. Recent research has investigated how the gender pay gap evolves through income distribution. Using harmonised data from the European Community Household Panel (ECHP) across ten European countries, Arulampalam et al. (2007) found that gender pay gaps are typically bigger at the top of the wage distribution, and that for some countries they are also bigger at the bottom of the wage distribution. However, the authors could not find a clear pattern in the existence of 'glass ceilings' and 'sticky floors' across different countries. Conversely, comparing the distribution of the gender wage gap in Spain and Sweden, De la Rica et al. (2008) found a U-shaped pattern for Spain which stands in sharp contrast to the pattern found for Sweden (see Figures 6.2a and 6.2b).[7] In Sweden, the gap is at its minimum at the bottom of the wage distribution, increasing continuously by 35 percentage points from the bottom to the top. Conversely, in Spain the gender gap is much higher at the bottom of the wage distribution, falls below average after the 25th percentile, and starts increasing sharply at the top quintiles. A similar U-shaped pattern is documented by Addis (2007) for Italy (see Figure 6.2c). One plausible explanation for the divergent pattern of the gender wage gap at different points of the income distribution (and one that is supported by the analysis of the care labour markets across different regimes which is presented in the following section) is that the high level of female employment created in the service industry by the welfare state in the Nordic countries, together with a generally more egalitarian wage policy, have contributed to shoring up the floor. The same mechanism does not seem to have been at work in the two Mediterranean countries.

While low levels of education are more of a penalty for women than for men in terms of hourly wage, the return to education is much higher for women than for men. These two facts account for the much sharper increase for women in the gap between the wages at the top and those at the bottom of the income distribution. This pattern is especially marked in the US, as documented by Gordon and Dew-

---

7   De la Rica et al. (2008) use the 1999 European Community Household Panel (ECHP) for full-time workers to derive quantile measures of the (unexplained) gender gap in Spain and Sweden at the end of the 1990s. They then compare the gender gap (in terms of the differences of logged gross hourly wages of male and female workers) at different points of the income distribution with the mean gap for the two countries (see Figures 6.2a and 6.2b).

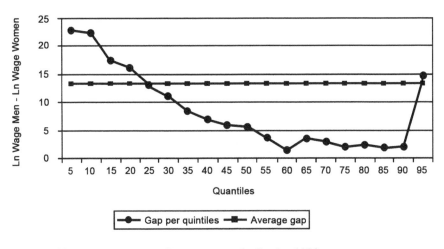

Figure 6.2a   Aggregate gender wage gap in Spain, 1999

Source: De la Rica et al. (2008), computed on ECHP 1999 database.

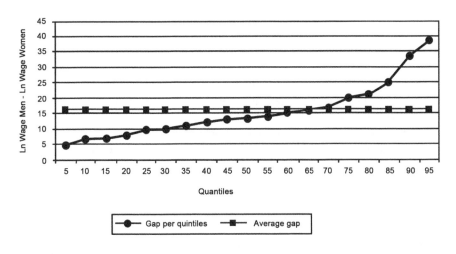

Figure 6.2b   Aggregate gender wage gap in Sweden, 1999

Source: De la Rica et al. (2008), computed on ECHP 1999 database.

Becker (2008), but it is also evident in Europe. Once again, institutional factors help to explain the widening gap. In the US, the greater increase in the 50–10 income ratio for women is consistent with a decrease in the real minimum wage, particularly in 1980–86, since women are roughly twice as likely as men to be paid the minimum wage, while decreased union density was identified as the main factor for men (Gordon and Dew-Becker 2008, pp. 6–7). This may also be true in

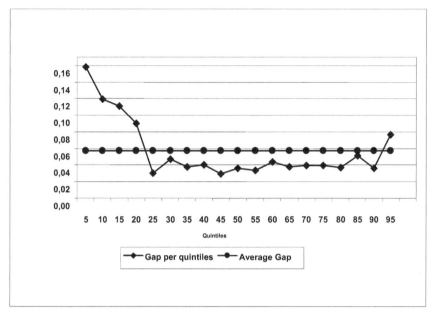

Figure 6.2c   Aggregate gender wage gap in Italy, 2002

Source: Addis (2007), computed on ECHP 2002 database.

Europe, where the widening of the within-gender pay differential may be explained more by the sluggishness of wage increases at the bottom of the distribution than by high increases at the top.

The pattern of the wage gap at the bottom of the distribution can be related to that of the female participation rate. If low-skilled women's wages fall through the floor at levels well below men's wages at the bottom of the wage distribution, and well below the average wage, it is plausible that they will have less of an incentive to participate in the labour market, since their wage will not cover the cost of domestic, unpaid work. Female labour supply will consequently be discouraged.

The elderly care sector is a labour-intensive, highly gender-segregated, low-pay sector. It is also highly segmented: qualified professional workers co-exist with less qualified, often irregular workers; wide disparities in working conditions divide staff employed by private contractors (or not-for-profit organisations) and staff employed by public institutions, and workers in home care from those in residential care, regular and irregular workers. We observe huge cross-country differences in care job quality and the degree of wage compression. In the Netherlands, for instance, care work is paid better than other low-paid sectors, while the opposite is true for the UK, where the minimum wage sets the level for care work pay. In Sweden, the cross-sector wage differential is much narrower than in the Mediterranean countries.[8]

Institutional and cultural factors and policy choices can explain these differences. Those countries aiming at a narrower wage dispersion have resorted to two main policies: technology and training, and public provision. Generally speaking, education and skill levels are mostly low for care workers in the Mediterranean countries, France and the UK, while they are reasonably high for skilled and semi-skilled workers in the vocational systems of Austria and Germany, and they are highest in Scandinavian countries (Simonazzi 2009). Public employment (the solution typically pursued by the Nordic countries) has been an important factor in determining job quality and setting a floor for lower wages. Conversely, a shift towards the contracting-out of previously publicly provided services for the sake of cost reduction is an important factor in job quality deterioration (as in the UK).

As argued above, working conditions in the care sector may discourage the domestic supply of care labour, but the high cost of market care can discourage demand. Faced with a sharp increase in the demand for care labour, all countries are experiencing problems in recruiting enough workers to meet demand. In some countries, the shortage of care workers has been met by a large influx of immigrant, mostly female, workers (Bettio et al. 2006). The magnitude of the labour shortage in the LTC sector, in total and across the skill spectrum, and the extent to which migrant workers are employed to fill the gap and the modalities of migrant involvement in the labour market differ widely across countries and across the various segments of the care labour market. Sweden and France seem to rely least on immigrant carers. In Sweden, substantial public spending has resulted in a largely native workforce, which is well-paid and highly trained. There is a small but growing number of foreign-born workers mostly employed by public agencies. In spite of a very different care system, native care workers are still predominant in France: care reforms and (tied) cash subsidies have been directed at supporting the female participation and employment rate. Conversely, the UK is one of the largest importers of professional healthcare workers, a large percentage of whom work in the long-term care system; since the beginning of this century, immigrants from Eastern European countries employed in unskilled, personal care have been on the rise, especially in the larger cities. Substantial cash benefits, little regulatory supervision and a tradition of home care have encouraged extensive use of foreign care workers in Austria and Germany, and especially in Southern European countries. Unlike in the UK, many of these workers are undocumented immigrants, hired informally by families through informal networks.[9] These

---

8   In Italy, for instance, using data from the 2002 Survey on Household Income and Wealth (SHIW), Addis (2007) estimates a 17 per cent wage penalty of the domestic sector compared to industry.

9   In the three Mediterranean countries, foreign (mostly female) workers provide an increasing share of home care: the underground economy covers one-third of the market in Spain, where language is less of a problem, since workers migrate from Latin American

workers often co-reside with the elderly person round the clock, and stay for a three-month period on a rotating basis. Foreign long-term care workers fill the gaps in the care chain; they are more likely to take jobs in the less desirable tasks or segments of the market; and they do not compete with professional care workers. However, since illegal carers are so very cheap to employ, they may raise serious competition against home service providers and prevent the formation of a more equitable and sustainable care system.

We can now try to pull these various threads together. Given the features of the care sector, we may expect female care workers to be heavily represented in the low quintiles of the income distribution. It could be argued that in many countries, relatively low wages at the bottom of the distribution may be a necessary substitution for the lack of publicly provided services, making it easier for working women to hire household help and carers for elderly dependants. However, among the lowest-paid there seems to be a thin line separating the opportunity cost of the female family carer and the cost of a paid carer. If care labour wages are too low to stimulate a sufficient supply of care labour, the increase in its price may be thwarted by the fall in demand brought about by the increase in the budget constraint, which pushes the carer back towards informal care provision. Immigration can provide yet another way out of the financial constraint of care, while introducing a third inequality gap besides income and gender: ethnicity.

Cash for Care (and Other Support Schemes)

Monetary transfers affect the care–employment trade-off through income and substitution effects.[10] Untied cash benefits soften the budget constraint, leaving the relative cost of formal to informal care (P_c/w) unaffected. Conversely, tied monetary transfers (for example, vouchers) reduce the market price of care, making paid care more affordable. We may thus have different effects on the formal/informal division of care according to the conditions regulating the disbursement and utilisation of cash transfers.

The size of the subsidy is clearly a crucial factor. Given their generally small size, cash allowances are unlikely to be the decisive factor in freeing up unpaid carers to participate in the labour market. They are more likely to be considered as an income subsidy which rewards previously unpaid carers or subsidises the cost of formal care. However, when combined with other sources of income, such as the dependent elderly person's pension, unconditional cash allowances can help in meeting the cost of paid care.

---

countries (Miguélez et al. 2006). More or less legal flows from bordering Eastern countries are supplying the market for informal carers in Greece and Italy.

10   The income effect is the change observed in the consumption of a good due to changes in purchasing power, while the substitution effect is the change in consumption of the same good due to variation in the relative price of goods.

In the case of untied monetary transfers, a flat-rate subsidy will be most effective in discouraging the market participation of women on low incomes, since even a low subsidy may compare not too unfavourably with the wage that they could earn on the market. The flexibility of working times, the possible wage penalty related to caring obligations, the need to resort to some form of paid care, combined with the probable old age of the carer, are likely to tilt the choice in favour of caregiving. Re-entering the labour market after the caregiving has concluded obviously becomes very difficult. For lower-middle-income families, conversely, the subsidy may be decisive in turning the choice in favour of buying the services in the market. A ready availability of cheap care labour, combined with unconditional cash allowances, can open the market opportunity to a large proportion of lower-middle-income families as well, even at relatively low levels of subsidies,.

All things considered, cash transfers are unlikely to be the key factor capable of changing the trade-off between care and paid work, but they may affect the care labour market by favouring the emergence of a supply of largely irregular, low-paid carers. The various European countries differ widely in their conditions regulating cash transfers for care. Leaving out the Scandinavian countries, where cash benefits are still very limited, we can distinguish different country patterns (see Table 6.2).[11] On the one hand we have countries (such as France and the UK) that are more restrictive in the use of monetary transfers to pay the family carer. In France, vouchers are provided to families for the direct recruitment of paid care workers. In the UK, direct payments are a relatively recent measure; the scheme is highly regulated, aimed at enhancing the elderly person's freedom and independence (Yeandle and Stiell 2007, p. 128). At the other extreme lie the Mediterranean and the Bismarckian countries. In Italy, both the state and families perceive the various allowances as forms of income subsidy that can be freely used to complement the family budget. In spite of the institution of long-term care insurance, Germany and Austria more closely resemble the Mediterranean countries with regard to its use. In both cases, the LTC insurance started from the premise that home care should take precedence over care in nursing homes. Hence, the allowance was by no means intended to reduce the quantity of care provided informally. The idea was instead to make caring more attractive, so that caregivers, especially women of working age, would continue to care rather than enter the labour market (Morel 2007, pp. 15–16).[12] By contrast, other countries (such as France and Belgium) resorted to tied cash benefits with the primary aim

---

11   See Simonazzi (2009) for a more detailed description of the various systems. See also Ungerson and Yeandle (2007) for an overview of the various cash-for-care schemes.

12   In the Netherlands, where elderly care was mainly institutionalised, a new policy taking the form of a 'personal budget' entitles dependent people to a care allowance to be used for the purchase of care services, whether informal (from relatives) or professional. The introduction of this benefit is part of a move towards providing care recipients with greater freedom in deciding how best to service their needs. It is also, as in other countries, a way of offering some form of remuneration to informal carers (Morel 2007, p. 19).

Table 6.2   Family eligibility and conditionality of monetary transfers

	Mediterranean/ Familistic	Continental/Bismarckian			Anglo-Saxon	Nordic
	Italy	Austria	Germany	France	UK	Sweden
Spouse	Yes	Yes	Yes	No	No	Nr
Other kin	Yes	Yes	Yes	No *	No	
Use of transfers earmarked?	No	No	No **	Yes	Yes	Nr

Notes:

* Family members can be paid if officially unemployed.

** The cash payment is subject to the definition of a care plan.

Nr = not very relevant.

Source: Simonazzi (2009).

of integrating low-skilled women into the regular labour market, while responding to the increasing need for care.[13]

Systems relying on in-kind provision (Sweden), contracting-out (the UK) and 'tied' cash allowances to be used to hire private carers (France) favour the formation of a formal and regular care labour market. Systems relying mostly on unconditional cash allowances (the Mediterranean countries, Austria and Germany) favour the informal market. In Austria, cash benefits, coupled with little regulatory supervision, a tradition of home care, and the permeability of the country's eastern borders (due also to historical ties) have encouraged a large influx of migrant carers, many of whom are illegal immigrants but are openly recruited by agencies for short-term, rotating care duties (Hermann 2006). In Germany, in spite of the prevalence of unconditional cash benefits, reliance on illegal foreign workers does not yet seem to have reached similar proportions (Kümmerling 2006). In regard to the Mediterranean countries, the limited amount of public involvement in care financing explains their failure to develop a formal private market of paid care for older people and the dominance of individual suppliers. The unconditional character of monetary transfers, in an unregulated labour market with a large grey economy, has led to the development of a large supply of irregular, often undocumented, immigrant carers to fill the gap in the supply of affordable care workers. We may conclude that cash-for-care schemes largely reflect the characteristics of care regimes, ending up by reinforcing their effects in terms of the division of care labour between formal and informal care and of the quantity and quality of care work. Thus, the conditions regulating the

---

13   I wish to thank an anonymous referee for providing information on the Belgian case.

trend towards subsidised home care may have important consequences for the future sustainability of the various care regimes.

The flow of cheap, legal carers since EU enlargement is changing the features of care regimes and care labour markets across Europe. We may envisage two possible outcomes. The first is an increase in the supply of cheap, regular labour, possibly on a temporary basis, in those countries where the formal care market predominates, as in the UK, France, and possibly Sweden. The second outcome concerns those countries which rely on untied monetary transfers or which have large informal markets. Here, greater freedom of movement within the enlarged Europe may have the effect of fuelling the informal/irregular care market. In Germany and Austria, reforms aimed at dealing with the financial difficulties of their insurance schemes will be decisive in determining in which direction the care regimes of these two countries will move: whether towards employing more immigrant carers, albeit on a formal basis, or towards the Mediterranean model, with its reliance on irregular migrant carers. The latter's capacity to move towards a more regulated care market will depend very much on how the cash benefits are disbursed and on the conditions regulating the formal and informal care markets. The case of Italy provides a good example. The irregular carers' pay is often extremely low compared with that earned by a regular worker, though much higher than what they could earn in their home countries. A new national contract for domestic workers (in March 2007) raised the cost to the family of an elderly dependant for a live-in minder on a regular contract to a level roughly comparable to the average female net earnings in industry and services (1,000–1,300 euros per month for the live-in carer, in addition to board and lodging costs, as compared to 950–1,250 euros for the industry take-home pay). With these new wages, even if social contributions can be deducted from tax, the regular-minder solution is no longer sustainable for lower-middle-income families, which used to rely on the extremely cheap supply of informal carers, and it is no longer competitive with residential care, especially if the latter receives a state subsidy. The risk is therefore that this form of work will be pushed back into the black market. If this is to be prevented, both the level and the conditions regulating the provision of monetary transfers need to be monitored: the level should be in line with what is considered a fair wage in the care market, and the transfer should be earmarked in order to guarantee that conditions are met.

However, our analysis has highlighted that in order to ease the trade-off between caregiving and labour market participation, measures in support of family carers on top of and beyond cash benefits are likely to be much more effective. European countries are introducing different schemes in support of the family carer: from support services such as respite care, counselling and a larger supply of home care providers in the community, through quasi-monetary provisions such as pension rights, social and accident insurance and tax exemption, to measures facilitating the reconciliation of caregiving with flexible participation in paid labour, such as training courses, rights to employment leave, and reduction of working time. While some of these measures, such as entitlement to pension contributions, reduce the opportunity cost of forgoing a paid job, and others, such as rights to work leave and respite care, can be equated to an increase in the opportunity cost, they all basically work by facilitating the reconciliation of care and paid work.

Conclusions

The shift to home care will undoubtedly increase the burden on the family carer. While the large cohorts moving into old age in the coming decades will challenge the fiscal sustainability of current health and long-term care systems, the simultaneous increase in female participation in the labour market will increase the opportunity cost of the family carer and make reconciliation more difficult. The increase in female employment will lead to the employment of more women in the care sector if public care policy tackles the issue of the trade-off between affordable market care and fair care pay and working conditions. This calls for a carefully targeted policy on publicly funded formal home care and on the conditions regulating cash-for-care schemes in support of informal care.

Unconditional cash benefits may either create 'incentive traps' attracting informal caregivers away from the normal labour market, or conversely, reliance on a low-quality, low-pay, irregular care market, if the relation between the opportunity cost of the family carer, the subsidy and the functioning of the care market are not controlled (Lundsgaard 2005). In fact, where labour markets are deregulated, or where service buyers are free to spend their benefits with no restrictions, the market has not been able to produce a sustainable solution in terms of the quantity and quality of care labour. Conversely, tied cash benefits may ensure, through substitution and income effects, a greater reliance on paid/regular care. Countries with more regulated labour markets have been more successful in securing an adequate supply of native workers to meet demand. However, cash-for-care is not the definitive solution to the trade-off between caregiving and employment. For this purpose, the provision of services in support of families may prove more effective.

References

Addis, E. (2007), 'Il differenziale salariale tra i sessi in Italia e il patto di genere', in A. Pinnelli, F. Raccioppi and L. Terzera (eds), *Genere, Famiglia e Salute*, Milan: Franco Angeli.

Arulampalam, W., Booth, A.L. and Bryan, M.L. (2007), 'Is there a glass ceiling over Europe? Exploring the gender pay gap across the wages distribution', *Industrial and Labor Relations Review*, vol. 60, no. 2, pp. 163–86.

Bettio, F. and Solinas, G. (2009), 'Which European model for elderly care? Equity and cost-effectiveness in home based care in three European countries', *Economia & Lavoro*, vol. 43, no. 1, pp. 53–71.

Bettio, F. and Verashchagina, A. (eds) (2008), *Frontiers in the Economics of Gender*, London: Routledge.

Bettio, F., Simonazzi, A. and Villa, P. (2006) 'Change in care regimes and female migration: The care drain in the Mediterranean', *Journal of European Social Policy*, vol. 16, no. 3, pp. 271–85.

Boeri, T., Del Boca, D. and Pissarides, C. (eds) (2005), *Women at Work. An Economic Perspective*, Oxford: Oxford University Press.

Bonsang, E. (2008), *Does Informal Care from Children to their Elderly Parents Substitute for Formal Care in Europe?*, Liège: University of Liège Centre for Research in Public Economics and Population Economics (CREPP), WP 2008/01.

Bosch, G., Lehndorff, S. and Rubery, J. (eds) (2009), *European Employment Models in Flux. A Comparison of Institutional Change in nine European Countries*, London: Palgrave Macmillan.

Carmichael, F. and Charles, S. (1998), 'The labour market costs of community care', *Journal of Health Economics*, no. 17, pp. 747–65.

Carmichael, F., Hulme, C., Sheppard, S. and Connel, G. (2008), 'Work–life imbalance: Informal care and paid employment in the UK', *Feminist Economics*, vol. 14, no. 2, pp. 3–35.

Crespo, L. (2008), 'Parental Caregiving and Employment Status of European Mid-life Women', mimeograph.

De la Rica, S., Dolado, J.J. and Llorens, V. (2008), 'Ceiling and floors: Gender wage gaps by education in Spain', *Journal of Population Economics*, vol. 21, no. 3, pp. 751–76.

Dolton, P., Marcenaro-Gutierrez, O. and Skalli, A. (2008), 'Gender Differences across Europe', in F. Bettio and A. Verashchagina (eds), *Frontiers in the Economics of Gender*, London: Routledge.

European Commission (2007), *Health and Long-term Care in the European Union*, special issue of *Eurobarometer*, December, <http://ec.europa.eu/public_opinion/archives/ebs/ebs_283_en.pdf> (accessed 8 May 2011).

European Commission (2008a), *Employment in Europe*, Luxembourg: European Communities.

—— (2008b), *European Union Labour Force Survey –Annual Results 2008*, Luxembourg: Eurostat, <http://epp.eurostat.ec.europa.eu/cache/ITY_OFFPUB/KS-QA-09-033/EN/KS-QA-09-033-EN.PDF> (accessed 10 May 2011).

—— (2008c), '*Long-term Care in the European Union*, DG Employment, Social Affairs and Equal Opportunities, Luxembourg: European Communities, <http://ec.europa.eu/social/BlobServlet?docId=3919&langId=en> (accessed 10 May 2011).

Fevang, E, Kverndokk, S. and Røed, K. (2008), *Informal Care and Labor Supply*, Institut zur Zukunft der Arbeit (IZA) Discussion Paper no. 3,717, September.

Glover, S., Ceri Gott, A.L., Porter, J., Price, R., Spencer, S. Srinivasan, V. and Willis, C. (2001), *Migration: An Economic and Social Analysis*, RDS Occasional Paper 67, London: Home Office.

Gordon, R.J. and Dew-Becker, I. (2008), 'Controversies about the rise of American inequality: A Survey', National Bureau of Economic and Social Research (NBER) Working Paper no. 13,982, April.

Hermann, C. (2006), *Elderly Care in Austria*, EU Project 'Dynamo' (Dynamics of National Employment Models), 6th Framework Programme.

Himmelweit, S. (2007), 'Policy on Care: A Help or a Hindrance to Gender Equality?', in J. Scott, S. Dex and H. Joshi (eds), *Women and Employment: 25 Years of Change*, Aldershot: Edward Elgar.

Jenson, J. and Jacobzone, S. (2000), *Care Allowances for Frail Elderly and their Impact on Women Care-givers*, OECD Labour Market and Social Policy Occasional Paper no. 41, Paris: OECD Publishing.

Kümmerling, A. (2006), *The Elderly Care Sector in Germany*, EU Project 'Dynamo' (Dynamics of National Employment Models), 6th Framework Programme.

Lewis, J. Campbell, M. and Huerta, C. (2008), 'Patterns of paid and unpaid work in Western Europe: Gender, commodification, preferences and the implications for policy', *Journal of European Social Policy*, vol. 18, no. 1, pp. 21–37.

Lundsgaard, J. (2005), *Consumer Direction and Choice in Long-term Care for Older Persons, Including Payments for Informal Care: How Can it Help Improve Care Outcomes, Employment and Fiscal Sustainability?*, OECD Health Working Papers no. 20.

Miguélez, F., Lope, A. and Olivares, I. (2006), *Elderly Care Sector in Spain*, EU Project 'Dynamo' (Dynamics of National Employment Models), 6th Framework Programme.

Morel, N. (2007), 'Care Policies as Employment Strategy. The Impact of Bismarckian Welfare State Institutions on Child- and Elderly-care Policy Reforms in France, Belgium, Germany and the Netherlands', Florence: mimeograph.

OECD (2002), 'Women at Work: Who are They and How are They Faring?', in *Employment Outlook*, Paris: OECD, ch. 2.

OECD (2005), *Trends in International Migration*, SOPEMI Report, Paris: OECD.

OECD (2009), StatExtracts, <http://stats.oecd.org> (accessed 10 May 2011).

Pinnelli, A., Raccioppi, F. and Terzera, L. (2007), *Genere, Famiglia e Salute*, Milan: Franco Angeli.

Pissarides, C., Garibaldi, P., Olivetti, C., Petrongolo, B. and Wasmer, E. (2005), 'Women in the Labour Force: How Well is Europe Doing?', in T. Boeri, D. Del Boca and C. Pissarides (eds), *Women at Work: An Economic Perspective*, Oxford: Oxford University Press.

Scott, J., Dex, S. and Joshi, H. (eds) (2007), *Women and Employment, 25 Years of Change*, Aldershot: Edward Elgar.

Simonazzi, A. (2009), 'Care regimes and national employment models', *Cambridge Journal of Economics*, vol. 33, no. 2, pp. 211–32.

Simonazzi, A., Villa, P., Lucidi, F. and Naticchioni, P. (2009), 'Continuity and Change in the Italian Model', in G. Bosch, S. Lehndorff and J. Rubery (eds), *European Employment Models in Flux: A Comparison of Institutional Change in Nine European Countries*, London: Palgrave Macmillan, pp. 201–22.

Spiess, C.K. and Schneider, U. (2003), 'Interactions between care-giving and paid work hours among European midlife women, 1994 to 1996', *Ageing and Society*, no. 23, pp. 41–68.

Ungerson, C. and Yeandle, S. (eds) (2007*)*, *Cash for Care in Developed Welfare States*, Basingstoke: Palgrave Macmillan.

Wolf, D.A. and Soldo, B.J. (1994), 'Married women's allocation of time to employment and care of elderly parents', *Journal of Human Resources*, vol. 29, no. 4, pp. 1,259–76.

Yeandle, S. and Stiell, B. (2007), 'Issues in the Development of the Direct Payments Scheme for Older People in England', in C. Ungerson and S. Yeandle (eds), *Cash for Care in Developed Welfare States*, Basingstoke: Palgrave Macmillan.

Chapter 7

Transnational Caregiving between Australia, Italy and El Salvador: The Impact of Institutions on the Capability to Care at a Distance

Laura Merla and Loretta Baldassar

Research on transnational caregiving relations (Baldassar et al. 2007a; Baldassar et al. 2007b; Merla 2010; Merla 2011) has shown that, despite living at a distance, migrant family members and their homeland kin exchange all the forms of care and support that are exchanged in proximate families (Finch 1989). Transnational care incorporates the provision of different 'types' of care, including moral and emotional support, financial assistance and practical support, all of which can be exchanged transnationally through the use of various communication technologies, as well as personal care and accommodation, which require co-presence and can only be exchanged during visits. Baldassar et al. (2007a) describe transnational caregiving practices as mediated by a dialectic encompassing the *capacity* of individual members to engage in caregiving and their culturally informed sense of *obligation* to provide care, as well as the particularistic kin relationships and *negotiated family commitments* that people with specific family networks share. This model illustrates the complex mix of motivations that inform transnational caregiving between migrant and 'homeland' kin. In this chapter, we will attempt to extend this analysis of transnational care dynamics through an application of the capabilities approach. Based on a comparison of transnational care practices of Australian migrants from El Salvador and Italy, we conceptualise the ability to exchange care across distance as a set of 'capabilities'. We examine the role institutions play in providing access to these capabilities.

Our use of the term 'capability' draws on Sen's work (Sen 1980; Sen 1985; Sen 1987; Sen 1993) and on Robeyns' interpretation of his work (Robeyns 2003; Robeyns 2007). The capabilities approach proposes a multi-dimensional approach to well-being that attempts to account for both non-financial and non-material constituents (Robeyns 2007). Quality of life is defined as one's freedom to live the kind of life which, upon reflection, one finds valuable. Capabilities refer to 'what real opportunities you have regarding the life you may lead' (Sen 1987, p. 36). They represent people's potential functionings, or freedom to be and do what they want to be and do. These functionings constitute what makes a life valuable.

Examples of capabilities include being well fed, taking part in the community, being sheltered, relating to other people, working in the labour market, caring for others and being healthy (Robeyns 2003, p. 63). This approach acknowledges that people differ in their capacity to transform capabilities into functionings, depending on personal, social or environmental factors, such as physical and mental handicaps, traditions, social norms, public infrastructure and so on. It is also important to note that people exercise considerable choice in their management of resources and capabilities. For example, the competing demands for time and finances of the local family versus the transnational family (private school fees or trips to the homeland). This tension led Singh (2006) to argue that the existence of a special kind of transnational family money needs to be acknowledged (Wilding and Baldassar 2009). These concerns further highlight the value of considering transnational family caregiving as a set of capabilities. Sen's capabilities approach is a framework of thought rather than a fully specified theory, and does not provide a definitive list of capabilities.[1] It thus allows for the design of context-sensitive definitions of the criteria that influence people's well-being.

In this chapter, we wish to underline that the ability to exchange care with one's ageing parents, especially when these parents live in a distant country, significantly impacts on migrants' well-being. In her attempt to apply the capabilities approach to gender equality, Robeyns (2003, pp. 71–3) acknowledges the importance of care. Her list of capabilities includes elements such as domestic work and non-market care (that is, being able to raise children and to take care of others), time-autonomy (being able to exercise autonomy in allocating one's time), mobility (being able to be mobile) and social relations (being able to be part of social networks and to give and receive social support), all of which are closely related to the exchange of care between migrants and ageing parents in the two studies that inform this chapter.

The first three sections of this chapter are dedicated to a description of our methodology, the migration histories of Italian and Salvadoran migrants in Australia, and the welfare structures of these migrants' home countries: Italy and El Salvador. We begin our results section with case studies of an Italian and a Salvadoran migrant's experiences of transnational care. We conclude with an analysis of the capabilities that influence the exchange of care across borders, and discuss the influence of institutions on these transnational caregiving-related capabilities.

Methods

The data for the El Salvadorian case are drawn from Merla's comparative research on transnational care practices of Latin American migrants living in Australia

---

1   This is a major point of divergence between Sen's and philosopher Martha Nussbaum's conceptions of the capabilities approach. According to Nussbaum's theory, there should be one universal general list of capabilities that can be translated into more details to suit the context (Nussbaum 2000).

and Europe, financed by the EC 6th Framework Programme – Marie Curie Outgoing International Fellowship (MOIF-CT-2006-039076 Transnational care) (Merla 2010; Merla 2011; Merla forthcoming).[2] The study focuses on migrants who occupy a low-qualified and/or low-remunerated position in Australia despite coming from a mix of working-class and professional backgrounds in El Salvador. Data collection in Australia comprised 27 life-history interviews and participant observation with Latin American migrants living in Perth, Western Australia. Among the 22 Salvadoran migrants interviewed, 17 were professionals in their home countries. The main aim of this research is to analyse the impact of low levels of social, economic and/or cultural capital on migrants' ability to exchange care with their elderly parents who live in their home country.

The discussion of the Italian case study is based primarily on data drawn from a larger collaborative study by Baldassar et al. (2007a), for which data collection comprised approximately 200 life-history interviews and participant observation with migrants and refugees in Perth, Western Australia, and their parents and other kin in Italy, the Netherlands, Ireland, Singapore, New Zealand and in the transit country of Iran. This research examines the dynamics of long-distance family relations, highlighting transnational caregiving as an important phenomenon of the migration process.[3] Additional data are drawn from Baldassar's previous ethnographic research, including approximately 50 interviews with families in Italy and Australia (Baldassar 2001).

Migration Histories

The majority of Salvadorans began arriving in Australia in 1982, under the United Nations Refugee Programme. Refugee status was granted to people who were identified by the UN High Commissioner for Refugees as being subject to persecution in their home country and in need of resettlement. The migration flows continued until the signing of a peace treaty in El Salvador in 1992, which put an end to the civil war that started in 1979. Between 1982 and 1993, a total of 9,993 Salvadoran refugees migrated to Australia, the majority arriving between 1988 and 1992 (Santos 2006, p. 80). In 2001, 1,200 Salvadorans lived in Western Australia (Office of Multicultural Interests 2005, p. 8). Salvadoran refugees included semi-skilled and unskilled workers, as well as professionals such as engineers, agronomists, doctors and teachers, but few of them were able to find a similar position in Australia. As Santos points out, for Salvadoran migrants: 'the need to learn the English language and to have their qualifications recognised in Australia proved insurmountable. Often this [need] results in [their] being downgraded in

---

2   This chapter reflects only the authors' views. The European Community is not liable for any use that may be made of the information contained herein.

3   See also Baldassar et al. (2007b).

their employment or becoming unemployed/underemployed for long periods of time' (Santos 2006, p. 83).

Italian migration to Western Australia has a considerably different history. Italians began arriving in significant numbers in the immediate post-Second World War period, although migration chains date back to the early 1920s (Baldassar 2004). The earlier and most numerous waves overwhelmingly comprised voluntary labour migrants. These migrants tended to congregate in certain occupations, including agriculture, small business, construction and food industries. On the whole, Italian labour migrants have obtained high levels of financial security, with some of the highest rates of home ownership in Australia. Their children and grandchildren have enjoyed increasing social mobility, with high rates entering the professional classes. The vast majority (91 per cent) of the 23,000 Italian-born people currently living in Western Australia arrived before 1986. Professional migrants from Italy have been relatively few in number, and most have arrived since the 1980s under the skilled migration scheme. These migrants tend to find jobs in Australia commensurate with their pre-migration employment.

Welfare Structures: Familialism in Italy and El Salvador

Blackman (2000) defines the Italian welfare regime as a family-oriented system, in which caregiving is largely provided within the family and community (see also Blackman et al. 2001). For families in Italy, there is a general expectation that elder care be provided within the family, such that public service provision of aged care is limited, though growing as neo-liberalism informs the development of the sector.

Martínez Franzoni (2008) characterises El Salvador as an informal-familialist welfare regime, in which families not only carry the full burden of care duties, but also turn into production units and social protection networks to compensate for the absence of the state and the weakness of formal labour markets. This not only includes the provision of personal 'hands-on' care, but also financial support, as pension benefits and free public health services are only available to a small proportion of the population. Remittances and extended family support are critical strategies to increase income and manage unpaid work.[4]

Both in Italy and El Salvador, women assume the quasi-exclusive responsibility of unpaid work in general, and care in particular (Martínez Franzoni 2005). This is reflected in our study. Italian migrants (from both the earlier labour and more recent professional cohorts), particularly daughters, report a very high sense of obligation to provide care, including personal (hands-on) care, to their kin. Many openly describe themselves as 'bad' daughters who have failed to live up to their parent's expectations because, by migrating, they are unable to provide the level

---

4   Poverty affects 43 per cent of the Salvadoran population (Martínez Franzoni 2008, p. 5), and remittances represent approximately 14 per cent of El Salvador's GDP.

of personal care that is culturally expected (Baldassar 2007b). The same sense of obligation to provide personal care is reported by Salvadoran daughters. Because of their difficult political and economic circumstances, all the Salvadoran migrants that were interviewed expressed a keen sense of obligation to provide financial and emotional support to their parents, especially to their mothers, with whom the majority reported sharing a special relationship (Merla 2010). More recent Italian professional migrants, in contrast, are more likely to be the recipients of financial support from their parents than vice versa (Baldassar 2007a).

Results

In this section, we propose to consider the following questions:

1. Which capabilities influence the capability to exchange care with parents living in a distant country?
2. What role do institutions play in facilitating access to these capabilities?

Our arguments will be based on the comparative analysis of our two samples, and we begin with two case studies in an effort to highlight the differences and similarities between Italian and Salvadoran migrants' experiences of long-distance care.

Case Studies

Amparo, Roberto and their three children had enjoyed a good socio-economic position before leaving El Salvador to go to Australia in 1989 under a political refugee programme. As their qualifications were not recognised in Australia, Roberto took the first jobs he could find, including distributing magazines to mailboxes and night cleaning in a shopping centre. Amparo stayed at home to care for the children. The family could not rely on the support of their kin back home, who were not happy about their decision to move to a far-away country. Also, Amparo did not want to worry them, so she kept her problems secret. She also felt bad about leaving her ill mother Salena behind, with whom she shared a particularly close relationship. Salena had refused to migrate with Amparo as she did not want to leave her other children. Migration did not prevent Amparo from staying in regular contact with her mother, mainly through telephone conversations. She could only afford to call Selena once a month, as she did not have access to cheap international telephone cards at that time. Telephone calls only went one way, from Australia to El Salvador, as the family back home could not afford them. Like the majority of Salvadoran elderly people, Selena relied entirely on her children's economic and practical help. The financial support Amparo provided to her mother did not stop with migration, and included the money from the sale of her house. She also sent money on birthdays and at Christmas, and began to send AU$200 every month once the money from the sale of her house had been spent. Amparo only saw her mother once again before she died. In order to cover her travel expenses of AU$3,100, Amparo had to take a cleaning job and Roberto worked extra hours. Roberto's brother lent her the AU$2,500 he had saved for his own trip to El Salvador. Travelling on her own was a real challenge because of her poor English. Amparo stayed in El Salvador for a month, spending all her time with her mother, caring for her at home and taking her to the doctor. Selena died a year after her daughter's visit. Amparo could not afford to attend the funeral.

Cecilia came from a wealthy Italian family. She has a university degree, and she was an only daughter, with brothers. She migrated to Australia with her husband in the mid-1970s to take up a well-paid position. Cecilia's parents were devastated at her decision to leave Italy and the passing of years did not bring acceptance of this decision. In fact, as her parents aged, she experienced an increasing sense of guilt at not being able to care for them in person. This sense of obligation was exacerbated by her parents' expressed wish that she return to Italy to care for them. As a result, Cecilia travelled frequently to Italy to be with them. Cecilia also benefited from financial assistance from her parents, not just in paying for all her regular return trips with her children, but also for the purchase of expensive items like her home and car. Her parents chose never to visit her in Australia, explaining that they found the prospect of air travel too frightening. Cecilia stayed in constant contact with her parents, even though their relationship was often fraught with tension. Regular phone calls, and more recently email and Skype contact, characterised this communication. When her father died, Cecilia was able not only to attend his funeral, but also to spend an extended period helping her mother adjust. In recent years, as her mother has become more frail, Cecilia and her brother, who lives near to her mother, have overseen the employment of a live-in carer. Cecilia and her parents refused the option of an aged care home. These have a negative connotation in Italy, and are viewed as a last resort for elderly people who have no family to care for them. A key issue for Cecilia was juggling her obligations of care to her parents with her obligations to care for her family in Australia, as well as her desire to have time for herself.

Analysis of the Capabilities

As these case studies show, the ability to exchange care at a distance is influenced by several factors, including mobility, social relations, time allocation, education and knowledge, paid work and communication. After providing a description of these capabilities, we will analyse the role institutions play in accessing and using these capabilities.

Mobility   All the migrants we interviewed emphasised the importance of being able to spend time with their parents during visits. The need for co-presence was represented by *mobility*, or the capability to travel between the home and the host countries, and to provide and receive accommodation during those visits. The mobility of the Salvadorans compared to the Italians represents one of the most significant differences between the two groups. The recent Italian professional migrants all enjoyed financial support from their parents, representing a flow of capital from home to host – the opposite direction to that normal for labour migration. The post-war Italian migrants, like the Salvadorans, sent remittances home, and this form of financial support was a central feature of their migration project, representing a family economic strategy. In more recent times, even the post-war Italian labour migrants have attained a level of wealth that permits them frequent visits home.

Hence, a key issue influencing the capability of mobility is the distribution of funds for the family in Australia or for visits to family back home. Finding time and money to spend on mobility and visits involves a negotiation of duties and commitments to both proximate and distant kin. Remittances are one of the key determinants of the (lack of) ability to travel. Migrants whose parents benefit from a pension and free health services in El Salvador have better opportunities to save money for a trip back home than those who regularly send remittances to their parents. Even when remittances are not regularly sent back home, the ability to finance travel is seriously affected by the precariousness of the economic situation of the Salvadoran migrants, especially in the early years following their settlement in Australia.

Social relations   Social relations and access to a social network that facilitates the transnational exchange of care can be crucial. Community groups or neighbourhoods, for instance, can provide financial support in cases of emergency (for example, urgent travel to see a dying mother), give useful tips on low-cost travel options or communication technologies, provide access to communication technologies (like the Internet or telephone) and offer practical and emotional support (such as bringing presents to distant kin during a visit to the home or host country). This kind of community support was especially evident in the working-class post-war Italian migrant group, due to high levels of social capital developed through extensive community ties. Informal loan arrangements and other favours helped smooth the difficulties of settlement and transnational caregiving. More recent professional migrants, like all professionals, tend to develop friendship and support networks through their employment and career networks, which often provide support of a similar kind although perhaps with less intensity of relations, and financial support is usually not needed.

Salvadorans have not developed similarly intense community ties. The Salvadoran association that was created in the late 1980s to provide support to newly arrived refugees ceased its activities after a few years. The Salvadoran community is split into several subgroups, mainly organised around Spanish-speaking churches (Catholic and Baptist), and are mixed with Latin American migrants from various origins. Still, these groups can provide financial and practical help to their members, but in the majority of cases, this support is based on personal friendships.

Time allocation   Time allocation refers to the capacity to take time to exchange care with one's family. This means being available for virtual caring practices, such as via Internet or telephone conversations, access to time off from paid work for travel, and having the time to investigate possible caring options (for example, migrants who arrange admission to a nursing home at a distance or oversee care arrangements with the help of local carers). Choosing a part-time job in order to be able to enjoy extended visits home and have the flexibility to return home if and when required at short notice was a common pattern with Italian women in the sample, reflecting the broader gender pattern of women in part-time work in order to sustain the caregiving needs of their families. Transnational caregiving is, in many ways, an extension of this family care duty. The research by Baldassar et al. (2007a) found that the greater ability to stay in touch provided by new technologies has increased the sense of obligation to stay in touch, and therefore the burden of care.

For Amparo, time allocation was less an issue, as she could not afford the cost of lengthy phone calls, did not use the Internet, and only visited her parents once. Also, like many of the Salvadoran wives who participated in this study, she stayed at home to care for her children, and only worked outside the home on a casual basis. In the Salvadoran case, time is more a concern for men who work long hours and have to negotiate leave with their employers. In addition, the precariousness of short-term employment contracts deprives them of certain leave options, such as long-service leave (three months' paid leave accessible to employees with ten years of continuous service). Most men accumulate their annual paid vacations, and only travel once they have saved enough time to make a one- or two-month trip back home.

As Amparo's case shows, not having access to a satisfying employment situation, and when unemployed, to unemployment benefits, can limit people's capacity to send remittances and to cover the costs of long-distance care, such as those incurred by visits or by the use of communication technologies.

Education and knowledge Education and knowledge cover two different dimensions. The first relates directly to the capability to exchange care at a distance, and includes the opportunity to develop one's knowledge of communication technologies and to learn the host country's language. In our case, this language is English, which is also essential for mobility, as it is the language used in airports. The second is indirectly related to transnational care. Having one's qualifications recognised, or having the opportunity to study, impacts on one's socio-economic situation through access to paid work and income, which in turn influences the ability to participate in transnational caregiving.

Communication Being able to communicate with distant kin and to send them gifts is essential for long-distance care. Italian and Salvadoran migrants have different levels of access to communication technologies, and different abilities to afford this access. These differences are even more pronounced in the two home countries, since access to communication technologies is far more limited in El Salvador than it is in Italy. Age is a factor in the communication divide, not only with regard to knowledge about how to use the technology, but also having the physical health to use it, to hear a phone call, to type an email, to read a letter and so on.

The Influence of Institutions on Transnational Caregiving-related Capabilities

Despite arguments in the literature that the role of the nation state is diminished in transnational settings, an analysis of transnational caregiving-related capabilities reveals very clearly that the capability of Italian and Salvadoran migrants in Australia to exchange care at a distance is strongly influenced by both home and host country formal institutional and informal policies. These include – but are not limited to – migration policies; employment; work–family balance, education and gender equality policies; airline and communication regulation, and the development of communication infrastructures. While the state impacts on all the transnational caregiving-related capabilities that we have identified, we only have space here to focus on mobility, time allocation and communication. We then compare the role welfare regimes play in differently organised states, such as those characterised by more communalistic structures and those defined by individualism.

It is worth beginning with a comment on overriding social policy. For decades, Australia has been dominated by various forms of multicultural policy. This has the advantage of facilitating all kinds of arrangements for the benefit of diverse social groups, particularly migrants, and is evident in proactive initiatives, including community building grants, bilateral country agreements (like reciprocal healthcare and dual citizenship) and an attempt to foster community cohesion and harmony. Unfortunately, the progressive possibilities implied in multicultural policy are not evident in Australia's language policy, which lags behind multilingual Europe. Multicultural policy in Australia has been proactive in offering English language classes to migrants, although their success is variable and most critics argue that the service is inadequate to the task. A related issue is recognition of overseas qualifications, and here we see many inequities, with preferences for certain countries reflecting legacies of White Australia policy and British colonial practices.

In contrast to multicultural Australia, Italy is currently experiencing enormous tensions about how to handle its growing immigration (including illegal) intake within a broader context characterised by a Fortress Europe (Marfleet 1999) mentality that is hostile to religious and cultural diversity. This said, Italy has a host of initiatives designed to assist its own migrants abroad, including provincial and regional associations that foster community and support through diaspora newsletters, tour groups and websites. As remittances are essential to El Salvador's economy, it is important that migrants remain in their host country and keep sending money to their relatives. As a consequence, the Salvadoran government has developed initiatives designed to assist its own migrants abroad, one of the most visible being the creation of a special office in the Ministry of Foreign Affairs to oversee expatriates and migrants (Benavides et al. 2004). Its main objectives are to promote the integration of Salvadoran communities in their host countries, and to support the participation of the Salvadoran communities and associations in the economic, social and cultural development of El Salvador (Dirección General de Atención a la Comunidad en el Exterior 1998). The office also offers subscription to a 'virtual community' where information on El Salvador and its expatriates is exchanged.

The capability to be mobile is influenced by migration and visa policies, leave policies and airline regulations. Visa regulations are essential in granting travellers the right to cross borders and remain in the visited country for a certain period, while leave policies such as (paid) career breaks or holidays ensure that employed people can travel without putting their jobs at risk. States can also regulate airfares to ensure that travellers can be mobile at a reasonable price. Political refugees can be subject to visa restrictions in Australia which may limit their ability to travel. Italy and Australia enjoy reciprocal arrangements, so that visas to travel are only required for visits longer than three months. In contrast, El Salvador citizens require both expensive visas and health insurance in order to visit, which are more expensive for elderly people, making it more difficult, time-consuming and costly for Salvadoran elderly parents to visit.

Employment and work–family balance policies influence the capability to have time to engage in transnational caregiving practices. Policies aimed at offering a better balance between paid and unpaid work (such as gender equality, childcare, elder care and leave policies) rarely take the particularities of transnational care into consideration. This is primarily due to a lack of awareness about the requirements of transnational caregiving, and the almost total absence of transnational structures. For example, while Australia makes available a number of Carer Pensions to support people who care for others within the country, there is no bilateral arrangement which facilitates transnational caregiving. There is even an absence of awareness at the most basic level, where, for instance, it is difficult to facilitate communication between a migrant child in Australia and their parent's doctor abroad. The USA is spearheading changes in this area, with the introduction of 'care managers' – people who are employed to negotiate care arrangements on behalf of translocal kin (family members living a long way away but in the same country). Some migrants are beginning to make use of this initiative.

The state plays a determinant role in the provision and access to communication technologies, through the development of communication infrastructures (such as a reliable postal system, telephone lines and Internet connections), through price regulations, and through the development of policies to tackle the digital divide, like education about new technologies. The differences between Italy and El Salvador in this respect are striking, as the 'ICT at a glance' World Bank statistics show.[5] In 2005, 14.1 per cent of Salvadorans had access to telephone lines, compared to 42.7 per cent of Italians. Internet users represented 9.3 per cent of the population

---

5   Accessible on the World Bank's website, <http://www.worldbank.org/> (accessed 8 May 2011).

in El Salvador, compared to 47.8 per cent in Italy. Finally, only 5.1 per cent of the Salvadoran population had access to a personal computer, compared to 36.7 per cent of Italians. It is also interesting to note that the cost of the Internet is almost similar in the two countries (US\$22.60 per month in El Salvador and US\$24.80 in Italy in 2006), a figure which is particularly salient considering that 19 per cent of the Salvadoran population live on less than US\$1 per day.

Baldassar et al. (2007a; 2007b) found that while the digital divide might affect the older generation negatively, limiting their access to technology, it had a positive effect on family communication in general by extending the networks of support to include extended family members of the younger generations like nieces and nephews and grandchildren who use the technology on behalf of the elderly and so expand the networks of care. There is some suggestion that this has transformed the older communication structure from a 'hub', where information flowed through key people (like mothers), to a new 'star' structure, where information flows in a crisscross pattern and involves many more people. These changes were evident in both the Italian and Salvadoran case: migrants who still have their parents exchange information over the Internet with nieces, nephews or siblings who are equipped with a computer and play the role of key informants. Migrant children also play a determinant role in families where first-generation migrants are not familiar with computers and/or Internet technologies.

This brings us to another institution that plays a key role in transnational caregiving: the family. In particular, it is important to consider the changing role and structure of the family and how it differs across countries and how it impacts on transnational interactions. In both the Italian and Salvadoran cases, extended family solidarity partly helped migrants overcome the difficulties they faced in participating in their parents' care. Transnational caregiving does not only flow from host to home country, as Cecilia's case showed. Nor is it limited within the nuclear family. Given the strong family structures that characterise these two countries, Salvadoran and Italian migrants can count on the support and help of siblings, uncles and aunts, nieces and nephews, and even cousins. Apart from providing emotional support to the migrants when they need it, family networks contribute to the exchange of information between parents and their distant kin.

In the Salvadoran case, this extended family support is particularly critical, given the limited resources and economic conditions (Merla 2011; Merla forthcoming). Kin support not only helps compensate for the lack of communication infrastructures by family members offering to put their own computers and Internet connections at the service of transnational caregiving, they also help overcome financial difficulties linked to the prohibitive costs of telephone communication between El Salvador and Australia. A typical example is a brother living in the United States who relays information between his parents in El Salvador and his sister who lives in Australia. In emergencies, family members living in El Salvador know they can call family in the United States at a lower cost and ask them to call the migrants in Australia and inform them of the situation. This help is particularly important for the Australian migrants' well-being; they feel reassured by their access to timely and reliable information, particularly about family members who are chronically or critically ill. Extended family networks also help migrants finance their trip to Australia, especially in cases of emergency. But in contrast to the more recently arrived professional Italians, this help is limited to visits home: not a single Salvadoran migrant reported receiving money to help cope with expenses that were not related to a trip back home. Even problems generated by visa regulations restricting the parents' chances of visiting their children in Australia can be partly overcome by family solidarity. An example is a son living in the United States who invites both his parents and his Australian sister to meet at his house in the USA.

Conclusion

In this chapter, we wish to highlight an obvious though often invisible fact: that the ability to exchange care with one's ageing parents across distance can significantly impact on migrants' well-being. The capabilities approach proved particularly useful in examining this issue in two ways. First, it makes the link between transnational caregiving and well-being clear. By defining quality of life as one's freedom to live the kind of life which, upon reflection, one finds valuable, it allows us to acknowledge that being able to exchange care across distance can impact on well-being. Second, it highlights the key determinants that influence people's capacity to transform available resources into capabilities, and in particular the role of the state in facilitating or limiting well-being.

The capability of Italian and Salvadoran migrants in Australia to exchange care at a distance is strongly influenced by both home and host country formal institutional and informal policies such as migration policies, work–family balance, the development of communication infrastructures, as well as the institution of the family. A focus on the capability to be mobile, to have time to engage in transnational caregiving practices and to communicate with one's distant kin reveals important differences between Italian professional migrants and Salvadoran refugees. Of particular significance is the unequal access to the Australian territory due to differing visa regulations, the uneven capacity to access a similar employment position to the one held in the home country due to differing migration statuses, and the significant limitation of Salvadoran migrants' capability to communicate with their distant kin due to a lack of communication infrastructures in their homeland.

We highlighted the family as a key institution that influences transnational caregiving. This role is particularly important for countries which could be defined as familialist regimes, such as Italy and El Salvador. In both these countries, extended family solidarity partly helps migrants overcome the difficulties they face in participating in their parent's caring. Family networks contribute to the exchange of information between parents and their distant kin, helping to compensate for the lack of communication infrastructure or the ageing parent's inability to make use of new communication technologies; they provide financial support for travel, and can even help overcome problems generated by visa regulations restricting the parent's ability to visit their children. A key finding of our study is that institutional policies, both in home and host countries, completely overlook the important impact transnational caregiving can have on the well-being of both caregivers and the cared-for. There is an absence of specific policies designed to support transnational caregiving. We recommend that states work together to identify and develop a set of policies that address the needs of transnational families and their caregiving obligations. This requires that policy makers think beyond the usual confines of the nation, which by definition results in domestic policy. Based on our findings, we would argue that transnational caregiving policy is particularly needed in the area of citizenship and visas (the rules that govern entry and residence) and related reciprocal country arrangements for health cover for travellers; employment and leave entitlements (to allow carers the time to travel for caregiving), and development of access to new technologies (the mode of transnational caregiving).

Most people have some personal experience of transnational caregiving, yet the issue is largely invisible. Identifying transnational care as an important capability for well-being seems a useful way to better acknowledge and draw attention to this important social phenomenon.

References

Baldassar, L. (2001), *Visits Home: Migration Experiences between Italy and Australia*, Melbourne: Melbourne University Press.

—— (2004), 'Italians in Western Australia: From Dirty Ding to Multicultural Mate', in R. Wilding and F. Tilbury (eds), *A Changing People: Diverse Contributions to the State of Western Australia*, Perth: OMI, pp. 266–83.

—— (2007a), 'Transnational families and aged care: The mobility of care and the migrancy of ageing', *Journal of Ethnic and Migration Studies*, vol. 33, no. 2, pp. 275–97.

—— (2007b), 'Transnational families and the provision of moral and emotional support: The relationship between truth and distance', *Identities*, vol. 14, no. 4, pp. 385–409.

——, Baldock, C.V. and Wilding, R. (2007a), *Families Caring Across Borders: Migration, Ageing and Transnational Caregiving*, London: Palgrave Macmillan.

——, Wilding, R. and Baldock, C.V. (2007b), 'Long-distance Care-giving: Transnational Families and the Provision of Aged Care', in I. Paoletti (ed.), *Family Caregiving for Older Disabled People: Relational and Institutional Issues*, New York: Nova Science, pp. 201–27.

Benavides, B.M, Ortíz, X, Silva, C.M. and Vega, L. (2004), 'Pueden las remesas comprar el futuro? Estudio realizaso en el Cantón San José La Labor, Municipio de San Sebastián, El Salvador', in G. Lathrop and J.P. Pérez Saínz (eds),

Desarrollo económico local en Centroamérica. Estudios de comunidades globalizadas, San José, Costa Rica: Flacso, pp. 139–80.

Blackman, T. (2000), 'Defining responsibility for care: Approaches to the care of older people in six European countries', *International Journal of Social Welfare*, vol. 9, no. 3, pp. 181–90.

——, Brodhurst, S. and Convery, J. (eds) (2001), *Social Care and Social Exclusion: A Comparative Study of Older People's Care in Europe*, Basingstoke: Macmillan.

Dirección General de Atención a la Comunidad en el Exterior (1998), *Hacia una estrategia de integración y vinculación con las comunidades salvadoreñas en el exterior para el siglo XXI*, <http://www.elsalvador.org/embajadas/eeuu/home.nsf/0/b6e300a5b0fff36285256afc006b8a46?OpenDocument> (accessed 10 May 2011).

Finch, J. (1989), *Family Obligations and Social Change*, Cambridge: Polity Press.

Marfleet, P. (1999), 'Nationalism and internationalism in the new Europe', *International Socialism Journal*, no. 84.

Martínez Franzoni, J. (2005), 'Regímenes de bienestar en América Latina: Consideraciones generales e itinerarios regionales', *Revista Centroamericana de Ciencias Sociales*, vol. 2, no. 2, pp. 41–77.

—— (2008), *Domesticar la incertidumbre en América Latina: Mercado laboral, política social y familias*, San José, Costa Rica: Universidad de Costa Rica.

Merla, L. (2010), 'La gestion des émotions dans le cadre du devoir filial: le cas des migrants salvadoriens vivant en Australie occidentale', *Recherches sociologiques et anthropologiques*, vol. 41, no. 1, pp. 55–76.

—— (2011), 'Familles salvadoriennes à l'épreuve de la distance', *Autrepart*, nos 57–8.

—— (forthcoming), 'Salvadoran migrants in Australia: An analysis of transnational families' capability to care across borders', *International Migration* (accepted for publication).

Nussbaum, M. (2000), *Women and Human Development: The Capabilities Approach*, Cambridge: Cambridge University Press.

Office of Multicultural Interests (2005), *Western Australia Community Profiles 2001 Census: Central and South American-born*, Perth: Office of Multicultural Interests.

Robeyns, I. (2003), 'Sen's capability approach and gender inequality: Selecting relevant capabilities', *Feminist Economics*, vol. 9, nos 2–3, pp. 61–92.

—— (2007), 'Social Justice and the Gendered Division of Labour: Possibilities and Limits of the Capability Approach', paper presented at the COST Action 34 Conference, Barcelona, 25–27 June 2007.

Santos, B. (2006), 'From El Salvador to Australia: A 20th Century Exodus to a Promised Land', thesis submitted in total fulfilment of the requirements of the degree of Doctor of Philosophy, Australian Catholic University.

Singh, S. (2006), 'Towards a sociology of money and family in the Indian diaspora', *Contributions to Indian Sociology*, vol. 40, no. 3, pp. 375–98

Sen, A. (1980), 'Equality of What?', in S. McMurrin (ed.), *The Tanner Lectures on Human Values*, vol. 1, Cambridge: Cambridge University Press; reprinted in A. Sen (1982), *Choice, Welfare and Measurement*, Oxford: Blackwell, pp. 353–69.

—— (1985), *Commodities and Capabilities*, Amsterdam: North Holland; reprinted in 1999, Delhi: Oxford University Press.

—— (ed.) (1987), *The Standard of Living*, Cambridge: Cambridge University Press.

—— (1993), 'Capability and Well-being', in M. Nussbaum and A. Sen (eds), *The Quality of Life*, Oxford: Clarendon Press, pp. 31–53.

Wilding, R. and Baldassar, L. (2009), 'Transnational family–work balance: Experiences of Australian migrants caring for ageing parents and young children across distance and borders', *Journal of Family Studies*, vol. 15, no. 2, pp. 177–87.

Chapter 8

A Good Step Forward, but Not Far Enough: The Provision of Care Credits in European Pension Systems

Athina Vlachantoni[1]

There is a broad literature documenting the gradual transformation of pension provision into a policy problem (Banks and Emmerson 2000; Barr 2002); however, only a small part of this literature considers the reasons why pension provision is a problem for women in particular (Ginn and Arber 1993; Ginn et al. 2001b). Pension provision, in insurance-based systems more so than in non-contributory systems, has always created a challenge for women, in that pensions were not designed with them directly in mind. Instead, and particularly in insurance-based systems, women were intended to be *indirect* beneficiaries of the pension system through the marital bond to their husbands (Thane 2000). Traditionally designed pension systems of both types have been challenged by changes in men's and women's partnership, family and work patterns, and such changes have in some systems been taken into account in recent pension reforms (see, for example, the re-organisation of credits in the Basic and Second State Pension of carers in the UK through the Pension Reform Act 2007). However, the basic design of entitlement in pension systems has continued to be problematic (Ginn and Arber 1996; Leitner 2001). This is because typical male working patterns, which tend to be full-time, continuous and with increasing incomes throughout the working life, are still the default reference point for the calculation of pension entitlements, thereby overlooking the gender differences in work and care duties (Jenson and Sineau 2001; Lewis 1998). And it is this continuous 'mirroring' of, and failure to address, the differences and inequalities in the division of paid/unpaid labour which ultimately constitutes the pension problem from a gender perspective.

Although women's participation rates in the labour market have increased significantly since the mid-1970s, certain important differences in the nature of men's and women's participation patterns have remained (OECD 2002; SPC 2000). More women than men interrupt their working lives in order to care for dependants, and more women than men work part-time, which impacts on their

---

1   I would like to thank the editors of this volume, the anonymous reviewers, as well as Silke Roth and Lisa Warth and the participants of the COST Action 34 'Gender and Well-being' conference in Madrid in June 2008 for their helpful comments.

earnings throughout their lifetime, and particularly in old age (Ginn et al. 2001a). Across the EU-25 in 2005, and notwithstanding country variations, only 7 per cent of all working men were in part-time employment, compared to 1 in 3 women. In addition, part-time work is concentrated among relatively low-paid occupational sectors, such as health provision, education and service provision, and female part-time workers are more likely to spend their whole working life in this type of employment, while men tend to work part-time either at the beginning or at the very end of their working life (Laczko and Phillipson 1991; EFILWC 2003). Finally, the impact of women's employment patterns on pension accumulation is also affected by a gendered pay gap that in 2006 was still estimated at 15 per cent on average for the EU-27 (Eurostat 2006).

Changes in labour markets and their different implications for men and women are only part of the complex challenge that faces modern pension systems. Population ageing and the resultant increase in the cost of pension provision are an integral part of the pressure which has demanded the recalibration of pension systems (Bonoli and Shinkawa 2005; ISSA 2003; SPC 2000). These phenomena, too, like changes in labour markets, have distinct gender implications. Women across Europe tend to live longer than men, thereby constituting the majority of older people, but also the majority of older people facing the risk of poverty (European Commission 2006a; European Commission 2006b; Zaidi et al. 2006). On the other hand, cost-reducing strategies that target rising state pension expenditures are also more likely to disadvantage women than men, because women tend to be more reliant on statutory pension provision due to their tendency to have irregular ties with the labour market (Luckhaus 1997; Ginn 2004).

As part of their efforts to adjust to changing demographic, social and economic circumstances, European pension systems have responded with reform packages which combine various adjustments, such as the tightening of eligibility criteria, the changing balance of elements comprising the pension income, and the expansion of people's working lives (Holzmann et al. 2003). Pension reforms across the European Union have increasingly included the provision of care credits towards the carer's pension contributions in the statutory pension system in recognition of their caring work. Care credits take the form of an amount of time in months/years that is 'credited' to the carer's working record as if the carer were employed in the labour market. Theoretically, such amounts of time can be credited to a carer's pension contributions irrespective of whether the care is provided to under-age children, elderly persons or sick or disabled persons. In practice, however, and as will be shown later in this chapter, the concept of care credits has been applied to the provision of childcare to a much greater extent than other types of care.

The provision of care credits is an inherently gendered issue of social policy. This is because historically, most of the care has been provided by female family members, and this has not changed even as more women have entered the labour market (Bubeck 1995; EFILWC 1995; Jenson 1997). Far from a greater equalisation of caring obligations between men and women, there is evidence that labour market changes have led to a 'modernisation' of the division of paid and unpaid labour (Orloff 2002), whereby women combine the bulk of unpaid work with work in the labour market, while men's contribution to unpaid and/or care work has largely remained the same (Gershuny et al. 1994; OECD 2002). Consequently, unless labour markets are able to cater for care providers and pension systems to compensate carers with alternative ways of building up pension entitlements, caring for dependants – be they children, disabled or elderly persons – indirectly contributes to gender inequalities in the accumulation of lifetime and retirement income (Luckhaus and Ward 1997).

Care credits can be understood as an example of compensation within a system of pension provision that is inextricably linked with contributions to the paid labour market – what is termed 'gainful employment' in the policy literature – and which is consequently prone to producing gender inequalities in terms of pension accumulation prospects. As a mechanism of compensation within pension systems, care credits are a concept with multi-faceted policy significance. Firstly, like other mechanisms of compensating for time spent outside gainful employment, such as credits for time spent completing military service, care credits recognise the diversity in the individual life course, particularly with regard to work and care patterns. However, and unlike the recognition of military service, which is compulsory for men in some countries, care credits also serve to recognise the individual right to make choices throughout the life course for which individuals are not, directly or indirectly, penalised by the welfare state. Such recognition of diversity is particularly important for women whose care and employment patterns are often incompatible with eligibility rules in social security systems. Secondly, care credits ensure the valorisation of unpaid care work in the context of social insurance, thereby attaching a symbolic value in policy terms to the act or caring for dependants (Jenson 1997). Thirdly, care credits ensure the valorisation of unpaid care work, not just in principle, but also in practice, by attaching a temporal value to the credit contribution towards the carer's pension contribution record. Finally, care credits function as a vehicle for promoting greater gender equality in terms of pension accumulation, because across the developed world, the majority of care work still tends to be undertaken by women.

As part of the efforts to adjust modern pension systems to changing demographic, social and economic circumstances, care credits represent a good step forward in the promotion of gender equality within pension systems. At the same time, however, we need to consider the *kind* of gender equality which care credits imply, and it is here – in the application of the concept in practice – that this chapter argues that care credits could go even further. The rest of this chapter engages with these issues in four stages. The following section reviews the European strategy on gender equality and its application in pension provision, distinguishing between formal and substantive gender equality. Next, we will compare the operation of care credits in European pension systems based on a number of parameters, such as the length of time for which they credit a carer's contributions, the type of care for which they are awarded and the extent to which they can be combined with other care-related measures such as parental leave. Following this description is a discussion of the implications of the variety in the provision of care credits for the kind of gender equality pursued. It is argued that, although in principle care credits are an illustration of substantive gender equality in pension provision and thereby represent a good step forward for the promotion of gender equality, their practical implementation could be further expanded. The concluding section draws together the background and main points of the chapter, emphasising the policy challenge that the current organisation of care credit provision poses for addressing an increasing demand for elder care in Europe.

The European Strategy on Gender Equality and its Application in Pension Systems

Since its inception, the strategy of the European Communities for equal opportunities has primarily referred to opportunities provided in the employment sphere as part of the EC's economic goals. Part of the reason for this relates to the development of social policy at the European level more broadly, and its characterisation as 'something of a poor cousin' to economic policies (Caporaso and Jupille 2001). The strategy has three fundamental elements: Article 119 of the 1957 Treaty of Rome (known as Article 141 since the 1997 Amsterdam Treaty), the 1975 Directive on equal pay and the 1976 Directive on equal treatment. Article 119 expresses the fundamental principle that men and women should have equal pay and benefits in employment. The 1975 Directive on equal pay broadened the principle to include equal pay for work of equal value (75/117/EEC 1975), while the 1976 Directive on equal treatment extended the principle of equal treatment into areas adjacent to employment, such as training programmes and working conditions (76/207/EEC 1976).

During the late 1970s and early 1980s, and through established bodies such as the European Parliament's Committee on Women's Rights, the Equal Opportunities Unit and the European Women's Lobby, women mobilised to extend the equality discourse to areas beyond the labour market, into areas such as social security, the provision of care, unpaid work, and protection from sexual harassment and domestic violence. Some of these areas have been incorporated in the EC's strategy through the extension of the fundamental principle of Article 119. Such examples include the 1979 Directive on Equality on Social Security (79/7/EEC 1979), the 1986 Directive on equal treatment in occupational pension systems (86/378/EEC 1986) and the Community Charter of the Fundamental Social Rights of Workers 1989 (known in short as the 'Social Chapter'). Nevertheless, in practice, the effectiveness of such extensions beyond the strict boundaries of employment has been challenged for two main reasons, which are relevant to the discussion of compensatory mechanisms within modern pension systems. First, the inherent focus of the equal opportunities discourse on employment has undermined the conditions that hamper women's entry into the labour market, particularly the unequal division of labour in the private sphere of the household. And second, the diversity of policies with regard to gender and social policy at the national level has acted as a filter for European Directives, thus limiting their scope of implementation in domestic contexts (Williams 2003).

Since the mid-twentieth century, traditionally designed pension systems around Europe have reflected the gender differences in employment patterns and in wages, in addition to the unequal division of unpaid and care labour in the private sphere (Falkingham and Rake 1999). As a result, the pension problem for women was accentuated in Europe when more and more women started to receive a pension in their own right as a result of labour market participation (Ginn et al. 2001b). The adverse effects of women's typical working patterns can be mitigated, or compensated for, in several ways, reflecting the application of substantive equality that takes men's and women's differences into account. The application of substantive equality can be distinguished from the application of formal equality, whereby the same rule applies to all cases irrespective of their differences. One such mechanism is the calculation of the pension income according to the best income years of employment rather than the last 10 or 15 years, which often discriminates against women (Rake 1999). Similarly, the pension accumulation prospects of part-time workers are not compromised when the latter are permitted to 'buy' additional pension contributions (for example, in France and Germany), or when they are not penalised for transferring their pension rights from one sector to another (for example, in Germany and Denmark) (European Commission 2006b).

The pursuit of greater gender equality within pension systems more specifically, as well as pension adequacy for both men and women, is part of a broader pension policy agenda that developed rapidly at the European level after 2001 (SPC 2000; EPC 2001; CEU 2003). Increasing labour mobility and the need to harmonise occupational pension provision across the Continent provided the stimuli for the establishment of the Open Method of Coordination (OMC) for Pensions, which was streamlined in 2006 with European-wide policies in the areas of social protection and social inclusion. This common European agenda pledges to 'ensure that pension systems are transparent [and] well-adapted to the needs and aspirations of women and men and the requirements of modern societies' (COM (2005) 706 final 2005). However, at the national level, the adaptation of the principle of gender equality within pension systems has varied greatly, taking one of two forms.

The first form that gender equality strategies take in European pension systems promotes gender equality in the formal sense of the term – that is, by trying to establish equality between women and men without necessarily taking gender differentiations in work, life and care patterns into account. Given that pension systems tend to reward full-time, continuous and highly paid employment records, women face a *de facto* disadvantage in terms of building adequate pension rights. The problem with such strategies goes to the heart of the broader gender equality agenda at the European level – namely, it lies with the focus on paid employment as the fundamental reference principle for establishing equality or 'sameness' between men and women. As Luckhaus and Ward note, 'sameness in this context

... has been taken to mean men and women in paid work: it does not extend to men or women engaged in unpaid work' (Luckhaus and Ward 1997, p. 242). An example of promoting this form of gender equality is the abolition of differences between men and women in terms of the retirement age (European Commission 2006b). The equalisation of retirement ages in the name of gender equality may be taking higher female life expectancy into account and providing women with a longer period in which to build pension contributions, but it does not take into account women's greater tendency to care for dependants in the family.

The second form of gender equality strategies has a compensatory character, which means that these strategies take account of the origins of the pension problem for women and the gender differences in typical working/caring patterns. The existence of differentiated retirement ages for men and women before these were deemed illegal by EC legislation is an illustration of such a compensatory mechanism. In many developed countries, albeit not always explicitly, the establishment of different retirement ages reflected the state's assumptions about women's and men's roles in society. Because of women's higher life expectancy on average, rather than in spite of it, earlier retirement was granted to women so that, first, the couple would enjoy their retirement simultaneously, because women were usually younger than their husbands, and second, widows would receive social protection earlier (Fredman 1996). In this way, the state could claim to recognise women's contribution to the household, which was more likely than their contribution to the labour market. In reality, the policy intention behind this measure was not entirely benign, as the difference in retirement ages also compensated for the relatively low wages of women who were in fact engaged in paid employment *in addition* to their unpaid work in the household (Arber and Ginn 1995). The age of retirement is an area where equal treatment is not immediately applicable under EC law; rather, member states are obliged to examine their legislation periodically and to establish whether the derogation from the equality principle is still justified in each case (79/7/EEC 1979). For the time being, certain member states still have different retirement ages for men and women (for example, Poland, Italy, Slovenia and Austria until 2024), but are in the process of gradually abolishing them (European Commission 2006b).

The principal compensatory measure in pension systems, and another application of equality of a substantive nature, remains the provision of care credits which count towards the carer's basic state pension contributions. The provision of such credits for childcare varies considerably between member states, while the provision of such credits for long-term sick/disabled adult family members who are in need of care or for elderly family members (within or outside one's own household, but not within care institutions) is a far rarer practice. The following section reviews the operation of care credits in the European member states, drawing contrasts which are discussed later in the chapter.

Care Credits in European Pension Systems

Drawing on the most recent information supplied to the European Commission by national governments (except for Bulgaria and Romania), Table 8.1 summarises the operation of care credits in the European countries (MISSOC 2006). The table reflects the variation in policy assumptions about the symbolic and monetary value of care credits in each country context, as well as their role in each country's broader framework of social security. Three kinds of variation are discussed in this section: firstly, variations according to the type of care credits provided; secondly, variations according to the specific characteristics of such provisions, and thirdly, variations according to the assumptions behind the provision of credits for childcare.

In the first instance, there are European countries which do not provide any explicit credits for carers of either children, disabled or elderly persons (such as Denmark, the Netherlands and Slovenia), countries which provide one type of credit but not another (for example, Cyprus and Lithuania provide credits for childcare, but not for family/elder care, whereas Finland provides credits for family/elder care, but not for childcare), and countries which provide credits for care provided to all kinds of dependent persons within the household (such as Germany and Poland). With the exception of Finland, all of the countries which offer care credits for the provision of one type of care but not for another provide credits for periods spent caring for children (including disabled children), but not for periods spent caring for other dependent persons within the household, whether disabled or elderly. It should be noted that the analysis here solely depends on MISSOC data, and that some countries may operate additional mechanisms of care valorisation which are integrated in their broader welfare system and which would be evidenced in a more detailed case-by-case investigation.

There are a couple of implications of this kind of variation. The first implication is that where care credits are not provided for any type of care, this does not necessarily mean that the activity of caring *per se* is not recognised elsewhere within the social security system. The second implication, evident in the majority of European countries, is the selective valorisation of care by recognising childcare, but not recognising care for long-term sick or elderly persons in need of care. We will return to this point later in the chapter.

The second kind of variation in terms of the nature and the generosity of care credit provision is more widespread across Europe. In certain countries, credits for childcare are provided for parts or for the whole of the periods during which maternity and/or parental benefits are received (for example, Spain, Hungary and Poland). Other countries exhibit greater generosity by extending the covered period beyond such leave: for instance, Austria and Sweden provide (up to) four years of contributions to carers for every child, while France and Luxembourg provide two years for every child. Finally, in some countries the provision of care credits contributes to pro-natalist policies, as the number of contribution years per child increases with the number of children (for example, Austria and Greece). For

Table 8.1   Credits for childcare and for family/elder care in European countries

	Credits for childcare	Credits for family/elder care
Austria	Child-raising periods (maximum of 4 years per child, 5 years for multiple birth) Period receiving maternity benefit	None
Belgium	Child-raising periods (2 years maximum)	None
Bulgaria	N/A	N/A
Cyprus	Child-raising periods (maximum 156 weeks per child up to 12 years old to women entitled to pension after 1 January 1993) Period receiving maternity and parental benefits	None
Czech Republic	Child-raising periods (for child up to 4 years old)	Periods caring for a close relative who is incapacitated
Denmark	None	None
Estonia	Child-raising periods (child up to 8 years old)	None
Finland	None	Periods caring for dependants
France	Child-raising periods (2 years per child – for mothers) Period receiving maternity benefit and parental leave (within a limit of 3 years)	None
Germany	Child-raising period (3 years for every child up to 10 years old)	Period caring for dependants
Greece	Child-raising period for mothers of children born after 1 January 2003: 1 year for 1st child, 1½ years for 2nd child, 2 years for 3rd child and thereafter (maximum 4½ years)	None
Hungary	Period receiving the pregnancy-confinement benefit and childcare fee	None
Ireland	Child-raising period (full basic pension if up to 20 years' caring for children under 12 years old)	Full basic pension if up to 20 years' providing care to incapacitated persons of any age

Italy	Period receiving maternity benefit Additional optional buy-out of up to 6 months per child	Period caring for dependants (1 month per year maximum)
Latvia	Child-raising period (child up to 8 years old)	None
Lithuania	Period receiving maternity benefit	None
Luxembourg	Child-raising period (2 years per child)	Periods caring for dependants
Malta	None	None
Poland	Period receiving parental leave	Periods caring for a dependent person
Portugal	Child-raising period (2 years per child) Period receiving maternity benefit	None
Slovakia	Child-raising periods (children up to 6 years old, or up to 7 years old if the child is long-term severely disabled) Periods receiving maternity and parental benefits	Period receiving the benefit for care for a sick relative
Slovenia	None	None
Spain	First year of parental leave for child-raising up to 3 years old.	None
Sweden	Child-raising period (4 years for each child, longer for disabled child)	None
Switzerland	Child-raising period (for one or more children up to 16 years old)	Period caring for relatives in ascending or descending line, brothers and sisters, helpless and living in the same household
The Netherlands	None	None
UK	Child-raising period (for children up to 16 years old) (towards basic pension and for carers with 20 years of contributions – 1978 Home Responsibilities Protection) Periods receiving carer's allowance, statutory maternity pay, statutory adoption pay	Period caring for dependants (towards basic pension and for carers with 20 years of contributions – 1978 Home Responsibilities Protection) Period receiving carer's allowance

Source: MISSOC (2006).

the countries which provide care credits based on the period for which parental/
maternity benefits can be received, this kind of variation also reflects the different
value attached to different types of care provided, as leave to care for dependants
other than children tends to be shorter. The third kind of variation specifically to
do with childcare relates to policy assumptions about the age at which a child
is assumed to require less intense care and supervision, and the point at which
a child's carer is presumed available and able to enter (or re-enter) the labour
market. For example, Latvia provides credits for the period up to when a child is 8
years old, Estonia until the child is 10 years old, and Ireland and Cyprus until the
child is 12 years old.

A different kind of variation, which is equally important but less readily
observable from Table 8.1, relates to the policy intention behind the introduction of
care credits, which, as with any policy measure, is difficult to disentangle from the
final policy outcome. For instance, the German welfare state, which pioneered the
concept of care credits, was said to have introduced credits in order to recognise
women's contribution to the provision of care for dependants (Hohnerlein 2000).
But there can be several intentions behind the introduction of care credits, relating
to the different elements which they consist of, such as the temporal value of the
credit or the extent to which it is explicitly targeted at female carers. Such elements
can encourage a more equal division of paid/unpaid labour, facilitate entry or re-
entry of the carer in the labour market, facilitate the individual accumulation of
pension contributions, encourage women to have more children and/or contribute
to the amelioration of poverty in old age. We would expect, for example, that a
carer would be under greater pressure to enter the labour market in order to make
up for years 'lost' to care in terms of pension contributions where the temporal and
monetary value of care credits is low. By contrast, where care credits are generous
contributions towards a carer's pension record, we would expect that the carer can
exercise greater choice between continuing to provide care or joining or rejoining
the labour force to add to their individual or their household's income.

Although these variations can tell us a great deal about the differences
between countries in terms of the provision of care credits and the kind of gender
equality they promote, the real value and effect of care credits on a carer's
pension contributions must be assessed in the context of the broader pension
system in which the credits operate. In this respect, categorisations of pension
systems which go beyond the widely used Beveridgean/Bismarckian dichotomy[2]
are useful reference points. For example, Ginn and Arber have categorised the
pension systems of Western Europe according to the extent to which they provide

---

2   Beveridgean pension systems, named after William Beveridge, the architect of
the modern welfare state in Britain, typically provide a flat-rate pension, financed through
flat-rate National Insurance contributions. Bismarckian pension systems are named after
Otto von Bismarck, the Chancellor who introduced old-age pensions in Germany. They are
also funded through contributions, but both the size of the contributions and the benefits are
earnings-related.

opportunities for women to build pension rights (Ginn and Arber 1992), and along the lines of these groups of countries, Leitner has stressed the importance of looking at women's particular social and economic roles when assessing pension systems from a gender perspective (Leitner 2001). The 'basic security model', exemplified by Scandinavian countries and the Netherlands, provides a citizen's pension which is not determined by a person's employment (or caring) record, and which is combined with state earnings-related and occupational pension protection to provide adequate income security in old age. In the 'income security model', exemplified by Continental and to a lesser extent by Southern European countries, earnings-related pension schemes provide the bulk of income security in old age, thereby disadvantaging those with weak ties to the labour market (Ginn and Arber 1994). Here, the financial importance of care credits may be greater than in Scandinavian countries, as the link between pension contributions and the labour market tends to be stronger, but this is only the case if compensation for caring is included. Finally, in the 'residual model', exemplified by the UK and Ireland, the minimum pension has to be supplemented by earnings-related and/or private pension provision in order to provide income security in old age. Therefore, it is probably in this model where care credits can make the greatest difference for the pension income of carers, because compensation for care tends to be included in minimum pension provision, but not in occupational or private pension provision.

Care Credits in Practice: One Good Step Forward, but Not Far Enough

In principle, the provision of care credits towards pension contributions is a mechanism that compensates carers for the time they have spent outside the primary locus for accumulating pension entitlements. In this sense, they represent a good step forward for gender equality in three distinct ways. Firstly, in so far as they recognise the existence of differentiated life courses for the purpose of pension accumulation, care credits are consistent with the application of substantive gender equality. This is a significant departure from gender equalisation efforts which often result in 'downward' equalisation for women's entitlements – a loss, in other words, of additional rights which women had in recognition of their differentiated contribution to society (Fredman 1996). Given the continuing differences between typical male and female life, care and work patterns, a substantive perspective on gender equality is more likely to be beneficial for women in pension accumulation terms.

Secondly, the idea of providing care credits towards pension records departs from the conventional link in European-level social policy between paid employment and the promotion of gender equality. This departure represents a good forward step in that it is an important recognition that any policy strategy aimed at the further application of gender equality must also take men's and women's contribution in the private sphere into account. Considering the development to date of gender equality strategies at the European level, as discussed earlier in this chapter, the greater incorporation of private-sphere activities in discussions of gender equality is a considerable change of direction, reflecting also the different ways in which member states choose to combine employment and family policies (see Kaufmann 2002).

Thirdly, care credits also depart from the inherent link in traditional pension systems between pension accumulation and paid employment. The implications, and benefits, of this departure are particularly important for women in country contexts where the combination of work and care is more difficult, resulting in a higher care penalty in terms of pension accumulation. The value of care credits, both symbolically and in financial terms, may also be higher in contexts where female labour in the informal labour market is more prevalent and also more likely to go unnoticed for the purposes of social security, for example in Southern European countries (Kilpelainen 2004).

For these reasons, care credits undoubtedly represent a good step forward for carers, but also for individuals (male or female) who tend to follow less typical life courses which may be rewarded to a lesser extent by traditional pension system structures. The recognition of care as an activity that is worthy of valorisation within pension provision should also be regarded as a sign that social policy is more responsive to societal norms. In addition, and as long as women tend to perform the majority of (unpaid) caring within households, care credits represent a step forward, particularly for women. Nevertheless, in terms of their practical implementation, care credits could go even further, in three distinct ways.

The first way is by addressing the wide variation in the provision of care credits across European member states, as illustrated in Table 8.1. This variation reflects the lack of a uniform approach to the valorisation of care provision for the purpose of pension accumulation, which creates inequalities between European member states. Admittedly, the variation between different pension systems in the degree to which they 'mirror' and perpetuate gender inequalities in the labour market is difficult to eliminate, particularly given the strength of the principle of subsidiarity, which protects nation states' freedom to design and implement domestic social policy. Such variations in the degree to which redistributive and non-redistributive elements are combined in the entitlement structure can make a difference for women's pension accumulation prospects (Leitner 2001). For example, the closer the link between earnings and pension income, the more women are disadvantaged, because female employment records tend to be shorter, interrupted and in lower-paid jobs. Women are also more likely to be disadvantaged when occupational pension schemes place high thresholds of eligibility in terms of one's years of service, earnings or the level of one's contributions (Ginn et al. 2001b). In addition, if greater homogeneity in the provision of care credits in Europe is deemed desirable, a question remains about the appropriate policy instrument to implement and monitor it, particularly as co-ordination efforts in fields of social policy across the EC are subject to subsequent adjustment at the national level.

Secondly, as long as periods spent caring for dependants are valued to a lesser extent than periods spent working in the labour market, the provision of care credits remains an inadequate mechanism of compensation. As a result, and in their current form, care credits are an instrument which partly mitigates but also partly maintains different kinds of inequalities in modern pension systems. One kind of inequality refers to the type of contribution individuals make to society, distinguishing fundamentally between productive and reproductive contributions, but also different combinations of the two which allow the combination of work and family obligations by both men and women. If women continue to provide most of the care for dependants, then they will continue to be in a relatively worse-off position within pension systems.

The third way in which care credits could go further in the manner in which they are applied is by encouraging their use by both men and women carers. The broader issue of concern here is whether modern welfare states actually promote female emancipation by recognising gender differences, or whether they perpetuate existing structures of gender inequalities and female subordination. In other words, do care credits serve, at least in part, to preserve women's and men's traditional roles in society, which carry specific advantages/disadvantages within current pension entitlement structures? As Luckhaus and Ward point out, this is a drawback only as long as women tend to use care credits more than men for the purpose of building up pension contributions (Luckhaus and Ward 1997). Where only female carers (and often only carers of children rather than of other persons in need of care) are encouraged to make use of care credits, the net benefit of compensatory mechanisms for women's pension security remains unclear.

Conclusion

Care credits continue to be the primary compensatory mechanism for those who devote a considerable part of their life to persons in need of care, be they children, elderly or long-term sick or disabled persons. As such, their inclusion in modern pension systems is a welcome policy which helps to mitigate differences in men's and women's typical life courses, but the way care credits are currently organised – for instance, rewarding the provision of childcare over other types of care – raises further challenges for policy makers. Two policy-relevant conclusions can be drawn from the review in this chapter.

Firstly, the application of care credits must be incorporated in a broader framework of social policies designed to compensate carers without simultaneously promoting caring as a woman-only activity. The balance of these goals can be achieved through incentives which are seen to reward caring in the context of pension accumulation, or through incentives which ensure that caring is not penalised in social security terms.

Secondly, policy makers have the opportunity to expand the remit of care credits to cover care provided to older persons as well. This is an important step in light of the increasing demand for elder care which results from both demographic change and population ageing (Pavolini and Ranci 2008). The current emphasis of care credits on childcare over other types of care, combined with the lack of a European-wide, uniform strategy to valorise care provision *per se*, suggests an underestimation of this demand at a critical time for the provision of long-term care. European policy makers are drawing attention to the impact of population ageing on the prevalence of chronic diseases, disability and dependence among older people, the concomitant increase in demand on formal care as more women enter the labour market, and the shift in the responsibility for providing care away from institutional care and towards home care (European Commission 2008). Against the background of these developments, the further expansion of the concept of care credits could be at the centre of a strategy to address this demand effectively via a top-down EC initiative and the equal recognition by pension systems of different types of care provided.

References

75/117/EEC (1975), *Council Directive 75/117/EEC of 10 February 1975 on the approximation of the laws of the member states relating to the application of the principle of equal pay for men and women*, Brussels: European Union.

76/207/EEC (1976), *Council Directive 76/207/EEC of 9 February 1976 on the implementation of the principle of equal treatment for men and women as regards access to employment, vocational training and promotion, and working conditions*, Brussels: European Union.

79/7/EEC (1979), *Council Directive 79/7/EEC of 19 December 1978 on the progressive implementation of the principle of equal treatment for men and women in matters of social security*, Brussels: European Union.

86/378/EEC (1986), *Council Directive 86/378/EEC of 24 July 1986 on the implementation of the principle of equal treatment for men and women in occupational pension schemes*, Brussels: European Union.

Anderson, M. et al. (eds) (1994), *The Social and Political Economy of the Household*, Oxford: Oxford University Press.

Arber, S. and Ginn, J. (1995), 'Gender differences in the relationship between paid employment and informal care', *Work, Employment and Society*, vol. 9, no. 3, pp. 445–71.

Baldwin, S. and Falkingham, J. (eds) (1994), *Social Security and Social Change: New Challenges to the Beveridge Model*, Hemel Hempstead: Harvester Wheatsheaf.

Banks, J. and Emmerson, C. (2000), 'Public and private pension spending: Principles, practice and the need for reform', *Fiscal Studies*, vol. 21, no. 1, pp. 1–63.

Barr, N.A. (2002), 'Reforming pensions: Myths, truths and policy choices', *International Social Security Review*, vol. 55, no. 2, pp. 3–36.

Bonoli, G. and Shinkawa, T. (2005), *Ageing and Pension Reform Around the World: Evidence from Eleven Countries*, Cheltenham: Edward Elgar.

Bubeck, D.E. (1995), *Care, Gender and Justice*, Oxford: Clarendon Press.

Caporaso, J.A. and Jupille, J. (2001), 'The Europeanization of Gender Equality Policy and Domestic Structural Change', in M. Green Cowles et al. (eds), *Transforming Europe: Europeanization and Domestic Change*, Ithaca, NY: Cornell University Press.

Clasen, J. (ed) (1999), *Comparative Social Policy: Concepts, Theories and Methods*, Oxford: Blackwell.

COM (2005) 706 final (2005), *Communication from the Commission to the Council, the European Parliament, the European Economic and Social Committee and the Committee of the Regions. Working Together, Working Better: A New Framework for the Open Coordination of Social Protection and Inclusion Policies in the European Union*, Brussels: European Commission.

Council of the European Union (CEU) (2003), *Joint Report by the Commission and the Council on Adequate and Sustainable Pensions*, Brussels: Council of the European Union.

Economic Policy Committee (EPC) (2001), *Budgetary Challenges Posed by Ageing Populations: the Impact on Public Spending on Pensions, Health and Long-term Care for the Elderly and Possible Indicators of the Long-term Sustainability of Public Finances*, Brussels: European Union.

European Commission (2006a), *Joint Report on Social Protection and Social Inclusion 2006: Synthesis Report on Adequate and Sustainable Pensions*, Brussels: European Union.

—— (2006b), *Joint Report on Social Protection and Social Inclusion 2006: Synthesis Report on Adequate and Sustainable Pensions (Horizontal Analysis)*, Brussels: European Union.

—— (2008), *Joint Report on Social Protection and Social Inclusion*, Brussels: European Union.

European Foundation for the Improvement of Living and Working Conditions (EFILWC) (1995), *Who Will Care? Future Prospects for Family Care of Older People in the European Union*, Dublin: EFILWC.

—— (2003), *Part-time Work in Europe*, Dublin: EFILWC.

Eurostat (2005), 'Gender Pay Gap in Unadjusted Form', European Statistics, <http://europa.eu/documentation/statistics-polls/index_en.htm> (home page) (accessed 8 May 2011).

Falkingham, J. and Rake, K. (1999), *Partnership in Pensions: Delivering a Secure Retirement for Women?*, CASEpaper 24, London: London School of Economics, Centre for Analysis of Social Exclusion.

Fredman, S. (1996), 'The poverty of equality: Pensions and the European Court of Justice', *Industrial Law Journal*, vol. 25, no. 2, pp. 91–109.

Gershuny, J.I. et al. (1994), 'The Domestic Labour Revolution: A Process of Lagged Adaptation?', in M. Anderson et al. (eds), *The Social and Political Economy of the Household*, Oxford: Oxford University Press.

Ginn, J. (2004), *Actuarial Fairness or Social Justice? A Gender Perspective on Redistribution in Pension Systems*, Moncalieri: Centre for Research on Pensions and Welfare Policies.

—— and Arber, S. (1992), 'Towards women's independence: Pension systems in three contrasting European welfare states', *Journal of European Social Policy*, vol. 2, no. 4, pp. 255–77.

—— and Arber, S. (1993), 'Pension penalties: The gendered division of occupational welfare', *Work, Employment and Society*, vol. 7, no. 1, pp. 47–70.

—— and Arber, S. (1994), 'Heading for Hardship: How the British Pension System Has Failed Women', in S. Baldwin and J. Falkingham (eds), *Social Security and Social Change: New Challenges to the Beveridge Model*, Hemel Hempstead: Harvester Wheatsheaf.

—— and Arber, S. (1996), 'Patterns of employment, pensions and gender: The effect of work history on older women's non-state pensions', *Work, Employment and Society*, vol. 10, no. 3, pp. 469–90.

Ginn, J. et al. (2001a), 'Cross-national Trends in Women's Work', in J. Ginn et al. (eds), *Women, Work and Pensions: International Issues and Prospects*, Buckingham: Open University Press.

—— (2001b), 'Engendering Pensions: A Comparative Framework', in J. Ginn et al. (eds), *Women, Work and Pensions: International Issues and Prospects*, Buckingham: Open University Press.

—— (eds) (2001c), *Women, Work and Pensions: International Issues and Prospects*, Buckingham: Open University Press.

Green Cowles, M. et al. (eds), *Transforming Europe: Europeanization and Domestic Change*, Ithaca, NY: Cornell University Press.

Hobson, B. (ed.) (2003), *Recognition Struggles and Social Movements*, Cambridge: Cambridge University Press.

Hohnerlein, E.M. (2000), *Policy Measures in German Public Pension System to Cope with Low Fertility*, National Institute of Population and Social Security Research Study Series 3, pp. 28-45.

Holzmann, R. et al. (eds) (2003), *Pension Reform in Europe: Process and Progress*, Washington, DC: The World Bank.

International Social Security Association (ISSA) (2003), *Ageing and Social Security: Ten Key Issues*, Geneva: International Social Security Association.

Jenson, J. (1997), 'Who cares? Gender and welfare regimes', *Social Politics*, vol. 4, no. 2, pp. 182–7.

—— and Sineau, M. (2001), *Who Cares? Women's Work, Childcare and Welfare State Redesign*, Toronto: University of Toronto Press.

Kaufmann, F.-X. (2002), *Family Life and Family Policies in Europe*, Oxford: Oxford University Press.

Kilpelainen, R. (2004), *Formal and Informal Work in Europe: Preliminary Findings Based on the ECHP Data*, Discussion Paper no. 8, EU Formal and Informal Work in Europe (FIWE) Project.

Laczko, F. and Phillipson, C. (1991), *Changing Work and Retirement: Social Policy and the Older Worker*, Milton Keynes: Open University Press.

Leitner, S. (2001), 'Sex discrimination within EU pension systems', *Journal of European Social Policy*, vol. 11, no. 2, pp. 99–115.

Lewis, J. (1998), *Gender, Social Care and Welfare State Restructuring in Europe*, Aldershot: Ashgate.

Luckhaus, L. (1997), 'Privatisation and pensions: Some pitfalls for women?', *European Law Journal*, vol. 3, no. 1, pp. 83–100.

—— and Ward, S. (1997), 'Equal pension rights for men and women: A realistic perspective', *Journal of European Social Policy*, vol. 7, no. 3, pp. 237–53.

Mutual Information System on Social Protection in the EU Member States and the EEA (MISSOC) (2006), <http://ec.europa.eu/employment_social/social_protection/missoc_tables_archives_en.htm> (home page) (accessed 8 May 2011).

Organisation for Economic Cooperation and Development (OECD) (2002), 'Women at Work: Who are They and How are They Faring?' *Employment Outlook 2002*, Paris: OECD.

Orloff, A.S. (2002), *Women's Employment and Welfare Regimes: Globalisation, Export Orientation and Social Policy in Europe and North America*, Paper 12, Geneva: United Nations Research Institute for Social Development Programme.

Pavolini, E. and Ranci, C. (2008), 'Restructuring the welfare state: Reforms in the long-term care in Western European countries', *Journal of European Social Policy*, no. 18, pp. 246–59.

Rake, K. (1999), 'Accumulated Disadvantage? Welfare State Provision and the Incomes of Older Women and Men in Britain, France and Germany', in J. Clasen (ed.), *Comparative Social Policy: Concepts, Theories and Methods*, Oxford: Blackwell.

Social Protection Committee (SPC) (2000), *Adequate and Sustainable Pensions: A Report by the Social Protection Committee on the Future Evolution of Social Protection*, Brussels: European Union.

Thane, P. (2000), *Old Age in English History: Past Experiences, Present Issues*, Oxford: Oxford University Press.

Williams, F. (2003), 'Contesting "Race" and Gender in the European Union: A Multilayered Recognition Struggle for Voice and Visibility', in B. Hobson (ed.), *Recognition Struggles and Social Movements*, Cambridge: Cambridge University Press.

Zaidi, A. et al. (2006), *Pension Policy in EU25 and its Possible Impact on Elderly Poverty*, CASEpaper 116, London: London School of Economics, Centre for the Analysis of Social Exclusion.

PART III
Gender and Well-being in the Labour Market

Chapter 9

Gender (In)equality in the Labour Market and the Southern European Welfare States

Sara Falcão Casaca and Sónia Damião

The decline of the male-breadwinner model and the increasing participation of women in the labour market are contemporary features in European societies, including those of the so-called Southern European countries. Within this group, it is worth noting that the female employment rate in Portugal is considerably higher than in its Southern European counterparts, which are commonly viewed as 'latecomers' in terms of their social provision and commitment to childcare/elder care facilities (see Cousins 2000; Flaquer 2000; Carlos and Maratou-Alipranti 2000; Simoni and Trifiletti 2004). The welfare state is regarded as playing an important role in the modernisation of gender roles, by either encouraging or discouraging women's involvement in the labour market and influencing the patterns of such participation (Addis 1999). Building on this viewpoint, this chapter will compare the policies and measures designed and implemented in Portugal, Spain, Italy and Greece with regard to the reconciliation of work and family life. The data under analysis were provided by official European and national databases, and the selected period covered the years following the accession of both Portugal and Spain to the European Economic Community in 1986, since Italy and Greece were already members at that time.

The first section briefly reviews some feminist contributions calling for the inclusion of a gender perspective in the classical debate on the welfare state; the second section is devoted to an analysis of the indicators of gender relations in the labour market, and finally, a comparative picture is provided of the different policies and facilities available in the countries under analysis, mainly concerning childcare facilities and leave arrangements.

Gendering the Welfare States: The Debate

Feminist scholars have been critical of the Esping-Andersen typology of welfare regimes because of its gender-blindness. Lister (1994) and McLaughlin and Glendinning (1994), for instance, suggest that in addition to the concept of *decommodification*, there is a need to incorporate the concept of *defamilialisation* in the analysis of the dichotomy between dependence and independence. According to this view, women's independence only occurs in a scenario in which they are free from family and caring obligations, as well as from domestic affairs and related responsibilities (see Lewis 1992; Orloff, 1993). Another feminist, Nancy Fraser (1994), lays emphasis on the need for a new gender order, in which the traditional gendered opposition between breadwinning (socially associated with the main role of men) and caregiving (socially viewed as the main role of women), reinforced during the industrial era of capitalism, is eradicated. Accordingly, the debate on welfare states needs to embrace a vision that is compatible with a new gender order and with the specificities of Southern European regimes concerning gender issues (see, for example, Addis 1999; Trifiletti 1999).

According to Jane Lewis (1992), in so far as non-paid work dimensions are added to paid work ones, it is possible to identify some variations among welfare states: those which are based on a *strong male-breadwinner model*, those which may be classified as a *modified male-breadwinner model*, and finally, those where a *weak male-breadwinner model* prevails (the model found in Scandinavian countries; see Chapters 3 and 11 in this volume for details, merits and shortcomings of this model). Other typologies have been developed by feminist writers; the common trend has been to associate the prevalence of traditional gender regimes with Ireland and Southern European countries, while more modern gender regimes are said to be found in Northern European countries.

However, despite the helpful contribution made by analytical frameworks to the debate on gender regimes and welfare states, especially in terms of historical research and comparative analyses of contemporary societies, the specific gender regimes in Southern European countries show how difficult it is to develop typologies. According to Trifiletti (1999), the Mediterranean family is quite different from that of the traditional breadwinner model, as the state does not guarantee a family wage, and families' strategies often follow a pragmatic orientation in order to ensure that at least one member provides as much as possible ('breadcrumb revenues') and has a secure job (see Flaquer 2000; Saraceno 2004). The reality is more complex, heterogeneous and multi-faceted than the one that is commonly portrayed in typologies; as a result, the hierarchical continuum, ranging from traditional gender roles to more egalitarian ones, is far from being linear and simple to figure out (see, for example, Daly and Rake 2003; Aboim 2007; Wall 2007).

Labour Market Participation and Fertility Patterns

As demonstrated in Chapter 4 of this volume, the Mediterranean countries have low female labour market participation rates and low fertility, making these countries highly unequal in gender equality terms and – it is claimed – not sustainable, since fertility is well below reproduction level. To improve the well-being of women (and increase fertility), EU member countries have implemented different policies to help women reconcile paid work and family life. Chapter 10 of this volume, studying Greece, maintains that such policies are central to changing gender roles, in particular for women.

According to our data, the weakening of the male-breadwinner model seems to be occurring at very different rates in the four countries under analysis. Portugal exhibited the highest female employment rate in 2006 (62 per cent) and the lowest difference in relation to men, whereas the gender gap was particularly noticeable in Greece (see Table 9.1). The participation of Spanish women in the labour market has increased significantly over the last ten years, with the rate doubling between 1986 and 2006 (for further discussion, see Tobío 2005).

Portugal also stands out as the country in which the employment rates of mothers of children under 2 years of age (69.1 per cent) and those of children aged 3–5 (about 71.8 per cent) are high. In addition to this, the participation of Portuguese women in employment tends to be continuous over their life cycle, since in general they do not interrupt their careers after childbirth – as shown by the marginal decline (0.2 percentage points) seen in Table 9.1 – in sharp contrast to the common trend in Italy and Spain. However, it is worth noting that these figures underestimate the real participation of women in paid work, as many women are involved in the informal market, as mentioned below.

Table 9.1 also displays the diverse ways of organising paid work by couples across the four countries. Whereas the dual full-time earner model is the main one in Portugal (67 per cent of all couples), the traditional male-breadwinner model is the predominant one in Italy, comprising 45 per cent of all couples, and is also widespread in Greece and Spain.

The participation of women in the labour market has become a topic of increasing interest, not only in academic circles, but also in political spheres, where it has emerged as a major economic and social issue. Demographic changes in Europe, such as low birth rates combined with the current retirement rates, mean that a large population tends to result in a reduced proportion of people of working age (15–64 years), and the financial sustainability of social insurance systems becomes a very critical issue (Eurostat 2006b). Some demographic changes are particularly critical in Southern European countries, in which fertility rates are very low in comparison with the EU average (see Figure 9.1).

The scarce financial resources of many families may account for such figures, as well as the lack of public care facilities and the inherent difficulties in combining paid work with family duties, which are traditionally very intensive and asymmetrically distributed in terms of gender, with women being largely seen as the main caregivers. In our view, a further obstacle to the increase in fertility lies in the high incidence of precarious, temporary jobs, as well as irregular and informal forms of work. Table 9.2 shows that the percentage of temporary contracts is particularly high in Spain (almost 37 per cent of working women are employed on temporary contracts) and in Portugal (21.7 per cent of working women). Precariousness is also closely related to the high prevalence of the informal sector, where such employment situations are estimated to be responsible for 15–30 per cent of the GDP of Southern European countries (cf. Flaquer 2000, p. 22); this

Table 9.1   Employment rates in Southern European countries (1986–2006)

	Greece		Italy		Portugal		Spain	
Employment rates evolution (aged 15–64 years)								
	Men	Women	Men	Women	Men	Women	Men	Women
1986	75.2	36.1	72.8	34.1	76.9	47.3	63.3	25.1
1996	72.6	38.5	66.4	36.1	71.0	54.2	62.5	32.8
2006	74.6	47.4	70.5	46.3	73.9	62.0	76.1	53.2
Female employment rate by the existence of children (women aged 20–40 years in 2003)								
Without children	56.6		60.4		76.6		61.7	
With children	52.7		49.7		76.4		51.2	
Mothers' employment (women aged 15–64 years in 2005), by children's ages								
Under 2 years of age	49.5		47.3		69.1		52.6	
3–5 years old	53.6		50.6		71.8		54.2	
Under 16 years old	50.9		48.1		67.8		52.0	
Organisation of paid work by couples (25–49 years) when at least one partner has a job (% of couples), 2003[1]								
Women and men in full-time employment	47.0		38.0		67.0		44.0	
Women in part-time and men in full-time employment	5.0		13.0		7.0		9.0	
Men: single earner	44.0		45.0		21.0		43.0	
Women: single earner	2.0		2.0		4.0		3.0	

Sources: Eurostat (2005); OECD (2007).

Note: [1] Some (marginal) percentages are not included in the table, covering the following situations: 'men and women in part-time employment' and 'women in full-time employment and men in part-time employment'.

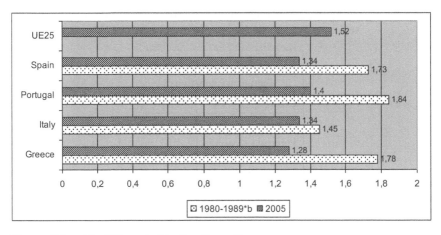

Figure 9.1   Fertility rates[a] in Southern Europe

Notes:

[a] The total fertility rate is the average number of children that would be born alive to a woman during her lifetime if she were to pass through all childbearing years conforming to the age-specific fertility rates of a given year.

[b] Average of the total fertility rates of the individual years within the respective period.

Sources: Eurostat (2006a; 2007); OECD (2007).

form of employment affects high proportions of women, who tend to work under difficult conditions and with long working hours (Trifiletti 1999), and is also largely connected to the persistence of traditional family businesses, in which a large number of women work, frequently without any pay (Cousins 2000).

Part-time employment is not very prevalent in the countries under analysis in Table 9.2, with Greece exhibiting the lowest percentages. Low wages, combined with economic necessity, the late development of the service sector and the traditional (labour-intensive) models of production, may account for such low figures (see, for example, Ferreira 1999; Perista and Lopes 1999; Cousins 2000; Casaca 2008). Even so, in Italy and Spain, about one-quarter of employed women work on a part-time basis, and the gender gap amounts to almost 20 percentage points in these two countries. It is also worth noting that working hours are very intensive for women in Portugal and Greece in particular (in both countries, about half of the female population aged 20–54 work about 40–44 hours a week), just as they are for men in all the countries under analysis (over 50 per cent of men perform more than 40 hours' paid work per week) (OECD 2007, p. 171).

Table 9.2   Temporary contracts, part-time work (% in total employment), self-employment and unemployment rates in 2006

	Men	Women
Temporary contracts		
Greece	9.0	13.0
Italy	11.2	15.8
Portugal	19.5	21.7
Spain	32.0	36.7
Part-time employment		
Greece	2.9	10.2
Italy	4.7	26.5
Portugal	7.4	15.8
Spain	4.3	23.2
Self-employment		
Greece	5.6	13.6
Italy	5.4	8.8
Portugal	6.9	9.6
Spain	6.4	10.9

Source: Eurostat Labour Force Survey.

Reconciliation of Paid Work and Family Life: An Overview of Childcare Provision and Leave Benefits

Childcare Services

Formal childcare is seen to have distinct configurations both within and between countries. Even though available data require some caution[1] in their reading and interpretation, the coverage rates shown in Table 9.3 give us information about

---

1   Various sources are available for this indicator, so data therefore need to be analysed with caution. Problems with regard to data comparability also result from the heterogeneity of the national childcare systems under analysis (differences in the type of childcare arrangements provided, the number of hours per day of each type of service, enrolment age and so on). The lack of available data does not allow for the calculation of full-time equivalents. Sometimes children are enrolled in more than one part-time programme, which brings with it the problem of double counting; on other occasions, the data include children who are cared for under paid parental leave. Childcare diversity can also be found within each country, as the responsibility for service provision may be

the relationship existing between the vacancies filled in childcare services and the total number of children in each age cohort. Portugal seems to exhibit a higher coverage rate of childcare services for children under the age of 3: 23.5 per cent in 2004, slightly above the rate displayed by Spain (20.7 per cent), and more than three times the rates displayed by Italy (6.3 per cent) and Greece (7 per cent). Portugal showed a gradual increase in the rate of childcare coverage until the end of the 1990s, at which time it was still below 12 per cent. More recently, however, the rate has increased more sharply, reaching 23.5 per cent in 2004. In the early 1990s, Spain, Greece and Italy displayed coverage rates of 2 per cent, 3 per cent and 6 per cent, respectively, of services for children below 3 years of age. Currently, in Greece and Italy, this indicator (provision of childcare services) is characterised by a certain stabilisation or stagnation, which places them in the lowest two positions within the EU-15.

Table 9.3   Childcare services coverage rates, by age (%)

	Children under 3 years of age				Children aged between 3 and compulsory school age			
	1990–95	1998–2000	2003	2004	1990–95	1998–2000	2003	2004
Greece	3	3	7	7.0	70	46	60	46.8
Italy	6	6	6	6.3	91	95	93	100.3
Portugal	12	12	19	23.5	48	75	75	77.9
Spain	2	5	10	20.7	84	84	98	98.6

Notes: 1998–2000 data refer to 1998 for Italy, 1999 for Portugal and 2000 for Greece and Spain; 2004 data for children aged under 3 refer exclusively to those in pre-school situations.

Sources: For 1990–1995: European Commission Network on Childcare and Other Measures to Reconcile Employment and Family Responsibilities (1996), in Torres et al. (2004); for 1998–2000: OECD (2001); for 2003: European Commission (2006), and for 2004: OECD, Family Database.

Starting from the lowest level of all the EU-15 countries in the early 1990s, Spain had recorded an increase of around 18.7 percent by 2004, and it has in fact doubled its childcare provision in recent years. Therefore, Portugal and Spain seem to stand out as the two Southern European countries with the highest provision of care services for children under 3 years of age, in part due to recent developments (even so, this level of provision still remains below the Barcelona

---

attributed to municipalities or regions, and different methods of data collection may be used (OECD Family Database; Plantenga and Siegel 2004; European Commission 2006).

targets).[2] Italy and Greece show an even greater deficit, which appears more significant if one takes into consideration the fact that women's employment rates in these two countries – especially those of mothers – are the lowest in the EU-15. This evidence might suggest that a weak demand for care services does not, in turn, encourage an increase in supply. On the other hand, the lack of childcare facilities does not appear to lead to a greater involvement of Italian and Greek women in the labour market.[3]

As far as childcare facilities for children between 3 years old and compulsory school age are concerned, Table 9.3 shows that the picture is different. Pre-school facilities, complemented or not by other daycare centres, are the main formal care solution for this age cohort. In the Portuguese education system, the pre-school level, which consists of a daily schedule of five hours of educational activities that can be extended to include some hours of care services, is non-compulsory. Pre-school education is also non-compulsory in the other Southern European countries, and in Greece it is only available for children over 4 years old. Compared to the facilities existing for younger children, care services for those aged 3–6 are broader, covering almost 100 per cent of this age cohort in Italy and Spain in 2003. Portugal displays a lower coverage rate, reaching 75 per cent in 2003, and Greece 60 per cent in the same year.

In 2005, the pre-school coverage rate for children of 4 years of age reached 84 per cent in Portugal and 57.8 per cent in Greece, while for children of 5 years of age it reached 87.1 per cent in Portugal and 82.5 per cent in Greece (see Table 9.4). The growth in pre-school facilities has been quite significant in Portugal over the last twenty years: the coverage rate was about 29.3 per cent in 1985/86, and reached 78.4 per cent in 2005/2006. Italy and Spain exhibit an almost total coverage of services for children aged 3–5, and Portugal has shown an interesting development with regard to the pre-school coverage rate for children aged 4–5 years. Greece only displays a satisfactory coverage rate for those children of 5 years of age, displaying the lowest figure (1.4 per cent) for the number of years expected in pre-school education for those children aged 3–5 years.

Pre-school education is often only a part-time service, so that working parents still need extra childcare facilities, which are less readily available (Plantenga and Siegel 2004). As a result, flexibility is an important issue when it comes to analysing the compatibility between childcare schedules and parents' employment (see also Wall 2004). In Portugal, private centres are usually open for 11 hours per day (OECD 2004, p. 95), but public services schedules do not meet the needs of

---

2   The Barcelona Targets in 2002 defined a set of quantified goals to be accomplished by all EU member states by 2010: to provide childcare to at least 33 per cent of children aged under 3 years, and to at least 90 per cent of children aged between 3 years and the compulsory school age.

3   It is important to note that official statistics do not reflect the care service provided by non-registered childminders, who usually have an important role to play in childcare provision in Southern European countries.

Table 9.4   Pre-school coverage rates (%), by years of age and expected years in education for children aged 3–5 years

	3 years of age			4 years of age			5 years of age			Expected years in education for children aged 3–5 years
	1998	2001	2005	1998	2001	2005	1998	2001	2005	2004
Greece	—	—	—	50	55.8	57.8	76	81.6	82.5	1.4
Italy	96.8	97.8	97.3	98.1	100	100	96.8	98.7	93.6	3.0
Portugal	54.5	63.4	61.4	65.8	76	84	73.1	85.3	87.1	2.3
Spain	72.5	89.7	94.6	99.8	100	99.3	100	100	100	3.1

Source: OECD, Family and Education databases, <http://www.oecd.org/els/social/family/database> (accessed May 2008).

many working parents (European Commission 2006, p. 41). Even though data are scarce, sources seem to suggest that childcare services and schools are even less flexible in the other Southern European countries (see, for example, Plantenga and Siegel 2004; Saraceno 2004).

The availability of services does not mean that they are affordable, however, since families usually find them very expensive. Consequently, the availability of childcare facilities does not necessarily imply that mothers' involvement in the labour market is made any easier. Only when welfare states assume the responsibility for childcare provision is there a reconceptualisation of care provision, with a shift from its being largely a family obligation to its becoming a social right (Leira 2002, p. 37). The extent to which childcare provision is defined as a social right differs from one welfare state to another across Europe (Leira 2002, p. 33).

In Portugal, the provision of public childcare is free, and the state also supports services provided by non-profit organisations (the so-called IPSS – private organisations of social solidarity – which are usually described as part of the voluntary sector). Parents pay an income-related fee, which amounts to 38 per cent of the cost of childcare in this solidarity network (OECD 2004, p. 105). Private (profit-oriented) facilities do not receive public subsidies, and consequently their prices are higher. According to Eurostat,[4] in Portugal the increase in childcare

---

4   Eurostat database – Population and Social Conditions, <http://epp.eurostat.ec.europa.eu> (accessed May 2008); OECD, Family and Education Databases, <http://www.oecd.org/document/0,3746,en_2649_201185_46462759_1_1_1_1,00.html> (accessed May 2008).

facilities has been underpinned by an increase in the number of private institutions, both for-profit and not-for-profit organisations. By 2005, 52.8 per cent of pre-school children were to be found at private pre-school facilities, clearly more than in other Southern European countries. In Spain, private pre-school children accounted for 35.2 per cent of all pre-school children, whereas in Italy the figure was 29.8 per cent and in Greece only 3.2 per cent in the same year.

As in Spain and Italy, in Greece parents pay an income-related fee, but access to such services tends to be difficult due to the lack of transparency (European Commission 2006, pp. 39–40). In Spain, childcare services are subsidised only for low-income families. In Italy, the cost varies according to the region, and the maximum fee for a public service is roughly equivalent to the amount that is charged by some private institutions. Although less expensive when compared to the private sector alternatives, public childcare services are expensive when compared with women's average earnings.

Leave Benefits

Leave benefits are part of a policy measure that seeks to facilitate the reconciliation of paid work and family life in the case of working parents, as they allow for career interruptions for family reasons, such as childbirth and childrearing. In general, leave arrangements may be divided into three distinct groups: *maternity leave* and *paternity leave*, which guarantee job protection during career interruption at the time of childbirth for employed mothers and fathers and are, generally, a form of paid leave, and *parental leave*, which guarantees job protection during leave taken for childcare purposes.

The employment protection inherent in maternity leave is, as Perista and Chagas Lopes (1999, p. 107) point out, an important right guaranteed to women, as long as the right to work is made a real possibility for mothers. In Southern European countries, maternity leave ranges from four to five months, with entitlement to full pay in Portugal, Spain and, albeit with a maximum limit, Greece; in Italy, it is only partly paid (80 per cent) (see Table 9.5). An added advantage to these maternity entitlements is that it may prevent women from exiting the labour market after childbirth, and as a result, can have a positive effect on the female labour supply, at least in the short term (Gornick et al. 1997, p. 48).

Paternity leave is shown to be extremely important, not only because it allows men greater involvement in family life, but also because it reflects a reconceptualisation of childcare, in which both mother and father are simultaneously waged workers and carers (see, for example, Perista and Chagas Lopes 1999; Leira 2002; Wall 2004). Portugal, and more recently Spain, exhibit more innovative paternity leave solutions than do Greece and Italy. The transfer of part of maternity leave to fathers has been made possible in the first two countries, in addition to paid and non-transferable paternity leave (five days in Portugal and 15 days in Spain). In 2004, the granting of a five-day paternity leave period was made compulsory in Portugal, and although the impact was not as

Table 9.5 Leave benefits in Southern European countries

	Maternity leave	Payment	Paternity leave	Payment	Parental leave	Payment
G	17 weeks (8 before and 9 after birth)	100% up to maximum of 43.44 euros per day (60.82 euros, with dependants)	2 days	100%	3½ months per parent (child less than 3½ years old)	Unpaid
IT	5 months (1 or 2 months before birth)	80%	Total or partial transferability of maternity leave if lone father or if mother is ill	80%	11 months for children under 8 years of age, shared between mother and father (6 months maximum for mother, or 7 if father claims at least 3 months)	Child under 3 years of age: 30% (6 months maximum) or 30% with limit if leave exceeds 6 months; child 3–8 years old: unpaid
P	120 days (plus 30 days per additional child in case of multiple births); 150 days option	100%, if 120 days; 80%, if 150 days	5 compulsory days in the first month after birth; transferability of maternity leave to the father if mother claims at least 6 weeks' maternity leave	100%	3 months per parent (child under 6 years of age); special leave: 2 years for mother or for father if child under 6 years of age (3 years if 3 or more children)	Unpaid (except first 15 days if claimed by father, which are paid 100%)
SP	16 weeks (plus 2 weeks per additional child if multiple births)	100%	15 days[1]; transferability to father of 10 weeks' maternity leave	100%	3 years (including maternity leave) for mother or father (child under 3 years of age)	Unpaid

Notes: [1] Ley de Igualdad, 24 March 2007. G – Greece; IT– Italy; P – Portugal; SP – Spain.

Sources: PF7: Key characteristics of parental leave systems, OECD Family Database, 2007; MISSOC – Mutual Information System on Social Protection (situation at 1 January 2007), European Commission; Labour Law (Portugal); Ley de Igualdad de 24 March 2007 (Spain); Perista and Chagas Lopes (1999).

widespread as expected, the take-up rate of this leave has increased since then (Moss and Wall 2007, p. 236). Recent changes have been introduced in the new Labour Code (2009), even though it will only be possible to evaluate their impact in future research.[5]

Parental leave is more focused on the reconciliation of work and family life, allowing mothers and fathers to take the responsibility for childcare. As Table 9.5 shows, in Southern European countries parental leave is unpaid in Spain and Greece, or involves a low level of wage compensation, which does not exceed 30 per cent of earnings, as in Italy. In Portugal, the first 15 days of parental leave are fully paid if claimed by the father – a policy mechanism that is clearly intended to promote a more equal division of family responsibilities between men and women.

The level of payment for leave is clearly related to its take-up rates (Leira 2002; European Commission 2006), and is therefore related to its effectiveness in promoting the reconciliation of work and family life. If the level of payment during the leave period is low (or zero), it may become a privilege of well-off families and be of no use to low-income families (Leira 2002, p. 82), while also exacerbating social inequalities. On the other hand, the payment level also affects the choice as to which parent will take up parental leave, thereby impacting upon gender roles (Leira 2002, p. 82; European Commission 2006, p. 48). The higher the earnings in the labour market, the higher the costs of taking up parental leave; thus, it is more likely that the parent with the lowest income, usually the mother, will stay at home to care for the child. In addition to this, the dominant organisational culture, in which employers still have a negative attitude towards men who take parental leave, may result in a low take-up rate for leave benefits, especially in the private sector (Perista and Chagas Lopes 1999; Leira 2002; European Commission 2006; Casaca 2008). Taking up leave for long periods may limit women's career opportunities, such as training or promotion, and reinforce gender discrimination in labour markets (Leira 2002). This situation may result in a negative long-term effect on women's earnings, and in turn, on the female labour supply (Gornick et al. 1997, p. 48). As a consequence, asymmetries between men and women with regard to family responsibilities and the labour market also run the risk of becoming a persistent phenomenon. In order to avoid this situation, commitment should also be oriented towards policy mechanisms that favour a more balanced share of parental leave between mothers and fathers. In addition to

---

5   The new Labour Code implemented in 2009 is designed to extend this period to ten days' compulsory leave. In addition, the father can also take a further ten days' non-compulsory leave to coincide with the mother's leave. With the aim of encouraging a more equal sharing of leave periods between both parents, the new law (Law No. 7/2009) establishes that parental leave may range from four to five months' full-paid leave, with 80 per cent of income replacement, or even 100 per cent if taken by the other parent (usually the father), or it may be extended to six months (83 per cent of income replacement, when both parents benefit from it and one of them exclusively takes one month's leave).

this, considering the aspect of wage compensation, leave benefits should be more financially attractive to men.

Conclusion

There are similarities in the trajectories and characteristics of Southern European states in regard to the promotion of a better balance between paid work and family life, but certain singularities need to be pointed out, too. Portugal reveals a low coverage rate of childcare facilities for children below 3 years of age, even though this is higher than in the other countries under analysis. This same trend is found in Spain, where, at the beginning of the twenty-first century, considerable growth was to be noted in care facilities for children below 3 years of age. Italy and Greece display the lowest rates of female employment, as well as the lowest childcare coverage rates and a lower pace of development. The growth in the provision of formal support to families in Portugal seems to be emerging more as a practical response to the prevalence of a dual full-time earner model (the country has the highest level of women's participation in the labour market in the cluster under analysis) and less as a strategy of anticipating those needs or as a reflection of any strong commitment towards *defamilialisation*. The development in childcare services has also taken place in tandem with the provision of more flexible solutions concerning time schedules, making it possible to respond better to families' needs.

A move towards *defamilisation* does not mean that informal care must be suppressed, but that there is an urgent need to eliminate 'the care penalty' or the 'invisible heart' (Folbre 2001) that has centred upon the under-valuation of care work mostly performed by women. This is particularly critical in the countries under analysis, as caregiving work is far from being shared equally within the families, and is still commonly seen as a women's obligation (including by women themselves) at the expense of their full economic and symbolic independence. We share the view that the dual-earner model combined with the dual-carer one, as well as with affordable, flexible and quality care services, is an appropriate future scenario for the societies under analysis.

Maternity leave guarantees employment protection to mothers. Due to European directives, southern countries do not vary much in terms of the duration and remuneration of this social benefit. Nevertheless, Portugal, and more recently Spain, have shown more innovative features than their counterparts, in particular with regard to the right of fathers to enjoy paid paternity leave (not transferable to mothers) and to the possibility of transferring part of the maternity leave to the father if both partners agree. In the case of parental leave, the low pay associated with this benefit and the weight of traditional gender ideologies contribute to the fact that it is mainly used by women, which may represent a regression in terms of the modernisation of gender roles and contribute towards greater discrimination against women in the labour market. Portugal shows some signs of innovation in this area, as part of the parental leave must be taken exclusively by the father and he is entitled to full remuneration.

To conclude: Portugal, and to a certain extent Spain, have displayed some important signs of change and innovation within the context of Southern Europe. In parallel with a more proactive, coherent and systematic state role in these issues, serious consideration also needs to be given to policies that seek to promote gender equality in the private sphere in order to truly encourage the modernisation of gender relations and guarantee full citizenship for both men and women.

References

Aboim, S. (2007), 'Clivagens e continuidades de género face aos valores da vida familiar', in K. Wall and L. Amâncio (eds), *Família e Género em Portugal e na Europa*, Lisbon: ICS/Imprensa de Ciências Sociais, pp. 35–91.

Addabbo, T. and Baldini, M. (2000), *The Gender Impact of Workforce Policies in Italy and the Effect of Unpaid Work*, Materiali di discussione, Bologna: Centro di Analisi delle Politique Pubbliche (CAPP).

Addis, E. (1999), 'Gender in the reform of the Italian welfare state', *South European Society and Politics*, vol. 4, no. 2, pp. 122–49.

Alcañiz, M. (2004), 'Conciliacion entre las esferas pública y privada: ¿Hacia un nuevo modelo en el sistema de géneros?', *Sociologia – Problemas e Práticas*, vol. 44, pp. 47–70.

Almeida, A.N., Guerreiro, M.D., Lobo, C., Torres, A. and Wall, K. (1998), 'Relações familiares: mudança e diversidade', in J.M.L. Viegas and A.F. Costa (eds), *Portugal: Que Modernidade?*, Oeiras: Celta Editora, pp. 45–78.

Bettio, F., Simonazzi, A. and Villa, P. (2006), 'Change in care regimes and female immigration: The "care drain" in the Mediterranean', *Journal of European Policy*, vol. 16, no. 3, pp. 271–85.

Bould, S. and Schmaus, G. (2008), 'The European Union Roadmap (2006–2010): Equal economic independence for women and men?', *Revista Sociologia e Politiche Sociali*, no. 11, pp. 35–57.

Carlos, M.P. and Maratou-Alipranti, L. (2000), 'Family policy and new family forms: The cases of Greece and Portugal', in A. Pfenning and T. Bahle (eds), *Families and Family Policies in Europe: Comparative Perspectives*, Frankfurt am Main: Peter Lang, pp. 34–49.

Casaca, S.F. (2008), 'Flexibilidade de emprego em Portugal e na União Europeia: Colocando a dimensão *género* no centro do debate', in F. Henriques (ed.), *Género, Diversidade e Cidadania*, Lisbon: Editora Colibri, pp. 131–54.

Cousins, C. (2000), 'Women and employment in Southern Europe: The implications of recent policy and labour market directions', *South European Society and Politics*, vol. 5, no. 1, pp. 97–122.

Crompton, R. (2006), *Employment and the Family: The Reconfiguration of Work and Family Life in Contemporary Societies*, Cambridge: Cambridge University Press.

Cunha, V. (2007), *O Lugar dos Filhos, Ideias, Práticas e Significados*, Lisbon: ICS/Imprensa de Ciências Sociais.

Daly, M. and Lewis, J. (2000), 'The concept of social care and the analysis of contemporary welfare states', *British Journal of Sociology*, vol. 51, no. 2, pp. 281–98.

Daly, M. and Rake, K. (2003), *Gender and the Welfare State*, Cambridge: Polity Press.

Damião, S. (2008), 'A Participação Feminina no Mercado de Trabalho e o Papel da Política Social: O caso de Portugal no contexto da Europa do Sul', master's degree thesis in Economics and Social Policies, ISEG, Technical University of Lisbon.

Direcção-Geral de Estudos, Estatística e Planeamento (DGEEP) and Ministério do Trabalho e da Solidariedade Social (MTSS) (2007), *Carta Social – Rede de Serviços e Equipamentos: Relatório 2006*, Lisbon: GEP, Centro de Informação e Documentação.

Esping-Andersen, G. (1990), *The Three Worlds of Welfare Capitalism*, Cambridge: Polity Press.

European Commission (2006), *Reconciliation of Work and Private Life: A Comparative Review of Thirty European Countries*, Luxembourg: Office for Official Publications of the European Communities.

Eurostat (2005), 'Reconciling work and family life in the EU25 in 2003', press release, 12 April 2005.

—— (2006a), 'Population in Europe 2005: First Results' *Statistics in Focus*, 16/2006.

—— (2006b), *The Social Situation in the European Union 2005–2006*, Luxembourg: Office for Official Publications of the European Communities.

—— (2007), *Living Conditions in Europe 2002–2005*, Luxembourg: Office for Official Publications of the European Communities.

Ferreira V. (1999), 'Os paradoxos da situação das mulheres em Portugal', *Revista Crítica de Ciências Sociais*, pp. 199–227.

Flaquer, L. (2000), 'Is there a Southern European model of family policy', in A. Pfenning and T. Bahle (eds), *Families and Family Policies in Europe: Comparative Perspectives*, Frankfurt am Main: Peter Lang, pp. 15–33.

Folbre, N. (2001), *The Invisible Heart: Economics and Family Values*, New York: The New Press.

Fraser, N. (1994), 'After the family wage,' *Political Theory*, vol. 22, no. 4, pp. 591–618.

Gabinete Estatístico e de Planeamento da Educação (2007), Portal da Educação, <http://www.min-edu.pt> (accessed 8 May 2011).

Gornick, J.C., Meyers, M.K. and Ross, K.E. (1997), 'Supporting the employment of mothers: Policy variation across fourteen welfare states', *Journal of European Social Policy*, vol. 7, no. 1, pp. 45–70.

Leira, A. (2002), *Working Parents and the Welfare State: Family Change and Policy Reform in Scandinavia*, Cambridge: Cambridge University Press.

Lewis, J. (1992), 'Gender and the development of welfare regimes', *Journal of European Policy*, vol. 2, no. 3, pp. 159–73.

Lister, R. (1994), 'She Has Other Duties: Women, Citizenship and Social Security', in S. Baldwin and J. Falkingham (eds), *Social Security and Social Change*, New York and London: Harvester Wheatsheaf.

McLaughlin, E. and Glendinning, C. (1994), Paying for Care in Europe: Is There a Feminist Approach?, in L. Hantrais and S.P. Mangan (eds), *Family Policy and Welfare of Women*, Loughborough: European Research Centre.

Moss, P. and Wall, K. (2007), *International Review of Leave Policies and Related Research 2007*, Employment Relations Research Series no. 80, London: Employment Market Analysis and Research.

Organisation for Economic Co-operation and Development (OECD) (2001), 'Balancing Work and Family Life: Helping Parents into Paid Employment', *Employment Outlook 2001*, Paris: OECD.

—— (2004), *Babies and Bosses: Políticas de Conciliação da Actividade Profissional e da Vida Familiar*, vol. 3, 'New Zealand, Portugal and Switzerland', Lisbon: Direcção-Geral de Estudos, Estatística e Planeamento.

—— (2007), *Babies and Bosses: Reconciling Work and Family Life*, Paris: OECD.

Orloff, A. (1993), 'Gender and the social rights of citizenship: The comparative analysis of gender relations and welfare states', *American Sociological Review*, no. 48, pp. 303–28.

Perista, H. and Chagas Lopes, M. (eds) (1999), *A Licença de Paternidade: Um Direito Novo para a Promoção da Igualdade*, Colecção Estudos 14, Lisbon: DEPP/MTS.

Pichio, A. (2006), *Unpaid Work and the Economy: A Gender Analysis of the Standard of Living*, London: Routledge.

Plantenga, J. and Siegel, M. (2004), 'European Childcare Strategies', position paper, Conference on 'Childcare in a Changing World', Groningen, the Netherlands.

Sainsbury, D. (ed.) (1999), *Gender and Welfare State Regimes*, Oxford: Oxford University Press.

Saraceno, C. (2004), 'A igualdade difícil: Mulheres no mercado de trabalho em Itália e a questão não resolvida da conciliação', *Sociologia – Problemas e Práticas*, no. 44, pp. 27–45.

Simoni, S. and Trifiletti, R. (2004), 'Caregiving in transition in Southern Europe: Neither complete altruists nor free-riders', *Social Policy and Administration*, vol. 38, no. 6, pp. 678–705.

Tobío, C. (2005), 'Change and reciprocity in intergenerational relationships: Spanish working mothers' discourse', paper presented at the 7th Conference of the European Sociological Association, Torun, Poland, September 2005.

Torres, A. (ed.), da Silva, F.V., Monteiro, T.L. and Cabrita, M. (2004), *Homens e Mulheres entre Família e Trabalho*, Estudos no. 1, Comissão para a Igualdade no Trabalho e no Emprego, Direcção-Geral de Estudos, Estatística e Planeamento.

Trifiletti, R. (1999), 'Southern Europe welfare regimes and the worsening position of women', *Journal of European Social Policy*, vol. 9, no. 1, pp. 49–64.

Wall, K. (2004), 'Development in Family Policy in Portugal in 2003', in *European Observatory on the Social Situation, Demography and the Family*, Working Paper 3–04, Lisbon: Instituto de Ciências Sociais.

—— (2007), 'Atitudes face à divisão familiar do trabalho em Portugal e na Europa', in K. Wall and L. Amâncio (eds), *Família e Género em Portugal e na Europa*, Lisbon: ICS/Imprensa de Ciências Sociais, pp. 211–58.

Chapter 10

Reconciliation of Work and Family in Greece: Policy Responses and Dimensions of Public Debate

Laura Alipranti-Maratou and Anna Nikolaou

Work and family are two realms of our lives that constantly interact with each other, at both the level of intimacy and the societal level. The different factors which have contributed to changes in male and female roles in the context of contemporary family life are shaped mainly by the overall process of development of Western societies and the shift to an industrial-consumer economy followed by a considerable increase of women in employment. As more and more women have entered the labour market, dual-career families have gradually started to become the norm. However despite the changes in social roles, the re-organisation of economic responsibilities has not been accompanied by a redistribution of domestic responsibilities between women and men.

As a response to these employment and care matters, this led, in the 1980s, to the appearance of reconciliation policies in the equal opportunities agenda of the European Union. *Reconciliation* is a concept that refers to the combination of paid and unpaid labour, or to the balance between paid work and caring responsibilities. In that context, measures aimed to facilitate the access of more women to the labour market, at the same time enabling them to reconcile maternity and care with professional life. The prime concern during that decade, however, was how women could actually combine their work and family responsibilities, and not how equal distribution of paid and unpaid labour could be achieved. During the 1990s, the reconciliation of work and family life gradually became a commitment to promoting gender equality in employment, which also coincided with the demands of business corporations for flexitime, a reduction of employment costs and an increase in competition (Hantrais 2000; Kaufman et al. 2002).

Since the 1990s, a number of structural socio-economic changes have occurred. These include the growing participation of women in employment, reforms in various sectors of economy, and radical technological changes and new technologies. Each and every one of these paved the way for new regulations of more flexible types of work that are predominantly directed towards working mothers (European Commission 2006).

In the case of Greece, the turning point for the development of coherent reconciliation policies was perhaps the transposition of the Open Method of

Coordination (OMC) guidelines, as defined in the Treaty of Amsterdam 1997, into national and regional policies.[1] The OMC was further officially defined and endorsed at the Lisbon Council in 2000.

Although in Greece reconciliation, equal opportunities and social policy have been closely connected in recent years with a commitment to promoting women's access to employment, the participation by women in the labour force has progressed at a slower pace than in most other European countries. Generally, policy making in these fields is characterised by fragmentary and often contradictory regulations, as the Greek state prefers to offer short-term solutions as an alternative to an integral social policy reform. Even though there is considerable discussion on incentives to strengthen women's work participation, partial development of family services and a lack of co-ordinated action create employment barriers. Also, despite efforts to modernise the social security system, some measures make it difficult for working mothers to stay in the labour market. Only limited state interventions have taken place, while at the same time family policy has not adjusted to emerging new social conditions. Public discussions are focusing on the reorientation of existing policies and the formulation of new and more coherent policy programmes which will include the gender dimension more explicitly.

With this in mind, in the remainder of this chapter we will examine family policies from a gender perspective. The increasing number of dual-career families, and therefore of working mothers, poses obvious policy demands, while the way in which policies are formed and promoted is highly indicative of dominant frames concerning gender equality. Certainly, institutional measures for the reconciliation of family and work are very important issues for public discussion between political parties, the General Secretariat for Equality, GGI and civil society, as is evidenced by relevant government action plans, recent legislative measures and mass media debates.

In the first section, we will present an overview of female employment in Greece as well as a list of existing policies and measures that are considered important for the reconciliation of work and family life. In the second section, we will present reconciliation policies in public debate. More specifically, we will present some of the findings of the MAGEEQ (Multiple Aspects of Gender Equality) project, a European collaboration which resulted in a study entitled *Policy Frames and Implementation Problems: The Case of Gender Mainstreaming.*[2] The overarching aim is to identify policy frames in public discourse on the issue of reconciliation of work and family based on the analysis of a range of public documents (laws, debates, policy texts). In other words, we will attempt a critical analysis of public discourse concerning reconciliation policy in Greece. As mentioned in various studies:

---

1   OMC allows member states to co-ordinate their employment policies and exchange knowledge, policy measures and good practices on social policy.

2   <http://www.mageeq.net/index.php?option=com_frontpage&Itemid=1> (accessed 8 May 2011).

in theory and in practice there are fundamental debates on what constitutes feminism, on developing normative feminist concepts, on identifying ideological and on constructing new strategies. Moreover in EU the main objective in terms of gender equality is to improve female participation in the labour market and to facilitate women's more active participation on it, rather than as an equality objective in its own right (Verloo et al. 2005, p. 6).

Female Employment and Reconciliation Policies: An Overview

Socio-economic developments in the EU countries have enhanced the social and productive role of women through rising educational standards and their increasing participation in the labour market. As a result, women are called on to combine work and caring responsibilities. Terms like 'dual-career families' and 'reconciliation of family and professional life' in policy texts reflect the need to try to unify notions which were considered in the past incompatible, to balance the obligations and the roles of men and women, and to redefine the boundaries between family and work lives (Hantrais and Letablier 1995; European Commission 2006; Lewis et al. 2008).

However, reconciliation, equal opportunities and family policy in Greece constitute fields that have recently been closely connected, with a commitment to promoting women's access to employment (Hrzenjak et al. 2005; Karamessini 2006; Mouriki 2008).

So, while dual-earner families have increased and despite the changes in social roles, the idea of gender equality in the domestic sphere has not been recognised as an issue. It is evident that re-organisation of economic responsibilities was not accompanied by a redistribution of domestic responsibilities in the context of two-working-parent families. Male participation in domestic tasks and everyday family and other obligations has only increased slowly (Maratou-Alipranti 1999; Symeonidou 2002; Davakis 2006; Koronaiou et al. 2007).

Moreover, since mentalities, perceptions and practices are not changing in everyday life and women continue to be the primary caregivers as well as remaining responsible for household tasks, coupled with the failure of European countries to develop innovative policies and specific measures for the promotion of equal opportunities and the reconciliation of work and family life, men's participation in the private sphere will continue to be limited (European Commission 2006; Symeonidou et al. 2007).

Female Employment: Structural Characteristics

Female employment has been the main factor in the steady growth of employment in the EU in recent years (European Commission 2008). During 2000–2006, the female employment rate went up each year, reaching 57.2 per cent in 2006 (see Table 10.1).

Table 10.1   Employment rates (women and men) aged 15–64 in EU member states, 2001 and 2006 (%)

	Women		Men		Gender gap	
	2001	2006	2001	2006	2001	2006
EU-27	54.3	57.2	70.9	71.6	16.6	14.4
Belgium	51.0	54.0	68.8	67.9	17.8	13.9
Bulgaria	46.8	54.6	52.7	62.8	5.9	8.2
Czech Republic	56.9	56.8	73.2	73.7	16.3	16.9
Denmark	72.0	73.4	80.2	81.2	8.2	7.8
Germany	58.7	62.2	72.8	72.8	14.1	10.6
Estonia	57.4	65.3	65.0	71.0	7.6	5.7
Ireland	54.9	59.3	76.6	77.7	21.7	18.4
Greece	41.5	47.4	71.4	74.6	29.9	27.2
Spain	43.1	53.2	72.5	76.1	29.4	22.9
France	56.0	57.7	69.7	68.5	13.7	10.8
Italy	41.1	46.3	68.5	70.5	27.4	24.2
Cyprus	57.2	60.3	79.3	79.4	22.1	19.1
Latvia	55.7	62.4	61.9	70.4	6.2	8.0
Lithuania	56.2	61.0	58.9	66.3	2.7	5.3
Luxembourg	50.9	54.6	75.0	72.6	24.1	18.0
Hungary	49.8	51.1	62.9	63.8	13.1	12.7
Malta	32.1	34.9	76.2	74.5	44.1	39.6
Netherlands	65.2	67.7	82.8	80.9	17.6	13.2
Austria	60.7	63.5	76.4	76.9	15.7	13.4
Poland	47.7	48.2	59.2	60.9	11.5	12.7
Portugal	61.3	62.0	77.0	73.9	15.7	11.9
Romania	57.1	53.0	67.8	64.6	10.7	11.6
Slovenia	58.8	61.8	68.6	71.1	9.8	9.3
Slovakia	51.8	51.9	62.0	67.0	10.2	15.1
Finland	65.4	67.3	70.8	71.4	5.4	4.1
Sweden	72.3	70.7	75.7	75.5	3.4	4.8
United Kingdom	65.0	65.8	78.0	77.3	13.0	11.5

Source: Eurostat Labour Force Survey, annual average.

However, in Greece, women's participation in the labour force has progressed at a slower pace than in most other European countries. The activity rate of the native-born population in Greece is below the EU level, and although it increased from 27 per cent in 1981 to 32 per cent in 1991, to 41.9 per cent in 2001 and then to 47.2 per cent in 2006, it is still the lowest rate among the 27 EU member states (see Tables 10.1 and 10.2).

Table 10.2   Economic activity rates by gender, Greece, 1961–2006 (%)

	Men		Women	
1961	73.8	(77.1)	33.5	
1971	66.3	(69.9)	24.1	(31.3)
1981	64.7	(70.8)	22.7	(29.8)
1982	70.9		29.6	
1983	70.8		33.1	
1984	70.0		33.4	
1985	68.8		34.2	
1986	67.7		34.1	
1987	66.6		34.0	
1988	66.6		35.2	
1989	65.6		35.1	
1990	64.7		34.9	
1991	63.5		32.6	
1992	63.5		34.2	
1993	63.6		34.7	
1994	63.7		34.9	
1995	63.6		35.6	
1996	63.3		36.5	
1997	62.2		36.1	
1998	60.5		39.4	
1999	59.8		40.2	
2000	59.7		40.2	
2001	71.4		41.5	
2006	74.6		47.4	

Sources: NSSG Census Results, 1961–81; Eurostat Labour Force Survey, 1983–2001.

The explanatory factors for women's lower economic activity rates point to the limited industrial development in the country, to high emigration during the period 1953–72, to high internal migration to urban centres, especially in the period 1961–81, to relatively low educational levels of older women resulting in high unemployment rates, and to traditional mentalities regarding gender social roles and to local labour market rigidities (Symeonidou 2004).

The recent increase in the employment rates (47.2 per cent in 2006) can be attributed to the fact that many new employment opportunities are now open to women, societal attitudes towards gender roles have changed, and employment opportunities among younger women (20–39 years old) with children (consistent with developments in other EU countries) has increased (Kikilias 2007). However, the gap in the employment rate between men and women persists as a result of a lower employment rate for women (see Table 10.2).[3]

It is important to analyse the participation in the labour force in relation to the family status and family responsibilities of women. Life cycle events are considered particularly significant in the study of women's economic activity and the evolution of family life. Thus, parenthood has a significant long-term effect on women's participation in the labour market and causes a drop in female activity, whereas these same factors tend to lead to an increase in the economic activity of men. This reflects women's predominant role as carers for children, elderly or disabled family members (European Commission 2008).

In 2006, the employment rate for EU-27 women aged 20–49 was 62.4 per cent when they had children under 12, compared with 76 per cent when they did not. The same figures for Greece were lower: 64.1 per cent for those without children and 57 per cent for those who had children under 12 years old (see Table 10.3).

These general tendencies also apply in the case of female activity rates in Greece by marital status. By looking at Table 10.4, it can be seen that single women's activity rates rose considerably, from 39.7 per cent in 1971 to 49 per cent in 2001, while activity rates for married women were much lower.

Married women have a lower participation rate as it is difficult for them to reintegrate into the labour market after childbirth. In Greece, very often marriage and children either postpone or terminally interrupt women's participation in the labour force, or lead women to informal types of work, as there is inflexibility in the Greek labour market (Symeonidou 2004).

Although childbearing leads to an increase in household duties and Greek women still have the primary responsibility for housekeeping and childcare, there was an increase in employment among younger women with children. This is consistent with what was happening in other EU countries. Women's employment seemed to be negatively affected only after the third child and in the younger age group (Symeonidou 2004).

---

3   At a national level, significant differences exist across the EU member countries, and range between 5 per cent in Finland and Sweden to more than 25 per cent in Greece and Malta.

Table 10.3 **Employment rates of women and men (aged 25–49) depending on whether they had children (under 12) in EU member states, 2006 (%)**

	Without children		With children		Difference	
	Women	Men	Women	Men	Women	Men
EU-27	76.0	80.8	62.4	91.4	-13.6	10.6
Belgium	75.5	81.7	69.3	92.2	-6.2	10.5
Bulgaria	74.7	76.6	61.5	81.2	-13.2	4.7
Czech Republic	83.2	87.1	53.4	93.9	-29.8	6.8
Germany	80.3	80.6	62.7	91.4	-17.6	10.8
Estonia	82.7	86.9	66.7	92.4	-16.0	5.5
Greece	64.1	82.5	57.0	96.8	-7.0	14.3
Spain	75.5	84.3	58.8	93.2	-16.7	8.8
France	73.7	76.6	65.9	91.1	-7.7	14.4
Italy	66.7	80.7	54.6	93.8	-12.1	13.1
Cyprus	82.1	87.8	70.8	95.7	-11.3	7.8
Latvia	82.1	80.9	68.4	91.2	-13.7	10.3
Lithuania	81.5	78.9	77.2	89.7	-4.3	10.7
Luxembourg	80.2	90.3	65.0	95.7	-15.3	5.5
Hungary	76.1	79.1	49.8	86.1	-26.3	7.0
Malta	68.7	88.6	32.6	94.0	-36.1	5.3
Netherlands	83.8	87.9	72.7	94.5	-11.2	6.6
Austria	83.6	87.7	68.5	92.9	-15.1	5.3
Poland	69.9	71.5	60.8	88.0	-9.2	16.5
Portugal	77.3	82.7	76.4	94.2	-0.9	11.5
Romania	70.7	76.9	66.3	85.4	-4.3	8.6
Slovenia	77.1	82.7	84.8	95.3	7.8	12.6
Slovakia	79.0	79.5	54.2	88.2	-24.8	8.7
Finland	78.9	79.5	70.6	92.7	-8.3	13.2
United Kingdom	82.9	84.1	63.1	91.0	-19.8	6.8

Source: Eurostat Labour Force Survey, annual average.

Table 10.4   Economic activity rates of women by marital status, Greece, 1971–2001 (%)

	Marital status			
	Single	Married	Widowed/ Divorced	Total
1971	39.7	23.7	15.8	25.9
1981	41.9	22.0	14.6	24.7
1983	41.7	34.5	14.9	33.1
1985	39.0	37.1	15.4	34.2
1987	37.5	37.4	14.9	34.0
1989	39.5	38.6	14.8	35.1
1991	38.9	34.7	15.1	32.6
1992	40.1	36.9	15.8	34.2
1996	44.9	39.3	16.2	36.2
2001	49.0	34.5	17.7	41.5

Sources: NSSG, Population Census, 1951, 1971, 2001.

In Greece, there is also limited part-time work, as legislation on part-time employment was not introduced until 1990 and seems to have had little impact as yet. Under the frame of the existing stereotypes and the weakness of reconciliation between family and professional life, women constitute the overwhelming majority of part-time employed workers in Greece (71 per cent). It is noticeable that in 2006, only 2.8 per cent of the total number of employed men worked part-time, while for women this figure rose to 10.5 per cent. This is accounted for by either an inability to find a full-time job, or because of care responsibilities for dependent family members (see Table 10.5) (Kikilias 2007).

Reconciliation Policies in Greece

As a member of the EU since 1981, Greece was obliged to comply with the directives that supported equal treatment of men and women: equal pay for work of equal value; equal access to employment; vocational training, promotion and working conditions, and so on. However, the provision of care to children and the elderly continue to be responsibilities that place a burden on the family, and particularly women (Maratou-Alipranti 1999; Symeonidou 2002). The under-development of the welfare state in Greece has traditionally burdened women, who had and still have to fulfil roles that in other societies are undertaken by the state (Maratou-Alipranti and Tastsoglou 2003; Naldini 2003; Petmesidou and Mosialos 2006).

Table 10.5   Part-time workers, Greece, 1983–2006 (%)

	Men	Women
1983	3.3	8.5
1984	2.7	7.6
1985	2.6	8.3
1986	2.6	7.8
1987	2.1	8.0
1988	2.3	7.4
1989	2.1	6.8
1990	1.9	5.7
1991	1.7	4.8
1992	2.8	8.4
1993	3.0	8.0
1994	3.0	8.0
1995	2.8	8.3
1996	3.2	8.9
1997	2.6	8.1
1998	3.3	10.5
1999	3.5	10.1
2000	2.6	7.9
2002	2.3	8.0
2006	2.8	10.5

Sources: Eurostat Labour Force Survey, 2005.

Recently, part of this excess demand has been channelled into the private sector (nurseries, homes for the elderly), and particularly into the expanding market for the provision of personal services due to the work of migrant women, who usually work illegally and without insurance (Maratou-Alipranti and Tastsoglou 2003; Maratou-Alipranti 2007).

Reconciliation policy is a relatively new area of social policy in Greece, as it first appeared in 1984. Parental leave was initially only offered in the private sector, but was extended to the public sector with Presidential Decree 193/1988. It allows for leave to cover dependent family members' needs, including natural or adopted children up to the age of 16 for whom parents maintain parental care rights, children over 16 who need special care for a medically recognised illness or disability, and spouses whose severe chronic illness makes self-care impossible.

So far, the most important provisions concern regulations covering maternity and parental leave, the operation of day-long schools and other facilitations for working mothers and fathers. However, state interventions have been limited, and overall family policy has not adjusted to emerging new social conditions. Moreover, while family policy has been of growing importance in Greece, until very recently the target was not gender equality (European Commission 2006; Davakis 2006; Mouriki 2008).

Women continue to be responsible for domestic work and taking care of small children (Maratou-Alipranti 1999; Symeonidou 2002; Koronaiou 2007). At the same time, short school hours, limited publicly funded childcare facilities for pre-school children, limited after-school childcare and holiday arrangements place the main burden of provision of childcare on couples and families (Moussourou and Stratigaki 2004). Despite some efforts to expand care services, the current insufficient childcare facilities which do not meet the present childcare needs constitute an employment barrier for women. Diverse studies and reports indicate that to a large extent, childcare in Greece is provided by close family members and other relatives or other people (Mouriki 2008, p. 22).

However, demographic trends (ageing population), changing family structures and lifestyles of women as well as the need to provide adequate care for the elderly, people with special needs, and families with small children, make the development of welfare services an imperative. Consequently, as these services are not met so far by local citizens, they are nowadays met by women migrants, who have become the main source of support in private family life (Maratou-Alipranti and Tastsoglou 2003; Maratou-Alipranti 2007; Papataxiarchis et al. 2008; Vaiou and Stratigaki 2008).

Table 10.6 describes regulations and provisions on maternity and parental leave to support working parents in relation to the upbringing of children in Greece.

Generally, one could say that Greece experiences a lack of an integrated and deliberate policy for promoting the reconciliation of family and professional life. Traditional dominant perceptions about gender roles, the inflexible welfare system, employers' mentality and the lack of flexible and personalised regulations are some of the factors which stand in the way of meeting the needs of the modern family (Stratigaki 2006).

Reconciliation of Work and Family Life and Public Debate in Greece[4]

In this section, we will present findings from the European collaborative study 'Mainstreaming Gender Equality' (MAGEEQ). The main purpose was to identify policy frames in public discourse on gender mainstreaming and equality. The member states which participated in the study were Austria, Greece, Hungary, the Netherlands, Slovenia and Spain. It was considered interesting to investigate the role played by the EU as a self-defined norm-setter (Verloo and Lombardo 2007, p. 31) in relevant policies, and although there is no strict competence on

---

4   This section analyses findings from Hrzenjak et al. (2005) and Pantelidou-Maloutas et al. (2004).

Table 10.6   Reconciliation policies in Greece, 2009

Public sector employees	Private sector employees
Maternity leave: 5 months (Law 2683/1999).	Maternity leave: 17 weeks.
Breastfeeding or continuous absence: 2 hours' reduction daily for children up to the age of 2, and a 1 hour reduction for children aged 2–4 years; or 9 months' paid leave to look after a newborn child (Law 2683/1999). Fathers can also make use of this provision if mothers do not.	Breastfeeding or continuous absence: 2 hours' reduction of working hours until the child's 1st birthday or 3½ months paid leave. Fathers can also make use of this provision if mothers do not.
Parental leave without pay: Each parent of a child under 6 years is entitled to unpaid parental leave up to 2 years after having completed 1 year of service (Law 2683/1999).	Parental leave without pay: Up to 3½ months for each parent (or 6 months for a single parent). The leave is unpaid, but it is counted as service time (for pension purposes). Working parents with children aged up to 3½ years.
	Specific provision of 6 months' paid maternity leave: For working women insured by IKA ETAM (Law 3655/2008, only for mothers).
Parental leave to attend school performances: Up to 6 days' annual leave with pay to attend school performances of school-aged children up to 16 years old (Law 2683/1999).	Parental leave to attend school performances: Up to 4 days' annual leave with pay to attend school performances of school-aged children up to 16 years old.
Parental leave for illness of a child (full-timers only): Up to 6 days' unpaid leave. The period of absence is considered as employment time for all purposes.	Parental leave for illness of a child (full-timers only): Up to 6 days' unpaid leave. The period of absence is considered as employment time for all purposes.
Paternity leave: None.	Paternity leave: In case of childbirth, the father is entitled to 2 days' paid leave for every child (2000, National General Collective Agreement).
Parental leave for up to 2 years for family reasons: Each parent of a child under 6 years is entitled to unpaid parental leave of up to 2 years after having completed 1 year of service. The leave does not count towards promotion or pension (Law 2085/1992).	

family matters, EU policy documents were selected on the grounds that they dealt with families (Meier et al. 2007, p. 110).

Description of the Research

The research involved the analysis of laws, parliamentary debates, policy plans and other public documents with respect to gender equality in three policy fields

– politics, family policy and domestic violence – and discussion of the issues of prostitution (Austria and Slovenia), migration (the Netherlands and Greece), homosexual rights (Spain) and anti-discrimination measures (Hungary) in specific national contexts (Verloo and Lombardo 2007, p. 21).

The aim was to identify policy frames in public discourse on these issues. Verloo defines a 'policy frame' as an 'organising principle that transforms fragmentary or incidental information into a structured and meaningful problem, in which a solution is implicitly or explicitly included' (Verloo 2005a, p. 20; see also Verloo and Lombardo 2007, pp. 32–3). The primary goal of the study was to uncover how policy frames reflect upon gender equality, which problem representation they use, and what blueprints or directions they offer for solutions (Meier et al. 2007, p. 110). The underlying idea was that the framing of policy issues, and especially divergences in the framing of policy issues, may facilitate or obstruct the transformation of gender relations. Here, we will focus on family policy and the various conceptualisations or variations in what is meant by 'reconciliation of work and family life' in public discourse.[5]

Although we illustrate data from a European project, we will focus on the Greek case. The data used cover the period after the World Conference on Women in Beijing (1995–2004). As mentioned above, in Greece the most important laws and provisions concerning family and gender issues during the period 1995–2003 aimed to ease the burdens on working parents and pregnant women and to enhance women's employment (Verloo et al. 2005, p. 133). Laws provide for, among other things, the operation of day-long public kindergartens and primary schools, parental leave, help at home for the elderly, regulation of flexible employment and informal types of work, the protection of pregnant women in the workplace, and the regulation of work hours. Most of these are explicit or implicit family policy measures aiming to reconcile work and family life. However, family policy in Greece is to a large extent connected to national demographic objectives and the support of families with many children, and it does not function as an equality tool (Maratou-Alipranti 2002; Stratigaki 2006).

Reconciliation Policy: A Multi-faceted Frame

An analysis of the documents (national and EU texts) established that the issue of the reconciliation of work and family life appears to be a major frame in the European discourse on family policy. Although family policy falls within the competence of national states, reconciliation seems to be a common concern of both the EU and member states, with the exception of the two new member states: Slovenia and Hungary (Meier et al. 2007, p. 118). In some EU texts, it is either implied or even explicitly stated that gender equality can be achieved through reconciliation policies. Gender equality is generally perceived as meaning the

---

5   For the methodology of critical frame analysis, see Verloo and Lombardo (2007). See also Verloo (2007).

greater participation of men in undertaking family duties and greater participation of women in the labour market. In their critical frame analysis of public documents, Meier et al. (2007, p. 118) explain the diversity of visions of reconciliation across Europe as follows: the importance of the reconciliation frame in the EU can be explained by the EU's historically strong focus on labour market policies combined with the absence of a clear competence in family policy; furthermore, the influence of EU policies can explain to a certain extent the strong tendency to frame family policy in terms of reconciliation in Spain (or Greece); in Slovenia, the reconciliation frame is of secondary importance, while in Hungary it has no particular importance; both countries offer periods of relatively long maternity leave, and diagnosis focuses on whether long maternity leave makes it difficult for women to (re-)enter the labour market; and in Austria the reconciliation frame is linked to difficulties women encounter when trying to (re-)enter the labour market after a long maternity leave.

Greece: Representations of the Public Discourse on Reconciliation Policy

In the Greek public discourse, reconciliation is at times represented as a problem or a dilemma (considering the limited options mothers have for pursuing a career), whereas at other times it is seen as a measure for the improvement of family life. Most documents portray the balance between paid work and caring responsibilities as a problem for women, who are also called upon to deal with it since their social role as caregivers is almost never disputed. In other words, the 'reconciliation frame' entails a fixed representation of women as responsible for the provision of care to dependent family members.

As a problem, reconciliation is seen to be primarily located in the organisation of intimacy and the unequal distribution of family roles, duties and responsibilities, although 'family life has not only been shaped by cultural norms and social customs, but by state regulations as well' (Meier et al. 2007, p. 111; Lewis 2009). Yet existing traditional perceptions of gender roles are seen as powerful mechanisms reproducing the problem. In reality, in many documents the regular use of rather 'mild' expressions like 'traditional gender stereotypes' and 'traditional values' draws attention away from the real cause of the problem, which is the inequality between men and women in the family (Hrzenjak et al. 2005).

Analysing the various documents, it was obvious that reconciliation of work and family life is rarely presented as a gender equality problem (it only surfaces as such in a few texts) in Greece. It is generally recognised as a social problem with several dimensions associated with the social organisation of the provision of care, the lack of an integrated family policy, and state support and the pressing need to modernise the labour market in order to facilitate the participation of more women in employment. These are the top-most elements of a common frame we called 'failing family policies' that was also found in the public documents of all the other participant countries and the EU (Hrzenjak et al. 2005). The particular frame depicts the lack of co-ordination and adaptation of family policy to the contemporary social and family needs as a major citizenship issue. Moreover, the conservative and narrow approach to family policy issues, as it appears in parliamentary debates, suggests that women's rising participation in the labour market has actually caused the problem of combining work and care. Women are explicitly or implicitly held responsible for the low birth rates, since it is frequently implied that having children hinders them from pursuing a career. The logical prognostic frame in this case is 'to stop the demographic decline'. In that context, the well-being of the family and an increase of the birth rate are seen as crucial objectives for the advancement of the nation in Greece, and also in Hungary and Austria (Meier et al. 2007, p. 120). The conservative approach also lays great emphasis on norms by bringing into the discussion a number of issues such as a crisis in the value orientations of societies, changes in the family structure and the institution of marriage, and a divergence from traditional family patterns (Pantelidou-Maloutas et al. 2004).

This view of family policy is predominantly based on the essentialist assumption that women's primary 'natural duty' is to have children. Young couples, but mostly women, are blamed for being preoccupied with their career priorities, while at the same time they are responsible for the reproduction of the nation and society.

On the other hand, there are 'voices',[6] mainly from the left wing, that stress that the demographic problem is associated with particular economic and social changes, and that women and emancipation should not be blamed for the declining birth rates in Greece. In fact, these voices suggest that it is a woman's prerogative to decide when and how many children she will have, and that it must be made possible for women to reconcile maternity with professional life.

In contrast, a more liberal approach to the issue of reconciliation voices a concern for the declining birth rate – resulting also in a decline in the labour force – and the implications of this for future economic growth. In that respect, 'reconciliation' is among, other things, seen as a policy measure against demographic and potential growth decline.

In simple terms, the economy, the social security system and so on need more children and a higher percentage of working women in order to face the challenges of international competition, growth and population ageing. Women's human capital seems to be indispensable for the labour market, and in that sense gender equality is conceptualised more as an 'economic resource' than a fundamental principle of democracy and a human right.

In Greece, reconciliation policies are implicitly present in legal measures and regulations, while they appear more explicitly in a number of government documents on labour issues, such as the National Action Plans for employment. In brief, governmental reports entail a number of measures for the reorganisation of the labour market and the social security system in order to facilitate the entry, retention and advancement of women in employment. This can be achieved

---

6   In our analysis, the voices include MPs (speakers in parliamentary debates), lawmakers and authors of public documents.

first by the expansion and improvement of care services, and second by the redefinition of gender roles within the family and the redistribution of family duties and obligations. The former suggests an integral social policy that can only be expressed by the welfare state (though in reality, Greece and other European countries seem to be making deep cuts in welfare), while the latter is simply an issue of men being urged to take up more caring and housework tasks.

In that context, reconciliation is represented as a number of labour reforms that entail flexible working hours, part-time jobs and informal types of work, all aiming at the elimination of discrimination against women in the labour market. In other words, public discourse constructs new types of female employment, which reflects more an anti-labour mentality than an equality policy. For example, although most texts (laws, policy plans) favour part-time employment as a proper measure for women with caring responsibilities, texts produced by civil society and policy making bodies stress that unemployment and gender inequality are hidden behind part-time and other informal types of employment.

In addition, it can be shown that informal types of work are not protected by labour legislation and are not subject to labour inspection; furthermore, they are not covered by the general collective agreements, and they have no contractual working hours, no paid leave or bank holidays, and maternity is generally not protected.

Although reconciliation is represented as an issue of intimacy, it appears that most policy proposals offer solutions away from the traditional family models concerning the organisation of intimacy (see also Meier et al. 2007, p. 118). For example, Greek texts portray the unequal distribution of caring responsibilities between women and men as an in-house private problem within family life, but prognoses usually focus on employment issues and work flexibility. Generally, most action measures seem to coincide with the European demand for more flexible labour markets.

Furthermore, the majority of sources tend to overlook social inequalities, hence reconciliation and gender inequality are usually dissociated from any other structural inequalities. There is no reference, for example, to minority ethnic groups or 'race'. From the selected texts, only one policy plan referred to immigrants as a gendered social category. Immigrants were presented as unskilled workers who could benefit from vocational training, but the pressing issues of naturalisation or social security rights were not discussed. On the other hand, some laws and policy documents produced by policy making bodies lay some emphasis on class inequalities that referred both to the exclusion from employment and a gender-neutral distinction between employed and unemployed. Class inequality only becomes gendered when it intertwines with different employment statuses and preferences between women and men. This is framed as both gender-based discrimination and choice. It is suggested that compared to men, women generally work in low-paid jobs and in low- or medium-skilled positions, hence gender discrimination is implied; or women mainly prefer to work part-time or to work in informal and illegal jobs[7] tailored to their family needs as caregivers, which is seen as a matter of preference. Class inequalities in terms of working hours, pay, social benefits and maternity rights also refer to the unique distinction that is often made in public documents between those working in the public sector, which is the privileged sector in Greece, and those who work in the private sector.

Actually, most public documents indicate that the problem is not the lack of reconciliation and gender equality policies in employment, but rather their ineffective implementation, especially in the private sector. At the same time, in the Greek public discourse, class inequality and family status (which refers to the support of single-parent families and families with many children or women with children and family obligations) are interlocking and inherently connected. Diagnosis suggests that single-parent families and families with many children are at risk of poverty due to the lack of coherent state family support policies. The prognosis emphasises the need to eliminate discrimination on the basis of family status, to prevent dismissal on the grounds of marriage or maternity, and to prohibit the loss of employment, seniority rights or allowances.

Finally, as reconciliation is seen as a family problem and a matter of intimacy, the redistribution of family roles is represented as a solution. Yet it is rarely explained how in principle this can take place, and how perceptions of gender will eventually change. As Moussourou and Stratigaki argue most persuasively, in the context of redefinition and redistribution of gendered social and family roles:

> an essential reconciliation of family and work life would have come to a full circle after the industrial revolution, in favour of men and women, and it would allow the endorsement of 'another type' of work and 'another' family life and a relationship between the two that would render unnecessary any reference to reconciliation. (Moussourou and Stratigaki 2004, pp. 76–7)

Until then, we will continue with models that are not always compatible, and with incongruities between official rhetoric and institutional practices.

Conclusions

As we have seen, female employment has increased slowly in Greece, and still remains low. Furthermore, economic development has increased opportunities for salaried employment, especially in the service industry, where women predominate. However, married women continue to work full-time after childbirth as the development of part-time jobs is very limited and there is no flexibility in the labour market to help mothers to combine work and family life.

---

7   'Illegal' here means employment not registered with the social security system and revenue office.

Besides, social policies do little to support the employment of women with family responsibilities and there are limited services and arrangements, leaving the main burden on couples and families, and particularly on mothers and women in general.

The basic premise in the idea of the reconciliation of family and work life is to develop structures harmonising professional and family life. It is also believed that the improvement of women's participation in the labour market will contribute to the prosperity of the national labour force and the economic development of the country.

However, the analysis of public documents for Greece, in the context of the MAGEEQ project, shows that reconciliation is mainly thought of as a number of labour reforms, with great emphasis on flexible employment such as part-time jobs and informal types of work, all aiming at the integration of women with caring responsibilities into the labour market. At the same time, 'reconciliation' is represented, to a large extent, as an issue of intimacy. It appears, however, that most policy proposals do not offer real solutions as to how equal sharing of responsibilities and gender equality in the domestic sphere can be achieved.

References

Charalambis, D., Maratou-Alipranti, L. and Hadjiyannis, A. (eds) (2004), *Recent Social Trends in Greece*, Montreal: McGill-Queen University Press.

Davakis, K. (2006), 'Family Policies from a Gender Perspective', in M. Petmesidou and E. Mosialos (eds), *Social Policy Developments in Greece*, Aldershot: Ashgate.

European Commission (2006), *Reconciliation of Work and Private Life: A Comparative Review of Thirty European Countries*, Luxembourg: Office for Official Publications of the European Communities.

—— (2008), *Report on Equality between Women and Men*, Luxembourg: Office for Official Publications of the European Communities.

Hantrais, L. (ed.) (2000), *Gendered Policies in Europe. Reconciling Employment and Family Life*, London: Macmillan.

—— and Letablier, M.T. (1995), *La Relation Famille–emploi: Une comparaison des modes d'ajustement en Europe*, Paris: Centre d'Etudes d'Emploi.

Hrzenjak, M., Jalusic, V., Sauer B. and Tertinegg, K. (2005), *Report: Policy Frames and Implementation Problems – The Case of Gender Mainstreaming. Description and Critical Analysis, Gender Inequality and Family Policy*, MAGEEQ (Multiple Meanings of Gender Equality) Research Report, Vienna: IWM.

Karamessini, M. (2006), 'Gender Equality and Employment Policy', in M. Petmesidou and E. Mosialos (eds), *Social Policy Developments in Greece*, Aldershot: Ashgate.

Kaufman, F., Kuijisten, A., Schulze, H. and Stromeyer, J. (eds) (2002), *Family Life and Family Policies in Europe*, vol. 2, Oxford: Oxford University Press.

Kikilias, E. (2007), *Employment and Unemployment in Greece, 2000–2005*, Athens: EKKE Bulletin *Epikaira Themata*, no. 1.

Koronaiou, A (2007), *The Role of Fathers in Balancing Professional and Family-private Life*, Athens: KETHI, Research Centre for Gender Equality.

Lewis, J. (2008), 'Policies for parents in France, Germany, the Netherlands, and the UK in the 2000s', *Social Politics*, vol. 15, no. 3.

—— (2009), *Work–family Balance, Gender and Policy*, Cheltenham: Edward Elgar.

—— et al. (2008), *Patterns of Development in Work/Family Reconciliation*, Oxford: Oxford University Press.

Maratou-Alipranti, L. (1999), *The Family in Athens: Family Models and Patterns of Life of Athenian Couples*, 2nd edn, Athens: EKKE, National Centre for Social Research.

—— (ed.) (2002), *Families and Welfare State in Europe: Trends and Challenges in the New Century*, Athens: Gutenberg/EKKE.

—— (2007), *Female Migration in Greece*, Athens: KETHI, Research Centre for Gender Equality.

—— and Tastsoglou, E. (eds) (2003), 'Gender and international migration: Focus on Greece', *The Greek Review of Social Research*, special issue, no. 110A.

Matsaganis, M. and Petroglou, A. (2001), *The social protection system and Women*, Athens: KETHI (in Greek).

Meier, P., Peterson, E., Tertinegg, K. and Zentai, V. (2007), 'The Pregnant Worker and Caring Mother: Framing Family Policies across Europe', in M. Verloo (ed.), *Multiple Meanings of Gender Equality. A Critical Frame Analysis of Gender Policies in Europe*, Budapest and New York: Central European University Press, pp. 109–40.

Mouriki, A. (2008), *Policy Priorities and Important Matters Arising from the Reconciliation of Family and Professional Life Issues*, Athens: EKKE (in Greek).

Moussourou, L. and Stratigaki, M. (eds) (2004), *Family Policy Issues: Theoretical Approaches and Empirical Investigations*, Athens: Gutenberg (in Greek).

Naldini, M. (2003), *The Family in the Mediterranean Welfare States*, London: Frank Cass.

National Statistical Service Greece, *Statistical Yearbooks, 1981–2001*, Eurostat Labour Force Surveys

Pantelidou-Maloutas, M., Hadjiyanni, A., Kamoutsi, F., Maratou-Alipranti, L., Thanopoulou, M., Tsiganou, J., Filiopoulou, M., Nikolaou, A. and Tsanira, E. (2004), *Country Study: Greece*, MAGEEQ Research Report, Vienna: IWM.

Papataxiarchis, E., Kafetzis, T., Topaòi, P. et al. (2008), *The Worlds of Domestic Work: Gender, Migration and cultural transformations in Athens of the Early 21st Century*, Athens: University of the Aegean (in Greek).

Petmesidou, M. and Mosialos, E. (eds). (2006), *Social Policy Developments in Greece*, Aldershot: Ashgate.

Stratigaki, M. (2006), *The Gender of Social Policy*, Athens: Metaichmio.

Symeonidou, H. (2002), *The Division of Paid and Unpaid Work in Greece*, Athens: EKKE.

—— (2004), 'Women's Employment', in D. Charalambis, L. Maratou-Alipranti and A. Hadjiyannis (eds), *Recent Social Trends in Greece*, Montreal: McGill-Queen University Press.

—— (2007), *Family Policies in European Union Countries: Reconciliation of Family and Professional Life*, Athens: A. Sakkoulas (in Greek).

Vaiou, D. and Stratigaki, M. (2008), *The Gender of Migration*, Athens: Metaichmio.

Verloo, M. (2005a), 'Mainstreaming gender equality in Europe: A critical frame analysis approach', *The Greek Review of Social Research*, no. 117, pp. 11–34.

—— (2005b), 'Reflections on the concept and practice of the Council of Europe approach to gender mainstreaming', *Social Politics*, no. 12, pp. 344–65.

—— (ed.), (2007), *Multiple Meanings of Gender Equality: A Critical Frame Analysis of Gender Policies in Europe*, Budapest and New York: Central European University Press.

—— and Lombardo, E. (2007), 'Contested Gender Equality and Policy Variety in Europe: Introducing a Critical Frame Analysis Approach', in M. Verloo (ed.), *Multiple Meanings of Gender Equality: A Critical Frame Analysis of Gender Policies in Europe*, Budapest and New York: Central European University Press, pp. 21–49.

——, Maratou-Alipranti, L., Tertinegg, K. and Beveren, J. (2005), 'Framing the organisation of intimacy as a policy problem across Europe', *The Greek Review of Social Research*, no. 117, pp. 119–47.

Chapter 11

Perceived Work–life Conflict among Swedish Dual-earner Families

Linda Lane and Margareta Bäck-Wiklund

Changes in work and family life during the past century have made balancing work and family roles more stressful for families, and more changes are expected. In 2000, the Lisbon European Council clarified the goals of the European Union for raising the employment of women and openly encouraged the replacement of the male-breadwinner model with some variation of dual earning. As dual earning becomes more prevalent, a growing proportion of families in the European Union are experiencing difficulty in finding a satisfactory balance between the demands of paid work and family life, and consequently are experiencing rising levels of work–life conflict.

The increase in number of dual-earner families has not substantially influenced traditional gender patterns. Indeed, the persistence of gender inequality appears to support arguments for women's double burden or 'second shift', with work in the labour market and responsibility for unpaid domestic work (Hochschild 1997). There is however, evidence that gender values are changing. The European Value Study (2000) found that most people believe sharing household tasks contributes to a successful partnership. Even in European countries where equality has not been a prioritised goal, research shows that women want equality (Apparala et al. 2003) and are more likely to express disagreement over the gender division of household work than men (Nordenmark 2008). Nevertheless, there remains a distinctive gap between the gender values individuals express and the actual gender division of labour they experience.

Men and women in dual-earner families face a dilemma: they must not only solve the problem of how their dearest possession – time – will be distributed between paid and unpaid work, but they must also decide which of the partners in the relationship will perform which tasks. In this discourse, Sweden, with its extensive family policy, emerges as a society at the forefront of the eradication of barriers to enable dual-earner families to combine work and family. However, despite welfare state generosity, recent research has found that Swedish dual-earner families experience higher levels of work–life conflict than dual-earner families in other European countries (Tang and Cousins 2005; Strandh and Nordenmark 2006; Van der Lippe et al. 2006).

In this chapter, our aim is to analyse and explain Swedish dual-earners' experiences of work–life conflict, with specific emphasis on women, and to provide insight as to why Swedish dual-earners are experiencing more work–life conflict. We will first investigate the importance of work and household demands in perception of work–life conflict, and then discuss our findings with reference to Swedish gender equality policy ambitions. We will begin with a brief overview of approaches to the study of work–life conflict, followed by a presentation of the Swedish institutional context. Next, we will present our data and methodology. In the subsequent sections, we will present and discuss our findings, and end with some concluding remarks.

Work–life Conflict

Research on the interaction between family and work takes a high priority in both a national and international context. Trying to understand the impact of work–life conflict on individuals as they attempt to combine work and family has received a great deal of attention (see, for example, Pleck 1977; Greenhaus and Beutell 1985; Higgins and Duxbury 1992; Voydanoff 2004). Early research on work–life conflict reflected the traditional view of work and family as two separate autonomous spheres, where men assumed the role of breadwinners and women the role of housewives. Consequently, research focused on understanding how changing work patterns affected perceptions of work–life conflict. However, as increasing numbers of married women entered the labour market, research on work–life conflict began to include studies of changing gender roles. Research on changing gender roles was concentrated around understanding the consequences of women's multiple roles – as wife, mother and worker outside the home – on their well-being and the well-being of their families (Pleck 1977).

Structural changes in the labour market, the development of new ways of organising work and the introduction of new technologies stimulated the emergence of women into the labour market. However, as work patterns and gender roles changed, it became increasingly difficult to sustain clear divisions between work and family. Boundaries between work and family became blurred as women and men found that work impinged upon their ability to participate fully in family activities, and conversely that family life could adversely affect their ability to do a good job at work. The development of open-system theories was an attempt to explain the consequences of these changes for individuals.

Open-systems theories hypothesised that work and family do not make up separate worlds. Events at work affect events at home, and vice versa (Dilworth 2004). Within this framework, work–life conflict is theorised as a form of inter-role conflict that occurs when the role pressures from work and family domains are mutually incompatible (Voydanoff 2004; Greenhaus and Beutell 1985). Work–life conflict occurs when there are high demands at work and in the family and there is not sufficient time available to meet all these demands (Higgins and Duxbury 1992). Work–life conflict has been shown to lead to various stress-related outcomes, and to interfere with one's ability to perform family and parental roles

(Bohen and Viveros-Long 1981). Small and Riley (1990) found that balancing work and family demands influences leisure activities, home management and marital satisfaction.

The cumulative demands of balancing roles in work and family domains can result in two types of conflicts: conflict from work to family, and conflict from family to work (Kinnunen and Mauno 1998). Work-to-family conflict occurs when the effects of work interfere with family life. Interference may be caused by working long hours, or non-standard hours, coping with stress of work intensification, or frustrations caused by stress, lack of job autonomy or expectations in unfulfilling jobs, all of which make it difficult for individuals to meet family expectations (Greenhaus and Beutell 1985). Conversely, family-to-work conflict occurs when the effects of family interfere with an individual's ability to perform their work. Important sources of family conflict are spousal disagreement about family roles, such as the gender division of labour and childcare responsibilities (Alvarez and Miles 2003; Lavee and Katz 2002). Although there is evidence of a strong correlation between the two types of conflict, individuals tend to report more work-to-family conflict than family-to-work conflict (Gutek et al. 1991; Frone et al. 1992).

A number of studies have shown that men and women experience work–life conflict differently. Pleck (1977) suggested that because of society's expectations concerning the gender division of labour, men experienced more work-to-family conflict, while women experienced more family-to-work conflict. Crouter (1984) found that dual-earner families, especially those with children, reported more family-to-work conflict, and Barnett (1994) identified the number and age of children as potential contributors.

In dual-earner families, an individual's perception of work–life conflict is assumed to be related to how they comprehend and value tasks assigned to them as men and women. Thus, work–life conflict may occur when expectations concerning levels of participation in household or work activities are not fulfilled. An important aspect is whether couples perceive the division of labour between them as being fair (Coltrane 2000). Fairness rests on two exchange norms: the *equity exchange norm*, when each partner in the relationship receives rewards and performs duties proportional to their contributions, and the *equality exchange norm*, when partners share rewards and duties equally regardless of contribution levels (Deutsch 1985). For example, in families adhering to an equity norm, husbands may feel entitled to the reward of undertaking less housework or childcare if they work longer hours in the labour market or earn more than their wives. However, in families practising an equality norm, duties such as housework and childcare are divided equally between partners regardless of work hours or earnings.

Gager (2008) argued that in the division of housework, women prefer an equality norm while men prefer an equity norm. However, simply referring to an equity or equality norm does not adequately explain the often contradictory alternative solutions couples in dual-earner families choose. It is not only who does what, how and when, but also whether or not the couple perceives the distribution of housework between them as fair that contributes to work–life conflict (Thompson

1991; Major 1993). Although couples' perceptions of fairness may include aspects of both equity and equality, or may be based on some other rule such as need, Dilworth (2004) argues that in the final analysis it is gender ideology that informs perceptions of fairness and expectations concerning what constitutes a fair share.

Researchers who study the effect of gender ideology on perceptions of fairness have analysed the concept in terms of those holding traditional views concerning gender roles, and those holding egalitarian views. Individuals with a traditional gender-role ideology hold beliefs that there are gender-defined appropriate tasks for women and men. From this perspective, the traditional family organisation is perceived as culturally appropriate, and may explain why women do more housework even when they work full-time (Greenstein 2000). Couples may perceive this obviously unequal distribution as fair even if doing so entails the equivalent of two full-time jobs for the woman, because it is in accordance with the couple's expectations. As Thompson (1991) argued, gender differences in expectations might explain why wives appear to lack a sense of unfairness when evaluating the household division of labour.

Individuals holding an egalitarian gender-role ideology believe that men and women are not predestined to perform certain tasks based on biological sex. Couples where both hold egalitarian views share more housework (Bianchi et al. 2000; Shelton and John 1996). The stronger the feelings individuals hold about equality, the more likely they are to disagree when they perceive the division of labour as unfair. When couples do not hold the same gender ideologies or do not hold them to the same extent, women may continue to perform more housework, since men seem to do more housework only when both partners hold egalitarian views (Greenstein 1996).

The type of tasks performed is also important to perceptions of fairness. Blair and Johnson (1992) found that the more often men perform traditional women's work such as cleaning, cooking and childcare, the fairer women perceived the distribution of housework to be. The more balanced the relative contribution of both partners, the higher the sense of fairness. Conversely, doing more than one's fair share of housework was associated with disagreement over the division of housework, high stress levels, marital dissatisfaction and lower levels of well-being (Lavee and Katz 2002; Lennon and Rosenfield 1994; Yogev and Brett 1985).

The way disagreements are articulated and their potential for affecting work–life conflict will depend on the woman's ability to negotiate a solution to her double-burden workload. Hobson (1990) claims that women have three alternatives: (1) exit – stop working and concentrate on housework, or alternatively leave the relationship; (2) loyalty – accept the relationship as it is and suffer the double burden of paid and unpaid work, or (3) voice – express disagreement and negotiate for a more equal distribution of household tasks. Gershuny et al. (2005) argued that the choice of exit, loyalty or voice would depend on factors such as the institutional context, stage in the life course and access to legal, economic and social resources.

The Swedish Institutional Context

The Swedish welfare state has for half a century pursued a gender equality policy that affords both women and men the opportunity to combine work and family. The foundation of the Swedish dual-earner model began with the enactment of the Equal Opportunity Act in 1980, and was consolidated and given additional institutional support by a number of amendments in the 1990s. The standpoint of the Swedish equality policy is egalitarianism, and as such, its goal is to change cultural perceptions of gender such that biology is not a decisive criterion for the division of labour in the household or the labour market. This policy was formulated in the knowledge that culturally determined gender norms and perceptions are historically and socially defined and are slow to change. However, this insight need not make gender equality a less legitimate goal, nor should it deter efforts that contribute to goal achievement. In this respect, the Swedish equality policy may be defined as aspirational, as it has a culturally defined goal with legitimate objectives for all members of Swedish society and comprises a frame of aspirational reference, something 'worth striving for' (Merton 1963, pp. 132–3).

Swedish equality encourages economic independence for both partners. Consequently, to reap the full benefits of the welfare system, one must participate in the labour market, with full-time wage-earning providing the best coverage and highest income security. A retreat to a single-breadwinner model is discouraged by relatively low universal replacement rates. The two most salient pillars of family policy are parental insurance and publicly financed childcare. Policies include over one year of almost full-income compensated parental leave, guaranteed high-quality childcare at affordable rates for children aged one year and older, and after-school care for schoolchildren up to the age of 9. In response to arguments for reducing gender imbalance in care work and for promoting modern parenthood, the government introduced 30 days' non-transferable designated father leave (the so called 'daddy quota') in 1995, and extended it to two months in 2001 (Bergman and Hobson 2002). The Swedish parental insurance system is flexible. Parents may combine parental leave with work, choosing to work fewer days per week, fewer hours per day or a combination of both until the child's sixth birthday.

Paid parental leave entitlements and income replacement are dependent on labour market participation, thus the availability and organisation of work are important concerns. Employment is usually a permanent full-time contract, although non-standard flexible arrangements are becoming standard in some sectors (Håkansson 2001). A noted consequence of flexibility is increased precariousness and job insecurity (Wikman 2002). Swedish workers are working longer hours than before. A survey from 2003 found that 15 per cent of women and 30 per cent of men reported working more than 45 hours per week on a regular basis. In addition, the survey found that between 1993 and 2001, the number of full-time working mothers in families with children aged 0–5 years increased from 20 to 27 per cent, and in families with children aged 6–12 years from 33 per cent to 49 per cent (Larsson 2007). Job demands such as work intensification and long commuting times also contributed to the pressure men and women experienced when trying to combine work and family life (Isacsson 2008). Theorell (2003) found that since the 1990s, job demands rapidly increased, regardless of the sector studied, while job resources such as control over work decreased for both sexes.

Family policy has not compensated for structural changes in the labour market, nor has gender equality policy made substantial changes in the gender division of labour. Consequently, Swedish dual-earners are finding it difficult to balance work with personal and family life, and are reporting more work–life conflict (Bygren et al. 2004). A number of comparative studies have explored perceptions of work–life conflict in Sweden. Tang and Cousins (2005) attribute conflict to efforts to balance work and family life, and to efforts to encourage men to participate more in housework and childcare. Strandh and Nordenmark (2006) suggest that large differences between gender values and actual performance of household and caring tasks may be contributing factors, while Van der Lippe et al. (2006) discuss conflict in terms of combination pressure, and find support for imbalance based on gender and cultural differences. The gender culture argument appreciates the idea that gender ideologies vary between cultures and across time and space, and permeate societies on a multitude of levels (Lane 2004).

Data and Method

Our data are from a survey of 32 service sector organisations in eight European countries conducted between December 2006 and June 2007 as part of the 'Quality of Life in a Changing Europe' project funded by the European Union Sixth Framework Programme. In this study, the data are restricted to 448 married/cohabitating Swedish respondents.

Satisfaction with one's work–life balance is about an individual's perception of his or her ability to successfully combine time and commitments at work with personal or family life. A lack of balance occurs when the demands of work and other aspects of life, including family life, are high and individuals do not have enough resources at home or at work to balance those demands (Voydanoff 2004; Greenhaus and Beutell 1985). *Demands* are those physical, psychological, social or organisational aspects of work and family life that require effort and are associated with physiological and or psychological costs. *Resources* are physical, psychological, social or organisational aspects of work and family that diminish the effects of work and family demands (Pierto et al. 2008).

The demands we experience and our perceptions of how they contribute to work–life conflict are a product of the attitudes we hold and the experiences we have throughout life. Experiences and attitudes may differ depending on individual characteristics such as age, gender, income and educational level, or by hours worked and commuting time. In addition, in dual-earner families, the demographic characteristics of a respondent's partner may also have an effect on the respondent's perceptions of work–life conflict. Therefore, we include a partner's educational level and hours worked per week in our analysis. A gender dimension is achieved by including the number of hours spent doing housework and caring for elderly family members and the number of children living in the household, all of which provide information on the domestic domain. Dual-earners who endorse egalitarian gender ideologies tend to share household and caring tasks more equally (Bianchi et al. 2000; Shelton and John 1996).

To provide insight into how respondents perceive the division of household labour, we included two single-item measures. The first question was 'How often do you and your partner have disagreements over housework?' The responses ranged from one – 'never/rarely' (once or twice per year) – to five – 'several times per week' – with mean scores of 3.6 (s.d. = 1.2) for women and 3.7 (s.d. = 0.9) for men. The second question assessed perceptions of performing a fair share of housework. The responses ranged from one – 'I do much more than my fair share' – to five – 'I do much less than my fair share' – with a mean score of 2.2 (s.d. = 0.9) for women and 3.2 (s.d. = 0.7) for men.

We used a number of scales in our analysis. The dependent variable, work–life conflict, was measured using a three-item version of a scale developed by Netemeyer et al. (1996) that included the question 'How often does it happen that you do not have the energy to engage in leisure activities with your spouse/family/friends because of your job?' (Cronbach's alpha 0.74).[1] Characteristics of work that employees must cope with, such as work intensification, were included in a work demand intensity scale, which we measured using a five-item scale developed by Karasek and Theorell (1990) which included the question 'Does your job require you to work fast?' (Cronbach's alpha 0.73). To capture employees' uncertainty in the labour market due to job flexibility, we used a four-item version of a scale developed by Kraimer et al. (2005) which included the statement, 'I am afraid of losing my job' (Cronbach's alpha 0.88). Career demands were measured with a three-item scale developed by Dikkers et al. (2004) that included the statement, 'In order to be taken seriously in this organisation, employees should work long days and be available all the time' (Cronbach's alpha 0.86). To capture contributions to work–life conflict from stress and concern over the care and well-being of children while at work, we included a three-item childcare flexibility scale based on Emlen et al. (2000). Statements and questions included 'Overall, how easy is it for you to find daycare for your children?' (Cronbach's alpha 0.72; see Table 11.1 on pp.8–9, notes to table are on p.10).

---

1   Cronbach's alpha coefficient (α) is a statistical measure used to check the internal consistency of the items included in a scale. A relationship coefficient of 0.7 or higher implies a relatively high level of internal consistency.

Table 11.1　Mean values (M), standard deviations (s.d.), scale reliabilities (α) and correlations among study variables

Variables	Women		Men								
	M	s.d.	M	s.d.	α	1	2	3	4	5	6
Work-life conflict	1.6	0.4	1.7	0.4	0.74						
1. Age	43.9	10.4	44.3	10.1	-	1					
2. Household income[a]	7.9	1.8	8.5	1.4	-	.10*	1				
3. Educational level[b]	5.1	1.2	5.5	1.1	-	0	.24**	1			
4. Partner's educational level	4.9	1.3	5.3	1.1	-	-.06	.22**	.36**	1		
5. Partner's work hours	36.7	7.6	42.6	7.7	-	.12**	-.17**	.03	-.03	1	
6. Children living at home (%)	60	0.7	65	0.8	-	-.06	-.04	-.02	.05	.04	1
7. Respondents' working hours	43.3	8.0	36.3	7.8	-	.13**	.34**	.27**	.20**	-.04	-.07
8. Work demand intensity	2.6	0.4	2. 7	0.4	0.73	0	-.02	.04	-.03	0	-.04
9. Career demand	2.6	1.0	3.0	0.9	0.86	.03	.16**	.04	.14**	-.03	.05
10. Commuting time (minutes one-way)	34.5	23.1	30.7	26.9	-	.09	.04	.02	-.09	0	-.12*
11. Job insecurity	2.1	1.1	1.8	0.9	0.88	-.03	-.15**	-.08	-.15**	-.04	-.05
12. Childcare flexibility	3.1	0.6	3. 1	0.6	0.72	-.02	.06	-.08	.05	-.08	.06
13. No. of hours' housework	12.9	7.5	8.9	4.9	-	.03	-.02	-.05	-.07	-.07	.14*
14. No. of hours' elder care	4.7	1.3	3.8	0.3	-	.16	-.03	.11	.08	-.07	-.10
15. Disagreements over housework[c]	3.6	1.2	3.7	0.9	-	.22**	.05	.04	.11*	0	.01
16. Fair share of housework[d]	2.2	0.9	3.3	0.7	-	.08	.14**	.14**	.21**	.12*	-.07
17. Health status[e]	1.9	0.7	1.8	0.7	-	.16**	-.06	-.08	-.08	.03	-.07

	7	8	9	10	11	12	13	14	15	16	17
Work-life conflict											
1. Age											
2. Household income[a]											
3. Educational level[b]											
4. Partner's educational level											
5. Partner's work hours											
6. Children living at home (%)											
7. Respondents' working hours	1										
8. Work demand intensity	.12*	1									
9. Career demand	.18**	.37**	1								
10. Commuting time (minutes one-way)	0	0	-.03	1							
11. Job insecurity	-.09*	.09*	.19**	.06	1						
12. Childcare flexibility	-.18*	-.19*	-.16*	-.06	-.09	1					
13. No. of hours' housework	-.18*	.04	-.01	.06	.04	-.07	1				
14. No. of hours' elder care	-.14	.11	-.09	.02	-.05	.80	-.09	1			
15. Disagreements over housework[c]	.03	-.09*	-.02	-.07	-.07	.07	-.17**	.27	1		
16. Fair share of housework[d]	.35**	-.01	.11*	-.01	-.08	.01	-.43**	.01	.26**	1	
17. Health status[e]	-.08	.20**	.11*	.09	.09	-.19*	.06	.39*	-.06	-.06	1

Notes to Table 11.1:

$n = 448$; ** $p \leq 0.01$ (2-tailed); * $p \leq 0.05$ level (2-tailed).

[a] Household income categories in Swedish kronor: 1 = 'Less than 1,500'; 2 = '1,500 to under 3,000'; 3 = '3,000 to under 5,000'; 4 = '5,000 to under 10,000'; 5 = '10,000 to under 15,000'; 6 = '15,000 to under 20,000'; 7 = '20,000 to under 25,000'; 8 = '25,000 to under 30,000'; 9 = '30,000 to under 50,000'; 10 = '50,000 to under 75,000'; 11 = '75,000 to under 100,000'; 12 = '100,000 or more'.

[b] Educational categories: 1 = 'Not completed primary school'; 2 = 'Completed compulsory education'; 3 = 'Further education'; 4 = 'Higher education not completed'; 5 = 'Higher education – first degree'; 6 = 'Postgraduate'; 7 = 'PhD or equivalent'; 8 = 'Other'.

[c] 1 = 'Never'; 2 = 'Rarely'; 3 = 'Fairly often'; 4 = 'Very often'.

[d] 1 = 'I do much more than my fair share of housework'; 2 = 'I do more than my fair share'; 3 = 'I do my fair share'; 4 = 'I do less than my fair share'; 5 = 'I do much less than my fair share'.

[e] 1 = 'Excellent health'; 4 = 'Poor health'.

Hierarchical multiple regression analysis was used to analyse the data in three steps. In the first step, we entered demographic variables, followed by work domain variables in the second step. In the final step, we entered household domain variables. The change in R^2 at each step of the hierarchical regression analysis was used to determine the variance explained by each group of variables. The beta values report the effect of the dependent variables on work-life conflict. Because gendered expectations about sharing work and domestic responsibilities may affect levels of work–life conflict, we analyse men and women separately.

Findings

Our goal was to investigate the importance of work and family demands for perceptions of work–life conflict. We began by examining the descriptive data. The mean scores presented in Table 11.1 indicate that respondents experienced moderate amounts of work–life conflict, with the score for men and women under the midpoint mark of the four–point scale. An ANOVA test to compare means found no difference between mean experiences of work–life conflict between women and men ($F = 3.54$, $p < 0.05$). However, we did find significant gender differences in a number of variables that may influence perceptions of work–life conflict. We found that male respondents lived in households with higher incomes ($F = 14.70$, $p < 0.001$). Gender differences in partners' educational levels revealed that male respondents had partners with the same educational level as themselves, while female respondents had partners that were less well educated than they were ($F = 14.84$, $p < 0.001$). Men experienced higher levels of career demands ($F = 15.32$, $p < 0.001$), but women experienced more job insecurity ($F = 6.75$, $p < 0.05$). In addition, not only did women spend more hours performing housework ($F = 38.35$, $p < 0.001$), they also perceived that they performed more than their fair share of housework ($F = 173.89$, $p < 0.001$). We found no significant difference in women and men's mean perceptions of how often they had disagreements with their partners about sharing of household work. However, the significant positive relationship between disagreements over housework and a fair share of housework ($r = 0.26$, $p < 0.01$), suggested a need for further analysis.

An evaluation of the frequency of disagreements over sharing of housework relative to performing a fair share of housework revealed that when women perceived that they did more than a fair share of housework, 19.6 per cent reported disagreement *very often* and 42.7 per cent reported disagreement *fairly often* with their partner over the sharing of housework. None of the men in this analysis reported experiencing disagreement over sharing of housework with their partner when they performed *more* than a fair share of housework. However, when men perceived that they did *less* than a fair share of housework, 33 per cent reported disagreement *very often*, and 41.3 per cent reported disagreement *fairly often* with their partner over the sharing of housework. Our analysis showed that when both women and men performed what they perceived to be a fair share of housework and their partners did the same, 92.1 percent of women and 89.2 per cent of men reported *rarely or never* experiencing disagreements over sharing of housework.

Table 11.2 presents the results of the multiple regression analysis. The analysis indicates that demographic variables contributed little toward explaining perceived work–life conflict. However in step three, we did find that age had a significant effect for men when both work and household domain variables were included.

The addition of work domain variables in Step 2 explained the most variance in work–life conflict, for women ($\Delta R^2 = 0.18$, $\Delta F = 11.93$, $p < 0.001$) and men ($\Delta R^2 = 0.37$, $\Delta F = 21.12$, $p < 0.001$). Change in variance is attributed to two variables: the intensity of the demands of work and career demands. Together they are responsible for observed change in perceptions of work–life conflict for both sexes, with work demand intensity providing the strongest relationship. In Step 3 as in Step 2, we found that two work domain variables – work demand intensity and career demands – had significant effects on perceptions of work–life conflict for both men and women. The analysis also showed significant effects of the number of work hours for women, but not for men. The analysis of household domain variables revealed that health status had a significant effect for both women and men, but the strength of the relationship was weaker for women. Gender-specific results included the significant negative effect of disagreements over sharing of housework for women's perceptions of work–life conflict and the significant positive effect of performing a fair share of housework for men's perceptions of work–life conflict. Step 3 also made significant contributions towards explaining variance in work–life conflict, for women ($\Delta R^2 = 0.04$, $\Delta F = 2.64$, $p < 0.05$) and for men ($\Delta R^2 = 0.07$, $\Delta F = 3.97$, $p < 0.01$); however, there was little difference in the contribution to variance change. Given that women have a greater responsibility for housework, even when both partners participate in the labour market, we expected a larger difference in variance between the sexes.

Table 11.2   Results of multiple regression analysis with work–life conflict as the dependent variable (standardized betas)

	Step 1		Step 2		Step 3	
	Women	**Men**	**Women**	**Men**	**Women**	**Men**
Demographic variables						
Age	.065	-.070	.032	-.056	.051	-.135*
Household income	.001	.088	-.030	.059	-.028	.100
Educational level	-.006	.078	-.006	.013	.004	.027
Partner's educational level	-.101	.140	-.066	.083	-.053	.086
Partner's average work hours	.029	.035	-.007	.059	-.021	.070
Children living at home	-.022	-.080	-.007	-.020	.015	-.018
$R2$	.016	.060				
F	0.701	1.769				
Work domain variables						
Respondents' working hours			.085	.100	.110*	.091
Work demand intensity			.330***	.482***	.289***	.451***
Career demand			.154*	.179*	.132*	.149*
Δ F					2.64*	3.976**

Commuting time	.074	.058	.067	.085
Job insecurity	.053	.001	.057	.005
R2			.431	.198
ΔR2			.371	.183
F			11.151***	5.884***
ΔF			21.129***	11.930***

Household domain variables

Childcare flexibility	-.086	-.045		
No. of hours' housework	-.061	.024		
Responsibility for elder care	.028	.061		
Disagreements over housework	.086	-.164*		
Fair share of housework	.122*	.029		
Health status	.256***	.132*		
R2	.506	.245		
ΔR2	.075	.047		
F	9.414***	4.882***		

Note: * $p \leq 0.05$; ** $p \leq 0.01$; *** $p \leq 0.001$.

Discussion

The effects of work domain variables on perceived work–life conflict were strong for both women and men. The significance of work demand intensity – that is, the need to perform more work in less time and at higher work intensity rates – was strong for both sexes. The result is also consistent with evidence that work demand intensity is increasing in response to changes in the way work is organised (Theorell 2003). Individuals respond to work demand intensity by trying to meet the new demands, which in turn may increase perceptions that work is demanding more energy and commitment at the expense of family life. Although not as strong, we also found significance for career demand pressure. Men and women in our study faced similar conditions in working life. Both wanted to get ahead in their jobs, and the pressure of meeting organisations' cultural norms such as working overtime and putting the organisation first reduced the amount of time available for other activities and increased perceptions of work–life conflict (Voydanoff 2004).

Gender differences become apparent in the analysis of household domain variables, where expectations individuals have concerning commitment to work and family are most clearly revealed. How partners in dual-earner families share work and household demands depends on the gender ideology they hold. It also depends on the power each partner can wield to demand a fair share of work from the other. For Swedish women, the experienced disparity between expectations as expressed in gender policy and the day-to-day performance of gendered tasks is a source of frustration that contributes to work–life conflict (see also Chapter 3 in this volume). They spend more hours per week performing household tasks than men do, and they perceive that they perform more than their fair share of these tasks. Because they value equality, Swedish women are more likely to report disagreement than other European women when their partners perform less than their fair share of household tasks (Nordenmark and Nyman 2003). Supported by the aspirational goals of gender equality embodied in Swedish policy, by social norms that do not stigmatise them for either quitting a job or a relationship and by family policies that reduce the risk of poverty, Swedish women claim the right to voice their concerns by disagreeing with their partners and expressing their desire for an alternative distribution of household tasks.

In Sweden, where gender equality is official policy and where family economy requires nearly full-time employment of both partners, there are social expectations that men share housework. Our findings show that men in our study find it difficult to live up to the expectations such a gender policy entails. Although they pay lip service to the idea, disagreement over who will perform which tasks and the actual sharing of household tasks in reality are perceived as an additional burden competing for their time and energy. Men prefer an equity norm, whereby they can lay claim to a breadwinner role, and buy out of housework because of their access to superior economic resources, but in the Swedish context, this is no longer regarded as an acceptable option. We conclude, in agreement with Bergman and Hobson (2002), that the pressure of expectations to live up to the idealised, gender-equal male role affects men's self-image, and that the loss of self-esteem this implies contributes to their experienced levels of work–life conflict.

A primary goal of Swedish welfare state policy is to make partners economically independent, but the price of independence is that when both are in the labour market, the home is under-prioritised. The male-breadwinner model has eroded in Sweden, but in reality, the majority of dual-earner families do not consist of self-sufficient full-time working partners who are economically independent from one another (Magnusson 2006; Bäck-Wiklund and Bergsten 1997). Consequently, underlying issues about the gender division of labour which includes unpaid household and care work, for which women remain primarily responsible, are ignored. Instead of the equality in Swedish gender policy promised to them, Swedish dual-earners are experiencing more work–life conflict than dual-earners in other European countries as they attempt to bridge the gap between the aspirational goals of gender equality policy and the need for practical solutions to the difficulties of combining work and family in everyday life.

Conclusions

In this study of Swedish men and women, our results suggest that work–life conflict is an integral part of the lives of Swedish dual-earner families. Time is the key element for understanding our findings. Men and women have limited time to meet the demands of work and family. Time spent meeting work demands necessarily restricts the amount of time spent on other demands, such as caring and housework. Swedish women and men experience high levels of labour market participation, and the welfare state provides economic and social support that enables both to combine the multiple roles of work and family life. Consequently, from a cumulative perspective, our results do not show significant differences in women's and men's perceived experiences of work–life conflict.

We found that the pressure of work demands is similarly associated with work–life conflict for both women and men. However, gender differences in perceived work–life conflict emerged when household responsibilities were included in the analysis. Despite an official egalitarian gender ideology, there is still a strong traditional gender division of labour that suggests that Swedish women in dual-earner families continue to experience a double burden of paid and unpaid work. The aspirational goals of Swedish gender equality policy are yet to be realised, leaving Swedish men and women in dual-earner families with a dilemma. On the one hand, when trying to live up to expectations of gender policy, dual-earner families find support from the extensive family policy arrangements available to them. On the other, dual-earners face many stressors in balancing work expectations, family life and social obligations which family policy alone is incapable of relieving. For example, the aspirational intentions of designated parental leave to involve fathers in the everyday caring activities of their children has not relieved women of the burden of childcare – although the number of fathers taking leave increased, the number of days taken by each father decreased. Also, even if parents of children under 8 years of age have the right to shorten their workday, non-standard employment contracts are gradually replacing the standard 40-hour work week. New working arrangements that include irregular and unpredictable work schedules demand employees' flexibility, but not in the way envisioned in the family policy. New ways of working mean that this is not an option for many parents. Thus, differences in fairness norms in combination with the absence of substantial changes in the gender division of labour mean that the dual-earner model may unwittingly contribute to work–life conflict.

References

Alvarez, B. and Miles, D. (2003), 'Gender effect on housework allocation: Evidence from Spanish two-earner couples', *Journal of Population Economics*, vol. 16, no. 2, pp. 227–42.

Apparala, M., Reifman, A. and Munsch, J. (2003), 'Cross-national comparison of attitudes towards fathers' and mothers' participation in household tasks and childcare', *Sex Roles*, vol. 48, nos 5–6, pp. 189–203.

Barnett, R.C. (1994), 'Home-to-work spillover revisited: A study of full-time employed women in dual-earner couples', *Journal of Marriage and the Family*, vol. 56, no. 3, pp. 647–57.

Bergman, H. and Hobson, B. (2002), 'Compulsory Fatherhood: The Coding of Fatherhood in the Swedish Welfare State', in B. Hobson and D. Morgan (eds), *Making Men into Fathers: Men, Masculinities and the Social Politics of Fatherhood*, Cambridge: Cambridge University Press, pp. 92–124.

Bianchi, S.M., Milkie, M.A., Sayer, L.C. and Robinson, J.P. (2000), 'Is anyone doing the housework? Trends in the gender division of household labor', *Social Forces*, vol. 79, no. 1, pp. 191–234.

Blair, S. and Johnson, M. (1992), 'Wives' perceptions of the fairness of the division of household labor: The intersection of housework and ideology', *Journal of Marriage and the Family*, vol. 54, no. 2, pp. 570–81.

Bohen, H. and Viveros-Long, A. (1981), *Balancing Jobs and Family Life: Do Flexible Work Schedules Help?*, Philadelphia, PA: Temple University Press.

Bygren, M., Gähler, M. and Nermo, M. (2004), *Familj och arbete*, Stockholm: SNS förlag.

Bäck-Wiklund, M. and Bergsten, B. (1997), *Det Moderna föräldraskapet: En studie av familj och kön i förändring*, Stockholm: Natur och Kultur.

Coltrane, S. (2000), 'Research on household labor: Modelling and measuring the social embeddedness of routine family work', *Journal of Marriage and Family*, vol. 62, no. 4, pp. 1,208–34.

Crouter, A.C. (1984), 'Spillover from family to work: The neglected side of the family interface', *Human Relations*, vol. 37, no. 6, pp. 425–41.

Deutsch, M. (1985), *Distributive Justice*, New Haven, CT: Yale University Press.

Dikkers, J., Geurts, S., Den Dulk, L., Peper, B. and Kompier, M. (2004), 'Relations among work-home culture, the utilization of work–home arrangements and work–home interference', *International Journal of Stress Management*, vol. 11, no. 4, pp. 323–45.

Dilworth, J.E. (2004), 'Predictors of negative spillover from family to work', *Journal of Family Issues*, vol. 25, no. 2, pp. 241–61.

Eby, L.T., Casper, W.J., Lockwood, A., Bordeaux, C. and Brinley, A. (2005), 'Work and family research in IO/OB: Content analysis and review of the literature (1980–2002)', *Journal of Vocational Behavior*, vol. 66, no. 1, pp. 124–97.

Emlen, A.C., Koren, P.E. and Schultze, K.H. (2000), *A Packet of Scales for Measuring Quality of Child Care from a Parent's Point of View*, Portland, OR: Regional Research Institute for Human Resources, Portland State University.

European Value Study (2000), *The European Value Study: A Third Wave 1999/2000*, Tilburg: Tilburg University, EVS, WORC.

Frone, M.R., Russell, M. and Cooper, M.L. (1992), 'Antecedents and outcomes of work–family conflict: Testing a model of the work–family interface', *Journal of Applied Psychology*, vol. 77, no. 1, pp. 65–78.

Gager, C.T. (2008), 'What's fair is fair? Role of justice in family labor allocation decisions', *Marriage and Family Review*, vol. 44, no. 4, pp. 511–45.

Greenhaus, J.H. and Beutell, N.J. (1985), 'Sources of conflict between work and family roles', *Academy of Management Review*, vol. 10, no. 1, pp. 76–88.

Greenstein, T. (1996), 'Gender ideology and perceptions of the fairness of the division of household labor: Effects on marital quality', *Social Forces*, vol. 74, no. 3, pp. 1,029–42.

—— (2000), 'Economic dependence, gender and the division of labor in the home: A replication and extension', *Journal of Marriage and the Family*, vol. 62, no. 2, pp. 322–36.

Gershuny, J., Bittman, M. and Brice, J. (2005), 'Exit, voice and suffering: Do couples adapt to changing employment patterns?', *Journal of Marriage and Family*, vol. 67, no. 3, pp. 656–65.

Gutek, B.A., Searle, S. and Klepa, L. (1991), 'Rational versus gender role explanations for work–family conflict', *Journal of applied Psychology*, vol. 76, no. 4, pp. 560–68.

Håkansson, K. (2001), 'Tidsbegränsade arbeten – språngbräda eller segmentering?', *VälfärdsBulletinen*, no. 2, Stockholm: Statistics Sweden.

Higgins, C.A. and Duxbury, L.E. (1992), 'Work–family conflict: A comparison of dual-career and traditional-career men', *Journal of Organizational Behaviour*, vol. 13, no. 4, pp. 389–411.

Hobson, B. (1990), 'No exit, no voice: Women's economic dependency and the welfare state', *Acta Sociologica*, vol. 33, no. 3, pp. 235–50.

Hochschild, A. (with Machung, A.) (1997), *The Second Shift*, New York: Avon Books.

Isacsson, G. (2008), *Commuting and Sickness Insurance Utilization*, Linköping: Väg- och transportforskningsinstitutet.

Karasek, R. and Theorell, T. (1990), *Healthy Work: Stress, Productivity and the Reconstruction of Working Life*, New York: Basic Books.

Kinnunen, U. and Mauno, S. (1998), 'Antecedents and outcomes of work–family conflict among employed women and men in Finland', *Human Relations*, vol. 51, no. 2, pp. 157–77.

Kraimer, M.L., Wayne, S.J., Liden, R.C. and Sparrowe, R.T. (2005), 'The role of job security in understanding the relationship between employees' perceptions of temporary workers and employees' performance', *Journal of Applied Psychology*, vol. 90, no. 2, pp. 389–98.

Lane, L. (2004), *Trying to Make a Living*, Med. 90, Ekonomisk-historiska institutionen Göteborg, Gothenburg: Göteborgs Universitet.

Larsson, J. (2007), *Om föräldrars tidspress – orsaker och förändringsmöjligheter*. Forskningsrapport no. 139, Sociologiska institutionen Göteborg, Gothenburg: Göteborgs Universitet.

Lavee, Y. and Katz, R. (2002), 'Division of labor, perceived fairness, and marital quality: The effect of gender ideology', *Journal of Marriage and Family*, vol. 64, no. 1, pp. 27–39.

Lennon, M. and Rosenfield, S. (1994), 'Relative fairness and the division of housework: The importance of options', *American Journal of Sociology*, vol. 100, no. 2, pp. 506–31.

Magnusson, E. (2006), *Hon, Han och Hemmet: Genuspsykologiska perspektiv på vardagslivet i nordiska barnfamiljer*, Stockholm: Natur och Kultur.

Major, B. (1993), 'Gender, entitlement and the distribution of family labor', *Journal of Social Issues*, vol. 49, no. 3, pp. 141–59.

Merton, R.K. (1963), *Social Theory and Social Structure*, Glencoe, IL: The Free Press.

Netemeyer, R.G., Boles, J.S. and McMurrian, R. (1996), 'Development and validation of work–family conflict and family–work conflict scales', *Journal of Applied Psychology*, vol. 81, no. 4, pp. 400–410.

Nordenmark, M. (2008), 'Bråk och rollkonflikter – jämställdhetens avigsida', in A. Grönlund and B. Halleröd (eds), *Jämställdhetens Pris*, Umeå: Boréa, pp. 111–36.

—— and Nyman, C. (2003), 'Fair or unfair? Perceived fairness of household division of labour and gender equality among women and men: The Swedish case', *European Journal of Women's Studies*, vol. 10, no. 2, pp. 181–209.

Pierto, L., Soria, M., Martínez, I. and Schaufli, W. (2008), 'Extension of the Job Demands-Resources Model in the prediction of burnout and engagement among teachers over time', *Psicothema*, vol. 20, no. 3, pp. 354–60.

Pleck, J.H. (1977), 'The work–family role system', *Social Problems*, vol. 24, no. 4, pp. 417–27.

Shelton, B. and John, D. (1996), 'The division of household labor', *Annual Review of Sociology*, no. 22, pp. 299–322.

Small, S.A. and Riley, D. (1990), 'Toward a multidimensional assessment of work spillover into family life', *Journal of Marriage and the Family*, vol. 52, no. 1, pp. 51–61.

Strandh, M. and Nordenmark, M. (2006), 'The interference of paid work with household demands in different social policy contexts: Perceived work–household conflict in Sweden, the UK, the Netherlands, Hungary and the Czech Republic', *British Journal of Sociology*, vol. 57, no. 4, pp. 597–617.

Tang, N. and Cousins, C. (2005), 'Working time, gender and family: An East–West European comparison', *Gender, Work and Organization*, vol. 12, no. 6, pp. 527–50.

Theorell, T. (2003), *Is Increased Work Influence Beneficial to Public Health?*, Stockholm: Statens folkhälsoinstitut.

Thompson, L. (1991), 'Family work: Women's sense of fairness', *Journal of Family Issues*, vol. 12, no. 2, pp. 181–96.

Van der Lippe, T., Jager, A. and Kops, Y. (2006), 'Combination pressure: The paid work–family balance of men and women in European countries', *Acta Sociologica*, vol. 49, no. 3, pp. 303–19.

Voydanoff, P. (2004), 'The effects of work demands and resources on work-to-family conflict and facilitation', *Journal of Marriage and Family*, vol. 66, no. 2, pp. 398–412.

Wikman, A. (2002), 'Temporära kontrakt & inlåsningseffekter', *VälfärdsBulletinen*, no. 1, Stockholm: Statistics Sweden.

Yogev, S. and Brett, J. (1985), 'Patterns of work and family involvement among single- and dual-earner couples', *Journal of Applied Psychology*, vol. 70, no. 4, pp. 754–68.

Chapter 12

What Makes French Employees So Happy with their Balance between Family and Work? The Impact of Firms' Family-friendly Policies

Ariane Pailhé and Anne Solaz

French fertility remains at a relative high level with respect to other countries in Europe. One explanation advanced is the family-friendly environment which allows mothers – even with young children – to continue working without mixed feelings. Furthermore, French people are satisfied with their balance between family and work: half are satisfied, one quarter very satisfied. Women are even a little more satisfied than men.

A family-friendly environment is created through different mediums. By developing public childcare facilities, financial support for private childcare, parental leave, family allowances or advantageous taxation represent one well-established medium. French family policy is designed to help women to have the number of children they want while continuing to work (Toulemon et al. 2008). A second medium is that of social and cultural norms (Bernardi 2003) which 'allow' mothers to continue working full-time even with young children. France has an intermediate position in the ranking of countries according to traditional gendered family norms (see Figure 12.A.1 in the Appendix).

Another medium that may help families to balance family and work is the workplace. Employers may contribute to the balance between family and work by being flexible about hours, by offering benefits in kind and/or financial benefits. The literature on the role of firms in work–life balance has been growing in recent years (Evans 2001, OECD 2002–2005). It shows that family-friendly programmes may contribute to enhancing job performance, reducing lateness, absenteeism, turnover or low job involvement. From the family point of view, a family-friendly work environment may help parents to juggle work and family schedules (Mesmer-Magnus and Viswesvaran 2006) which will enhance satisfaction with work–family balance. However, there are huge differences between firms in terms of family-friendly benefits and services, according to the size and gender composition of the workforce and the economic sector (Lefèvre et al. 2008). These differences result in large inequalities between individuals depending upon where they work.

The aim of this chapter is to analyse the determinants of satisfaction with work–family balance. It focuses on the meso level – that of the firm. The chapter will analyse (1) whether employers' family-friendly policies have an impact on individual satisfaction with the balance between work and family, (2) the relative impact of firms' family-friendly policies compared to individual and family characteristics, and (3) which types of programme are the most effective in increasing satisfaction with regard to work–family balance. As the determinants of job satisfaction differ according to gender (Clark 1997), the analysis will be conducted separately for men and women.

The empirical analysis is based on rich information provided by the Enquête Familles et Employeurs ('Families and Employers Survey'), a matched employer–employee survey carried out in 2004–2005 by the French Institute of Demographic Studies (INED). This cross-matched dataset offers a very rich source of information on both individual and family characteristics, as well as the characteristics of firms. It allows us to build a typology of firms according to their family-friendly policies, and to investigate the possible links between working in a particular type of establishment and the level of satisfaction with work–family balance.

The chapter is organised as follows. First, the previous research and background are described, followed by a typology of firms according to their family-friendliness. Some common factors affecting work–family satisfaction are then noted, before the method and the model's results are presented.

Background

There is a huge economics literature on self-perceived job satisfaction. The initial purpose was to link job satisfaction and observable phenomena such as resignations (Levy-Garboua et al. 2007), absenteeism or worker economic performance in management studies. The second purpose was to evaluate well-being, and then, indirectly, 'utility'. Indeed, according to Argyle (1989), job satisfaction, family satisfaction and marriage are the three most important predictors of well-being.

Beyond overall job satisfaction, various components of job satisfaction are studied in the literature. These include satisfaction with the amount of pay, work responsibilities, the work itself, promotional opportunities or co-workers. Less research has been conducted on job satisfaction with work–family balance. Using a survey of federal government employees, Saltzstein et al. (2001) showed that the quality of the work–family balance is one determinant of job satisfaction, whatever the family situation (single/in couple, with children/childless), the age and the partner's employment status (unemployed/employed). Our argument is that work–family balance may contribute to overall job satisfaction, and hence to well-being.

Satisfaction and Gender

Satisfaction indicators are always a mix of feelings about reality and expectations. Both are dependent on many factors and differ according to gender. The paradox of job satisfaction was pointed up by Clark (1997) in a pioneer work: 'though women's job content, wage and promotion opportunities are worse than men's, they report higher job satisfaction scores'. After controlling for selection bias, this paradox remains. It is assumed that the reason for this lies in the different expectations in well-being: women expect less from work, and will be more satisfied than men, all others things being equal.

According to the hypothesis of 'incompatibility of roles', women and men may perceive the problem of balancing paid work and family differently (Lehrer and Nerlove 1986).

The quality of the balance is essential in determining satisfaction with the work–family balance. In France, most women work full-time while having young children, and the 'dual burden' weighs mainly on their shoulders. As they bear the larger share of domestic and parental tasks while working, they are much more concerned about work–family balance. They may have more expectations than men because they may have more to gain from a better balance. As women bear a heavier share of the family tasks, they should be less satisfied than men.

However, satisfaction also depends on feelings about reality which are shaped by cultural factors and gender norms. The strong social pressure that allocates child-raising to women explains the division of labour between spouses (Shelton and John 1996). Role theory explains why women specialise in child-raising tasks by pointing to the substantial social rewards they receive when they participate in mothering, whereas men receive far fewer such rewards for fathering (Van der Lippe 1994). These social rewards may enable women to feel better about the way their employment and family life balance out.

However, this paradox is far from being universal in Europe. In a comparative study on 12 European countries using the ECHP data, after controlling for job characteristics, Davoine (2006) found that women were less satisfied in Portugal, whereas there was no gender effect in Finland, Denmark and the Netherlands, which are countries where the female labour force participation rate is very high. One explanation may be that with the emergence of almost universal female employment, holding a job is not seen as a privilege, so women are as demanding as men, or even more so. Another explanation might be that if female employment is the rule, then the institutional and business environment may have adapted to provide some help in terms of childcare facilities, work schedules and so on.

Factors Affecting Satisfaction with Work–family Balance

Time spent in paid work outside the family can therefore conflict with that spent with the family, at home. Perception of work–family balance derives from assessing the relative demands and resources associated with work and family roles

(Voydavnoff 2005). Work–family balance is at the intersection of two domains, family and work, which both have constraints and amenities (see Figure 12.1).

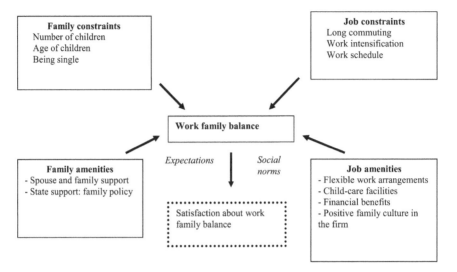

Figure 12.1   Components of work–family balance satisfaction

On the family side, one can assume that the larger the number of children and the younger they are, the higher the demands. The combination of work and family life may be eased through spousal and family support. Hence, according to Erdwins et al. (2001), spousal support is one of the largest determinants of work–family conflict. Grandparents or other relatives are also a resource for childcare. The availability of subsidised childcare facilities or subsidised childminders is also a key determinant. In France, collective and private care arrangements are well-developed for children under 3 years old, and 97 per cent of children are enrolled at school at the age of 3 (Blanpain 2006). As these facilities are available for most working parents, we do not focus here on the role they play.

On the employment side, work–family balance may be altered by long commuting, long or atypical work schedules and work intensification. Family-friendly programmes or policies may increase satisfaction with work–family balance. Those programmes and policies may include flexible working arrangements with regard to work schedule (for example, flexitime, telecommuting, compressed workweek, job-sharing), sick leave, childcare assistance (childcare referral services or on-site childcare) or cash benefits. A family-friendly culture at work may also play a key role concerning satisfaction with work–family balance. The perceptions of a supportive work/family culture and of supportive supervisors and co-workers may be determining factors, according to the literature on human resources management. Moreover, a condition for using family-friendly benefits would be that there are no negative career consequences associated with the use of such benefits.

Method

Data

The originality of our approach lies in the fact that it combines individual determinants, household determinants and firm determinants thanks to a matched survey of individuals and their employers. The dataset used here comes from the Enquête Familles et Employeurs conducted by INED in 2004–2005.[1] The objectives of this survey were to describe the work–life balance in France from the point of view of both individuals and employers, and to understand the correlation between the working lives and family behaviours of men and women. The 'Family' section was carried out by means of face-to-face interviews on a sample of approximately 9,500 respondents. The dataset contains rich sets of background information on individuals and households as well as a detailed description of the respondents' current work situation. The 'Employer' section took the form of a postal survey to the workplaces of the 'Family' survey respondents (2,673 respondent establishments with over 20 employees). The questionnaire covered the establishments' human resources management (work organisation, personnel management, working environment and general characteristics).

We use a matched sample: our sample was made up exclusively of men and women in couples with at least one child under the age of 25 living at home (more than half the week) working in an establishment with at least 20 employees. After excluding individuals with missing information, the sample included 988 women and 964 men. Sample characteristics are given in Table 12.A.1 (see Appendix).

As we have seen, work–family balance is a multi-faceted concept. For some people, work–family balance may be simply the feasibility of combining childbearing and employment. For others, it may be the possibility, for instance, of taking parental leave. For others, it may be flexible work schedules that enable them to take care of their children, or the possibility of having totally fulfilling private and professional lives.

Therefore, we propose a single measure of job satisfaction in terms of work–family balance which is a general satisfaction indicator. The following question was used to build our variable of interest:

> How satisfied are you with your job in terms of reconciling your family with your working life?
>
> 1. Very dissatisfied

---

1   See <http://www-efe.ined.fr> (accessed 8 May 2011).

2. Slightly dissatisfied
3. Fairly satisfied
4. Very satisfied.

The question was included in a series covering other components of job satisfaction: income, job interest and schedules.

Typology of Employers According to their Family-friendly Policy

The aim of the typology was to synthesise the huge amount of information about family-friendly policy obtained through the 'Employer' section of the survey. It avoided building ad hoc synthetic indicators and constraining the weight of any variable.

For that purpose, we ran a classification analysis using 21 variables related to the work–family balance. These 21 variables cover benefits in cash and in kind related to children and proposed by the employer, and the availability of work schedule adjustments. The analysis also included two variables measuring the degree of availability of part-time work schedules and the choice of day off. Table 12.1 gives their distribution.

Table 12.1   Description of the family-friendly variables chosen

Variables	Items	Frequency
Number of paid days off when a child is ill	0	32.0
	1–3	13.4
	4–6	22.6
	>6	32.0
Number of additional weeks off for maternity leave	0	91.8
	1–3	4.5
	>3	3.7
The establishment proposes childcare	Yes	7.8
The establishment gives access to holiday camps for children	Yes	40.2
The establishment offers a childbirth bonus	Yes	65.8
The establishment offers financial benefits for childcare	Yes	27.6
The establishment offers financial benefits for child education	Yes	32.0

The establishment offers financial benefits for disabled children	Yes	26.5
Full wage during maternity and paternity leave	Yes	70.6
Work schedule adjustments for the start of the new school year	Yes	85.9
Work schedule adjustments for children (school, kindergarten)	Yes	39.1
Work schedule adjustments for a sick child	Yes	71.7
Work schedule adjustments for long commuting	Yes	23.6
Possibility to work at home for private reasons	Yes	11.9
Some jobs are defined as part-time	Yes	49.3
Part-time accepted at employee's request	No	8.3
	Sometimes	42.1
	Always	49.6
Possibility to choose days off (gained by French reform of working hours)	No	19.5
	Constrained	14.7
	Need agreement	53.7
	Free	12.1
Availability is a requirement for promotion	Never	2.2
	Sometimes	34.0
	Often	31.4
	Always	9.4
Holiday vouchers	Yes	50.0
The employer subsidises health insurance	For all	55.0
	For executives	8.0
	No	37.0
The employer provides health services	Yes	31.6

Note: Sample = establishments of 20 employees or more.

Source: Enquête Familles et Employeurs, INED, 2004–2005.

We used a mixed method of classification which consisted of using first a hierarchical upward classification, followed by a consolidation. The method of hierarchical upward classification involves grouping together classes successively by aggregation. At each step, the two groups formed by the preceding iteration were merged. At the first step, the aggregation consisted of creating n-1 classes, with n being the number of individuals. At the second step, n-2 classes were created, and so on. Seven classes were determined, which could be grouped into either six or three groups. We obtained the following three (see Figure 12.2).

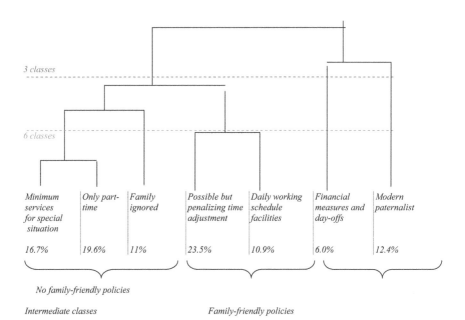

Figure 12.2   Classification tree

Two types of establishment provided extensive measures to help their employees. The class called 'modern paternalist' (12 per cent of establishments) included firms in which everything was done to keep employees at work. Almost all types of family-friendly measures were implemented more frequently by organisations belonging to this class. For instance, childcare centres in the workplace were available more frequently than on average (five times more), as were financial contributions to childcare (90 per cent, compared to 30 per cent on average). Additional pay for maternity and paternity leave was the rule. However, work schedule adjustments did not exist.

Additional covariates confirmed that this type of firm had strong schedule constraints: work schedules were extended; night and Sunday work were more common.

Six per cent of organisations belonged to the class called 'Financial measures and days off'. It was characterised by an institutionalisation of the days off. The duration of maternity leave was extended beyond the legal minimum. Paid days off for looking after sick children were plentiful. Moreover, employees were free to choose their days off obtained under the 'reduction of working hours' policy. Part-time work was available on request. Moreover, half of these establishments offered financial contributions for childcare or education. Measures in kind such as holiday camps or holidays vouchers were also largely provided.

These establishments opened five days a week. The sectors represented were finance (banking and insurance) and central administration. The firms were relatively large (half had more than 500 employees, and one third more than 1,000) and were more likely to be in Paris and its suburbs. The proportion of highly qualified employees was large.

At the other end of the scale, we found groups of establishments which provided very few such services.

In the class called 'Family ignored', which represents 11 per cent of the organisations, family constraints were completely ignored. All the measures described above were less prevalent than elsewhere. None of these establishments offered part-time work. Promotion was dependent on workers' availability. Some benefits were available, but the links to work–family balance were not as strong. For example, members of the managerial staff were more likely to benefit from subsidised health insurance. Help with housing might also be provided. The introduction of additional covariates showed that the proportion of men was high in such establishments (half had more than 75 per cent male workers). The construction sector and small businesses (half with 20–50 employees) were over-represented.

The class called 'Only part-time' was very similar to the previous one. It differed essentially in the availability of opportunities to work part-time. A very common measure, such as offering flexible schedules at the start of the new school year, was not available. The construction and metallurgical industries were over-represented. These firms had an international or European market.

The class called 'Minimum services for special situation' comprised 17 per cent of the organisations. Employers in this category provided few measures except in the case of a sick child or for the start of the new school year. In most cases, days off were granted for sickness. The childbirth bonus existed in three-quarters of these establishments. This category was quite heterogeneous. Large French corporations, but also non-profit organisations were over-represented. They might be open at night or on Sunday (25 per cent of cases). The retailing and manufacturing industries were highly represented here. They were more likely to have trade unions and a human resources department.

The intermediate classes provided only some kinds of services.

In the class called 'Possible but penalising time adjustment', work schedule adjustments were more often possible to adapt to school or kindergarten schedules, or for long commuting. For instance, 97 per cent of firms allowed this kind of adjustment in the case of a sick child. Numerous firms allowed employees to take part-time work, but employees who did so were penalised in terms of the progress of their career: promotion was linked to availability (in half of cases, 'often' or 'always'). Twenty-four per cent of establishments belonged to this class, in which, on average, employees were relatively young.

Lastly, the 11 per cent of organisations belonging to the class 'Daily working schedule facilities' were characterised by schedules and working time facilities. Family measures tended to fit the employee's situation, and they were barely institutionalised. Daily working schedule facilities were provided to fit school and kindergarten schedules or for long commuting. This class was similar in numerous respects to the previous one, but offered some additional measures, like the possibility of working at home. Working at home for private reasons was allowed three times more than on average. The number of days off allowed in case of a sick child was higher (more than six days off in 70 per cent of cases). There was likely to be access to a health centre, but no health insurance subsidies were available. These establishments were mainly in the state public sector (60 per cent of the employers in this category were state organisations, whereas state organisations only accounted for 13 per cent of employers overall), and particularly in the education sector (45 per cent of the employers in this category were educational organisations, compared to 8 per cent of employers overall). Most employees were highly qualified. They often worked less than 35 hours a week (teachers). The majority of employees were women, including in managerial positions.

Multivariate Analysis

As mentioned above, roles and values are a huge factor in satisfaction with work–family balance, and the determinants are gender-specific. For this reason, two separate estimations were performed for women and men.

Our sample was made up exclusively of employees. For some people, and especially women, the probability of being employed was correlated with their potential satisfaction with work–family balance. In other words, work–family balance dissatisfaction might be a reason for quitting the labour market. In our original dataset, 36 per cent of housewives with children reported that their previous work frequently came into conflict with their family life. This proportion fell to 17 per cent among working women. Those who were not included in our sample – people not in the labour force – may be self-selected into this state, and hence not be representative.[2] Since only very few men are out of the labour force, we only corrected for selection bias for women.

---

2   Another self-selection process would be that the women's preference for one type of firm might be linked to the better conditions of work–family balance in this sector. While controlling for a maximum of characteristics of job status, we expected to minimise unobserved heterogeneity, and then this selection problem. Again, as in France, the unemployment rate is high especially for women, job mobility low, and job choice is rather limited. Moreover, work–family balance is not the first reason cited for choosing a

Since women who worked were selected non-randomly from the population, estimating the determinants of wages from the sub-population who worked might introduce bias. We tested for selection bias following the classical Heckman's two-step procedure (Heckman 1979). This procedure estimates, in a first step, the probability for being in work[3] relative to being out of the labour force by introducing at least one specific covariate called an 'instrumental variable' or 'exclusion variable' (a variable that explains the probability of working, but not work–family balance satisfaction). The unemployed, students and retirees were excluded from our sample. The explanatory variables were age, age squared, education level, number of children, and a dummy variable if the person had at least one child aged under 3 years, a dummy variable for living in a couple, and dummy variables for being a disabled person. We used two instruments – the mother's activity status during adolescence and immigrant status – as the exclusion variables. The estimations show the expected effects of education (higher probability of participation for the higher levels) and of children (negative and significant). Being an immigrant reduced the probability of being employed, while having a mother who worked continuously during the subject's own adolescence increased it. The detailed results of this first step are presented in Table 12.A.2 in the Appendix.[4]

In a second step, we estimate an ordered probit on the scale of satisfaction with work–family balance. The ordinal dependent variable required the use of ordered probit regression.

Covariates

In addition to individual characteristics (age and education), variables related to the four dimensions influencing satisfaction related to work–family balance were introduced as explanatory variables:

Family constraints:
- number of children under 18 living in the household
- a dummy variable indicating the presence of children under 3 in the household

---

job. Usually, wages, geographical proximity, the interest of the job and job security come first. So we can assume that the family-friendly policy of a firm acts as a bonus, but does not influence the job search process directly, after controlling for some job characteristics.

3   Our sample included only wage-earners working in establishments with at least 20 employees. We did not control for potential selectivity of being employed in an establishment of more or less than 20 employees. We assumed that establishment size was a random process – in other words, that people do not choose to work in an establishment according its size, especially in a context of high unemployment

4   The estimations show the expected effects of education (higher probability of participation for the higher levels), and of children (negative and significant). Being an immigrant reduces the probability of being employed, while having a continuously working mother increases it. The detailed results are presented in Table 12.A.2 in the Appendix.

- a dummy variable indicating that the respondent was single

Family resources:
- a variable indicating the proximity of the respondent's mother[5] – whether the time taken to travel from the respondent's to his or her mother's home was less than 90 minutes; this variable was a proxy for external help to take care of the children

Employment constraints:
- number of hours worked per week
- schedules:
  - non-standard work schedule – whether the respondent works on evenings, Saturdays or Sundays (regularly or occasionally)
  - strict control of working hours (clocking in and out)
  - schedules fixed by employer
- commuting duration (less than 30 minutes/between 30 minutes and 1 hour/ more than 1 hour/no regular journey)
- quality of job:
  - work under pressure

Employment resources:
- monthly wage (in logarithm)
- schedules:
  - reduced number of working days (four days or less worked per week)
  - regular time schedule (same schedule every day)
  - the possibility to change the schedule

Employer characteristics:
- branch (transportation/finance and real estate/others)
- state public sector
- size of the firm (less than or more than 50 employees)
- work family culture (from the employee's family-friendly employer classes' point of view)
  - acceptance from female colleagues and supervisors of employee's absence for family reasons
  - acceptance from male colleagues and supervisors of employee's absence for family reasons

---

5   We did not use information on the proximity of the mother-in-law since this information was not available for all respondents.

Results

Descriptive Statistics

There was not much gender difference in satisfaction about work–family balance (see Table 12.2).

Table 12.2   Distribution according to the level of satisfaction (%)

	Satisfaction			
	Very dissatisfied	**Slightly dissatisfied**	**Fairly satisfied**	**Very satisfied**
Female	5.0	14.7	54.5	25.7
Male	5.8	13.6	57.6	23.1
1 child under 18	4.1	15.8	55.7	24.0
2 children	6.4	13.5	57.0	23.1
3 or more children	6.7	14.1	54.9	24.3
Single	5.4	14	56.6	24.1
Couple	5.8	15.1	52.0	27.1
Private	6.1	15	57.8	21.1
Public	4.0	12.5	52.7	30.8
Classes				
Minimum services for special situation	5.4	15.8	57.7	21.2
Only part-time	7.8	15.6	55.4	21.2
Family ignored	9.2	10.8	60.8	19.2
Possible, but penalising time adjustment	8.0	13.7	56.7	21.7
Daily working schedule facilities	0.5	15.0	49.0	35.5
Financial measures and days off	2.5	10.5	58.2	28.9
Modern paternalist	4.7	14.4	55.3	25.6

Source: Enquête Familles et Employeurs, INED, 2004–2005.

This result confirms that work–family balance satisfaction is a large and complex concept. Respondents were not asked about their domestic or parental workload. If they had been, women should have been more dissatisfied than men because of the unequal division of work between women and men. Reconciling family and work does not involve partners in the same manner. The usual parental and domestic tasks are mainly performed by women (Algava 2002; Brousse 2000). In the case of exceptional events such as a sick child, it is mainly the mother (58 per cent in our sample) who takes care of him or her, compared to 9 per cent of fathers. This gender-neutral result also shows that, since satisfaction is a subjective concept, it integrates prevailing social norms which are very strong and gender-oriented on this subject.

The number of children under 18 years old in the household does not affect the frequency of satisfaction items, neither does the single/couple situation, except couples who declare more often being 'very satisfied'. On the other hand, working in the public or private sector does make a difference, with people working in the public sector reporting much more often being 'very satisfied'.

These first results show that the distinction between very and fairly satisfied is crucial, and that we cannot merge the positive and negative items. We will therefore keep the complete scale in the model. They also show that work–family balance satisfaction is more sensitive to job and workplace characteristics than to family characteristics.

Multivariate Analysis

The results of the multivariate analysis are shown in Table 12.3.

Table 12.3   Determinants of satisfaction with work–family balance

	Men			Women		
	Parameter		**T-Stat**	**Parameter**		**T-Stat**
Individual characteristics						
Age	0.079		1.34	0.067		0.94
Age²	-0.001		-1.02	-0.001		-0.80
Education high (ref. = no)	0.008		0.06	0.217		1.03
Education medium	0.002		-0.01	0.091		0.54
Education low	-0.111		-1.04	0.166		1.10
Family characteristics constraints						
Single	0.251		1.47	0.018		0.16
No. of children	-0.028		-0.64	-0.148	*	-1.66
Child < 3	0.124		1.25	-0.258	*	-1.45
Resources						
Parents close	0.122		1.47	0.137	*	1.72
Job characteristics						
Monthly wage log	-0.011		-0.09	0.069		0.63
Weekly hours	-0.026	***	-4.45	-0.014	**	-2.22

Non standard schedule	-0.251	***	-2.75	-0.273	***	-3.22
Regular time schedule	0.389	***	4.66	0.278	***	3.50
Schedule fixed by employer	-0.324	***	-3.41	-0.282	***	-3.30
Check-in control by time clock	0.222	***	2.37	-0.117		-1.33
Availability to change	0.256	**	3.06	0.259	***	3.18
Work less than 4 days per week	0.198		1.45	0.216	**	2.33
Commuting < 30 minutes (ref. >90 minutes)	0.436	***	3.22	0.536	***	3.78
Commuting =30–90 minutes	0.287	**	1.95	0.316	**	2.11
Commuting = no usual trip	0.254		1.24	0.687	***	3.27
Managerial responsibilities	-0.099		-1.14	-0.094		-0.91
Working conditions						
Work under pressure	-0.496	***	-6.1	-0.500	***	-6.45
Family-friendly work environment						
Female colleagues and supervisor family-friendly	0.158		1.42	0.245	*	1.89
Male colleagues and supervisor family-friendly	0.225	**	2.23	0.027		0.28
Firm characteristics						
Minimum services for special situation (ref. = only part-time)	-0.167		1.36	0.121		0.89
Family ignored	0.270	*	1.66	0.002		0.01
Possible, but penalising time adjustment	-0.004		-0.03	0.605		0.42
Daily working schedule facilities	-0.064		-0.36	0.442	**	2.57
Financial measures and days off	-0.031		-0.21	0.268	*	1.64
Modern paternalist	-0.086		-0.57	0.158		1.03
State public sector	0.234	*	1.86	0.027		0.25
Firm size < 50 employees	-0.137		-1.31	0.113		1.17
Finance and real estate sector	0.487	**	2.06	0.163		0.88
Transportation	-0.321	**	-2.02	0.147		0.60
Lambda				0.203		0.63
Pseudo R2	0.124			0.105		
N	964			988		

Note: * significant at 10%; ** significant at 5%; *** significant at 1%.

Individual characteristics Whatever the gender, work–family balance satisfaction was not sensitive to individual characteristics such as education or age. The amount of the variance explained by a model containing only individual variables is very small.[6] The traditional u-shaped relation between age and job satisfaction was not found for work–family balance satisfaction. This may be explained by the restriction of our sample to working parents aged 20–49, and its homogenous nature. Education level was significant without controlling for selection bias (the more educated were more satisfied), but this no longer applied once selection bias had been controlled for.

Family characteristics Being a single parent had no impact. For women, as expected, having a very young child (under 3 years old) had a negative impact on satisfaction with work–family balance. Indeed, family constraints were highest with very young children. Work–family balance satisfaction also depended on the number of children under 18 living in the household. For men, neither the number of children nor having a young child played any role in their level of satisfaction with work–family balance. This reflects the fact that fathers' involvement with children is still low in France.

For men and women, family resources increased satisfaction. Having a grandmother living nearby – that is, external help to take care of the children – increased satisfaction. It was a bonus for reconciling family and work.

Job characteristics Introducing job characteristics in the model significantly increased its explanatory power. While wage level had no direct impact on satisfaction, the number of hours worked was a major factor. Long working hours decreased satisfaction with work–life balance for both sexes. However, as Harriet Presser emphasises: 'it really matters which hours people work, not just the number of hours people work'.[7] Indeed, having non-standard schedules (working at night or at weekends) is really prejudicial for work–family balance. Although some studies show that parents can replace each other in case of a non-standard schedule, and thus reduce costly childcare, satisfaction is reduced. Working only four days a week was also a means to improve work–family balance for women; it was not significant for men (and also less common). Commuting time was also important. The shorter the commuting time, the higher the level of satisfaction with work–family balance.

Conversely, having regular schedules was a bonus in terms of work–family balance. Schedules might be fixed by the employer or by the employee, depending on the type of job. Obviously, if the employer fixed the working schedules, satisfaction was reduced. Interestingly, clocking on and off had a positive effect on male satisfaction. It allowed employees to track the exact amount of hours

---

6   This table is not presented here.
7   This passage comes from Prof. Presser's lecture: <http://www.news.harvard. edu/gazette/2004/05.27/15-24_7.html> (accessed 8 May 2011).

worked; it objectified the hours worked in a country where the number of hours spent at work, rather than productivity, is a sign of job involvement. Moreover, some days off could be obtained in compensation for extra hours worked. Lastly, being able to change the working schedule to cope with an unexpected event significantly increased satisfaction.

The indicators of stress on the workplace also played a role. Working under pressure significantly reduced the level of satisfaction, particularly for men. For men, a poor work atmosphere also had a strong negative impact, whereas it did not matter for women. More objective indicators, such as the indicator for managerial position, had no significant impact.

Family-friendly work environment   Gender differences may stem from social norms prevailing in the workplace and the family-friendly climate at work. To control for possible social norms, we introduced some indicators of the attitudes of peers and supervisors towards parental involvement. The results show that peers' attitudes were crucial. When male colleagues or supervisors thought that an absence for a family reason was normal, men were more satisfied with their work–family balance. The result was the same for women with female colleagues and supervisors.

Firm characteristics   Since our regression contained many covariates, we limited the firm control covariates to those which were significant: state public sector, real estate and financial sector, and transportation sector. Other things being equal, the establishment size was not significant. As Lang and Johnson (1994) conclude on job satisfaction, 'firm size, contrary to prevailing wisdom, only acts as a moderator,' and then indirectly through other characteristics of the job and firm.

The family-friendly classes of establishments were significant overall for women. The reference class, 'Only part-time', was the group of establishments which offered the lower family-friendly benefits and services. For the male regression, the class 'Family ignored' was the only significantly different one. In that class, some benefits were available, such as subsidies for health insurance, but these were less closely linked to work–family balance. Thus, in their appreciation of work–family balance, men seemed to take into account some factors not directly linked with family or children. For them, working in the state public sector had a positive impact, and working in the finance and real estate sectors was even more positive. For women, working for the much more family-friendly types of employers did play a role. Working in firms where both benefits in kind and flexible working schedules were available was positive. This emphasises the fact that a family-friendly environment increases the satisfaction of mothers, but not that of fathers. One explanation may be that women are the main users of such amenities, since mothers assume the majority of parental tasks.

Conclusion

Recently, French companies have become aware of the need to introduce measures to enhance their employees' work–life balance in order to improve both their well-being and their involvement in work. Employers wish to get involved, sometimes even beyond the expectations of the employees. Many intend to invest more than they do at present. Their participation is very diverse, as shown by the family-friendly typology of firms. However, the measures chosen are not always well targeted, and only rarely constitute a coherent and deliberate policy on the part of companies.

Work–family balance satisfaction may be explained by a multitude of factors. Among those assessed in this chapter, the characteristics of the job were the most important, whether the respondents were men or women. Aspects of family life – both constraints and positive factors – played a small part, whereas job characteristics, especially working conditions, were essential. All the schedule flexibility covariates (regularity, opportunities to change working hours, and so on) were highly significant.

To capture the possible additional effects of the family-friendly atmosphere of a firm, we constructed a typology of seven classes of firms using objective indicators about the family measures they provide to their employees. We also derived subjective indicators of the family-friendly atmosphere using a question about the absence of negative judgement of peers (colleagues and supervisors). The results showed that the judgement of one's same-sex peers was a key aspect of work–family balance satisfaction for both women and men. Only some family-friendly objectives introduced into firms' practices played an additional role. The classes characterised by benefits and services were found to have little effect on work–family balance satisfaction, whereas the classes characterised by flexible schedules were significant for women's satisfaction. Since women assume the majority of parental tasks, they are also the main users of such amenities (for example, scheduling arrangements).

The debate about work–family balance usually focuses on parents' responsibilities, and in particular on mothers of young children. The increasing importance placed on firms' practices usually focuses on this infant period, both in the public debate and in employers' discourses. The provision of childcare by firms often appears as *the* solution to help parents to reconcile work and family. However, this chapter shows that parents need help all along the life cycle – not only when they have children under the age of 3 – and that childcare provision is not the unique solution. Schedule flexibility plays a far greater role in work–family balance satisfaction than financial or in-kind facilities.

Thus, further deep thought needs to be devoted to changing work organisation, workload and schedules in order to improve work–life balance effectively. The flexibility of work styles and schedules needs to be improved, as does French corporate culture, which interprets long working hours as a sign of motivation. This is a point put forward in the OECD report on work–life balance (OECD 2007). Thinking about and taking coherent measures at the level of the company, in collaboration with civil unions and social partners, is then necessary to improve working parents' well-being.

Companies can help to improve their employees' well-being by proposing diverse measures and scheduling arrangements. However, it is difficult, and doubtless ineffective in the short term, to force organisations to bear the whole responsibility for achieving progress in this area. The state has an important role to play, especially since the practices of companies are so diverse. It is important to pursue the development of formal childcare arrangements beyond those organised by firms. Fighting against the traditional norms regarding parental roles, both at work and within the family, is a more difficult issue which needs time to address. In this domain, public policies have an important role to play in helping to break the trend.

References

Algava, E. (2002), 'Quel temps pour les activités parentales?', *Etudes et résultats*, no. 162, Paris: Direction de la recherche, des études, de l'évaluation et des statistiques (DREES), March.

Argyle, M. (1989), *The Social Psychology of Work*, London: Penguin.

Bernardi, L. (2003), 'Channels of social influence on reproduction', *Population Research and Policy Review*, vol. 22, nos 5–6, pp. 527–55

Blanpain, N. (2006), 'Scolarisation et modes de garde des enfants âgés de 2 à 6 ans', *Études et résultats*, Paris: Direction de la recherche, des études, de l'évaluation et des statistiques (DREES), no. 497.

Brousse, C. (2000), 'La répartition du travail domestique entre conjoints reste très largement spécialisée et inégale', in *France, portrait social 1999–2000*, Paris: Institut national de la statistique et des études économiques (INSEE), pp. 137–51.

Clark, A. (1997), 'Job satisfaction and gender: Why are women so happy at work?', *Labour Economics*, no. 4, pp. 341–72.

Davoine, L. (2006), *Les déterminants de la satisfaction au travail en Europe: l'importance du contexte*, working paper, Paris: Centre Etude de l'Emploi, no. 76.

Erdwins, C.J., Buffardi, L.C., Casper, W.J. and O'Brien A.S. (2001), 'The relationship of women's role strain to social support, role satisfaction, and self-efficacy', *Family Relations*, vol. 50, no. 3, pp. 230–38.

Evans, J.M. (2001), *Firms' Contribution to the Reconciliation between Work and Family Life*, Labour Market and Social Policy Occasional Papers no. 48, Paris: OECD.

Heckman, J. (1979), 'Sample selection bias as a specification error', *Econometrica*, January, pp. 153–62.

Lang, J.R. and Johnson, N.B. (1994), 'Job satisfaction and firm size: An interactionist perspective', *Journal of Socio-Economics*, vol. 23, no. 4, pp. 405–23.

Lefèvre, C., Pailhé, A. and Solaz, A. (2008), 'Les employeurs, un autre acteur de la politique familiale?', *Recherches et prévisions*, no. 92, pp. 21–31.

Lehrer, E. and Nerlove, M. (1986), 'Female labor force behavior and fertility in the United States', *Annual Review of Sociology*, no. 12, pp. 181–204.

Levy-Garboua, L., Montmarquette, C. and Simonnet, V. (2007), 'Job satisfaction and quits', *Labour Economics*, no. 14, pp. 251–68.

Mesmer-Magnus, J. and Viswesvaran, C. (2006), 'How family-friendly work environments affect work/family conflict: A meta-analytic examination', *Journal of Labor Research*, vol. 27, no. 4, pp. 555–74.

OECD (2002–2005), *Babies and Bosses: Reconciling Work and Family Life*, Paris: OECD.

—— (2007), *Babies and Bosses: Reconciling Work and Family Life. A Synthesis of Findings for OECD Countries*, Paris: OECD.

Saltzstein, A.L., Ting, Y. and Saltzstein, G.H. (2001), 'Work–family balance and job satisfaction: The impact of family-friendly policies on attitudes of federal government employees', *Public Administrative Review*, vol. 61, no. 4, pp. 452–67.

Shelton, B. and John, D. (1996), 'The division of household labor', *Annual Review of Sociology*, no. 22, pp. 299–322.

Toulemon, L., Pailhé, A. and Rossier, C. (2008), 'France: High and stable fertility', *Demographic Research*, vol. 19, no. 16, pp. 503–56.

Van Bavel, J. (2006), 'Field of Education and Postponement of Parenthood in Europe', paper presented at 'Social Exclusion and the Changing Demographic Portrait of Europe' conference, European Association for Population Studies, Budapest, 6–8 September 2006.

Van der Lippe, T. (1994), 'Spouses and their division of labour', *Kyklos*, vol. 30, no. 1, pp. 43–62.

Voydavnoff, P. (2005), 'Toward a conceptualization of perceived work–family fit and balance: A demands and resources approach', *Journal of Marriage and Family*, no. 67, pp. 822–36.

Appendix

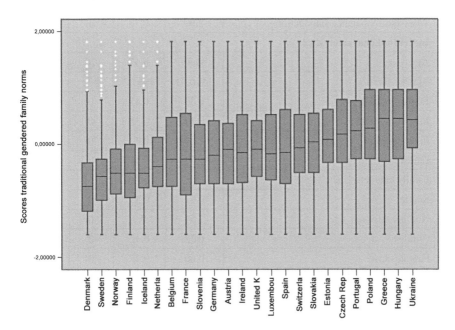

Figure 12A.1   Factor scores on traditional gendered family norms, box plot by country

Source: Van Bavel (2007).

Table 12.A.1   Description of variables

Variable	Mean	S.D.	Min.	Max.
Work-family balance satisfaction	2.99	0.78	1	4
Individual characteristics				
Age	38.36	6.67	20	49
Age2	1516.31	496.67	400	2401
Education high	0.33	0.47	0	1
Education medium	0.17	0.38	0	1
Education low	0.32	0.47	0	1
Education = no (ref.)	0.32	0.47	0	1
Family characteristics				
Single	0.11	0.31	0	1
Number children	1.59	0.9	0	8
Child < 3	0.23	0.42	0	1
Parents close	0.66	0.47	0	1
Job characteristics				
Monthly wage (log)	7.27	0.55	0	10.03
Weekly hours	36.29	8.49	1	75
Non-standard schedule (night, evening, Saturday, Sunday)	0.63	0.48	0	1
Regular schedule	0.52	0.50	0	1
Schedule fixed by employer	0.61	0.49	0	1
Check-in control by time clock	0.28	0.45	0	1
Availability to change	0.56	0.50	0	1
Work less than 4 days per week	0.20	0.40	0	1
Commuting < 30 minutes	0.64	0.48	0	1
Commuting =30–90 minutes	0.22	0.41	0	1
Commuting >90 minutes (ref.)	0.14	0.35	0	1
Commuting = no usual trip	0.06	0.23	0	1
Managerial responsibilities	0.27	0.44	0	1
Work under pressure	0.45	0.50	0	1
Family-friendly work environment				
Female colleagues and supervisor family-friendly	0.83	0.38	0	1
Male colleagues and supervisor family-friendly	0.72	0.45	0	1

Firm characteristics				
Minimum services for special situation	0.19	0.4	0	1
Only part-time (ref.)	0.11	0.32	0	1
Family ignored	0.06	0.24	0	1
Possible, but penalising time adjustment	0.16	0.36	0	1
Daily working schedule facilities	0.10	0.30	0	1
Financial measures and days off	0.12	0.32	0	1
Modern paternalist	0.22	0.42	0	1
State public sector	0.27	0.45	0	1
Firm size < 50 employees	0.19	0.39	0	1
Finance and real estate sector	0.04	0.2	0	1
Transportation	0.04	0.21	0	1

Table 12.A.2   Probability of being employed (Probit model)

	Women	
	Parameter	**T-stat**
Variables		
Age	0.178	3.220***
Age2	-0.003	-3.460***
No. of children	-0.463	-10.560***
Child < 3	-0.927	-9.610***
Education high (ref. = no)	1.061	10.700***
Education medium	0.609	5.570***
Education low	0.518	5.370***
Single	0.243	2.170**
Exclusion variables		
Working mother during adolescence	0.167	2.220**
Immigrant	-0.712	-5.640***
Disability	-0.117	-1.160
Constant	-2.017	-2.060**
Pseudo R2	1,640	
N	1,640,000	

Note: * significant at 10%; ** significant at 5%; *** significant at 1%.

Index

COST is supported by the EU RTD Framework Programme

SETTING SCIENCE AGENDAS FOR EUROPE

ESF provides the COST office through an EC contract

COST – the acronym for European Cooperation in Science and Technology – is the oldest and widest European intergovernmental network for cooperation in research. Established by the Ministerial Conference in November 1971, COST is presently used by the scientific communities of 35 European countries to cooperate in common research projects supported by national funds.

The funds provided by COST – less than 1% of the total value of the projects – support the COST cooperation networks (COST Actions) through which, with EUR 30 million per year, more than 30 000 European scientists are involved in research having a total value which exceeds EUR 2 billion per year. This is the financial worth of the European added value which COST achieves.

A "bottom up approach" (the initiative of launching a COST Action comes from the European scientists themselves), "à la carte participation" (only countries interested in the Action participate), "equality of access" (participation is open also to the scientific communities of countries not belonging to the European Union) and "flexible structure" (easy implementation and light management of the research initiatives) are the main characteristics of COST.

As precursor of advanced multidisciplinary research COST has a very important role for the realisation of the European Research Area (ERA) anticipating and complementing the activities of the Framework Programmes, constituting a "bridge" towards the scientific communities of emerging countries, increasing the mobility of researchers across Europe and fostering the establishment of "Networks of Excellence" in many key scientific domains such as: Biomedicine and Molecular Biosciences; Food and Agriculture; Forests, their Products and Services; Materials, Physical and Nanosciences; Chemistry and Molecular Sciences and Technologies; Earth System Science and Environmental Management; Information and Communication Technologies; Transport and Urban Development; Individuals, Societies, Cultures and Health. It covers basic and more applied research and also addresses issues of pre-normative nature or of societal importance. Web: http://www.cost.eu

Neither the COST office nor any person acting on its behalf is responsible for the use which might be made of the information contained in this publication. The COST office is not responsible for the external websites referred to in this publication.